Personal +
Community
Health

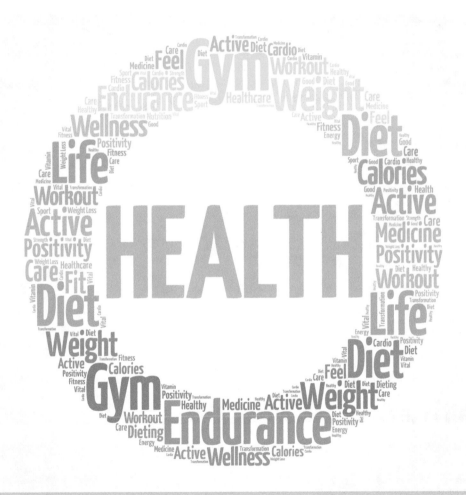

Dr. Joni Boyd + Dr. Shelley Hamill

Second Edition

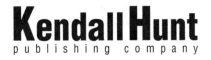
Kendall Hunt
publishing company

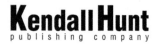

www.kendallhunt.com
Send all inquiries to:
4050 Westmark Drive
Dubuque, IA   52004-1840

Copyright © 2016, 2018 by Kendall Hunt Publishing Company

ISBN 978-1-5249-8521-9

Contents

Acknowledgments

First and foremost, I want to thank my God for the opportunity to fulfill my goals and dreams. I want to thank my husband, Timothy; my children, Timmy Jr., JohnieMae, Grace, and Titus, for your motivation for me to continue, even when times are tough. Thank you to June, Sheila, and Courtney for your support throughout all my endeavors. Thank you to my mentor, co-author, and friend, Shelley. Your guidance and friendship only compliment the passion for excellence and collegiality that make you awesome to work with.

+ Joni M. Boyd

I am grateful for the opportunity to continue on this journey and am most thankful for the support of those behind the scenes and in front. Mom, thank you for the life lessons and providing the strong foundation. Dibbrell, as always, for the love and support. In addition, Joni, my co-author, friend, and colleague, it has been wonderful to continue our adventures in publishing together. I might not have started down this road without your encouragement and support, so thank you! I look forward to our future endeavors.

+ Shelley Hamill

This second edition has had many people supporting our efforts through reviewing and editing. We are extremely grateful for the contributions of the following individuals:

>Dr. Kelly Boyd, Associate Professor, East Strausburg University
>Dr. Irene Cucina, Professor, Plymouth State University
>Karin Evans, MA, RD, Instructor, Winthrop University
>Dr. Danne Kasparek, Emeriti faculty, Winthrop University
>Bethann Rohaly, MS, Instructor, Winthrop University
>Jennifer Vickery, MS, Instructor (retired), Winthrop University

And finally, Caylee King and Matthew Edwards, our wonderful graduate assistants who have been invaluable in the process. Not sure we could have done this without you. Thank you!

+ Joni & Shelley

Welcome to Personal and Community Health!

This course is designed as an introduction to personal health with a focus on what each of us can do to work towards achieving optimal health. Each chapter has a foundation of content information, possible strategies for us to utilize, and resources for students to access using a bar code scanner.

The authors, in collaboration with other faculty, staff, and students, created this text with the intent of making it relevant for students. We wanted to design it so, at the completion of each chapter; students would know where to access further information.

Each chapter opens with either an activity or pre-assessment for students to begin determining where they are in their journey towards optimal health. While there may be a tremendous amount of information about each topic, this course is designed as an overview. If you wish to delve further into certain topics, we encourage you to take additional courses that specifically focus on that area of interest.

This is the second edition of this text. We have made revisions based on peer reviews, student feedback, and our own experiences from teaching our courses. We believe each improvement has made this text even more user applicable. We hope you agree.

Dr. Joni Boyd + Dr. Shelley Hamill

Chapter 1 +

Foundations

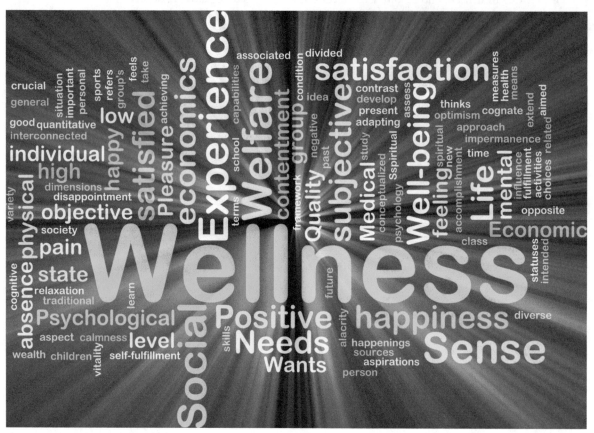

© Kheng Guan Toh/Shutterstock.com

PERSONAL OBSERVATIONS

Directions: As you begin this journey in exploring personal health, use Figure 1.1 on page 5 and answer the following questions:

1. In which dimensions of life are you most well?

2. In which dimensions are you least well?

3. Comment on the pattern you see in your inventory.

4. How do you feel about what you see?

5. What improvements, if any, would you like to see?

6. List two or three immediate steps you could take to make your wheel more round and make these improvements.

7. What is health literacy?

8. What role do you play as a consumer in your wellness?

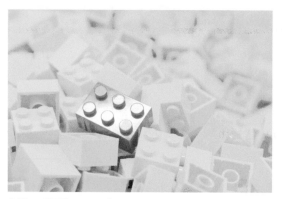

© ThamKC/Shutterstock.com

What is health? Have you thought about what it means to be healthy? Perhaps it just means not being sick or maybe having the energy to do what you want to do. Maybe, it includes more than just the physical aspects and includes other areas like mental health or social health. Many sources have defined health as being of sound mind and body. The World Health Organization defines **health** as a "state of complete physical, mental, and social well-being and not merely the absence of disease or infirmity". Yet, as comprehensive as that may sound, the definition of health today has evolved to include not just the physical and mental aspects, but also emotional, spiritual, and environmental components as well. Instead of looking at what health is, we have moved the focus on what is **wellness**. Wellness is seen as a life philosophy about making informed healthy choices, which can lead, over time to a healthy life-style. So how do we learn to make those healthy choices towards a healthier lifestyle? We learn by becoming health literate.

Health Literacy

"Health literacy is the degree to which individuals have the capacity to obtain, process and understand basic **health** information needed to make appropriate **health** decisions" (HRSA). In order to make healthy choices, we need to have the knowledge about what those choices are. We also need to have the skills that help us deal with the pressures associated with making the healthier choice rather than the choices our peers might make. Becoming health literate individuals is one of the goals we should all strive to achieve.

DIMENSIONS OF WELLNESS

"Wellness emphasizes an individual's potential and responsibility for his or her own health. It is a process in which a person is constantly moving either away from or toward a most favorable level of health. Wellness results from the adoption of low-risk, health-enhancing behaviors. The adoption of a wellness lifestyle

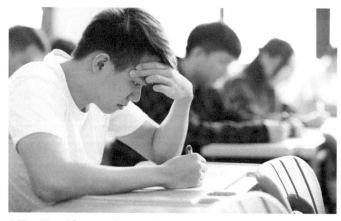

© Tom Wang/Shutterstock.com

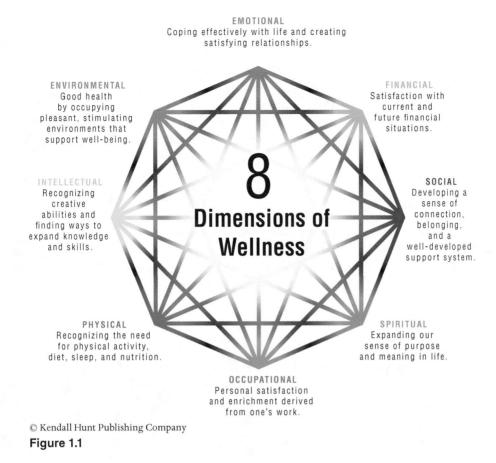

© Kendall Hunt Publishing Company

Figure 1.1

requires focusing on choices that will enhance the individual's potential to lead a productive, meaningful, and satisfying life."[1]

It is the complex interaction of each of the eight dimensions of wellness, (see Figure 1.1), that will lead us, over time, to a higher quality of life and better overall health and well-being. Constant, ongoing assessment of our behaviors in the following dimensions is key to living a balanced life.

Emotional

"A person who is emotionally healthy is able to enjoy life despite unexpected challenges and problems. Effectively coping with life's difficulties and unexpected events is essential to maintaining good health. Equally important to good personal wellness is the ability to understand your feelings and express those feelings or emotions outwardly in a positive and constructive manner. 'Bottled-up' negative emotions can affect the immune system and result in chronic stress, which in turn can lead to serious illnesses such as high blood pressure and can potentially lead to a premature death."[1]

Intellectual

"The mind can have substantial influence over the body. To be intellectually healthy, it is essential to continue to explore new avenues and interests and to regularly engage in new and ongoing learning opportunities and experiences. The more 'unknowns' an individual faces or explores, the more opportunities he or she has to learn and grow intellectually."[1]

Social

"Social health is our ability to relate to and interact with others. Socially healthy people are able to communicate and interact with the other people they come in contact with each day. They are respectful and caring of their family, friends, neighbors, and associates. Although reaching out and communicating with others may be difficult or uncomfortable initially, it is extremely important to our social health and their overall sense of wellbeing."[1]

Spiritual

"Spiritual health helps us achieve a sense of inner peace, satisfaction, and confidence. It can help give the sense that all is right with the world. A person's ethics, values, beliefs, and morals can contribute to their spiritual health. Good spiritual health can help give life meaning and purpose."[1]

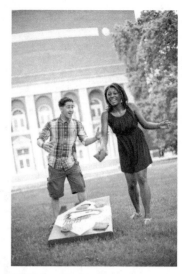

© Winthrop University

Physical

"Ensuring good physical health begins with devoting attention and time to attaining healthy levels of cardiovascular fitness, muscular strength and endurance, flexibility, and body composition. When coupled with good nutritional practices, good sleep habits, and the avoidance of risky social behaviors such as drinking and driving or unprotected sexual intercourse, a physically healthy body results. This is the component that is most often associated, at first glance, with a person's health."[1]

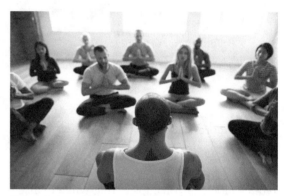

© Rawpixel.com/Shutterstock.com

Occupational

"Attaining occupational wellness begins with determining what roles, activities, and commitments take up a majority of our time. These roles, activities, or commitments could include but are not limited to being a student, parenting, volunteering in an organization, or working at a part-time job while pursuing your degree. It is when each of these areas are integrated and balanced in a personally and professionally fulfilling way that occupational wellness occurs."[1]

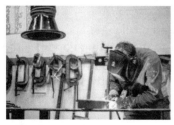

© Winthrop University

Environmental

"A person's health and wellness can be substantially affected by the quality of their environment. Access to clean air, nutritious food, sanitary water, and adequate clothing and shelter are essential components to being well. Our environment should, at the very least, be clean and safe."[1]

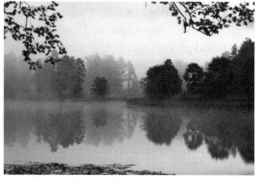

Courtesy of Shelley Hamill

FINANCIAL WELLNESS

"Financial wellness has an impact on an individual and society as a whole. The first step to gaining financial wellness is financial responsibility. There are numerous ways to be financially responsible, some of which include:

- Have a monthly budget and do not overspend
- Wait for items to go on sale
- Use coupons
- Avoid credit card debt (pay the balance every month)
- Use credit cards only in emergency situations
- Save at least 5 percent of net income in case of an emergency
- Do not get a car loan for more than five years (three- or four-year notes are even better)
- Always pay your bills on time
- Shop and trade at resale stores
- Pay off a mortgage early
- Check out books from a library instead of purchasing them from a bookstore
- Carpool
- Ride your bike
- Eat at home
- Go for a hike instead of going to a movie"[1]

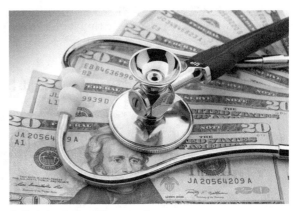

© Christian Delbert/Shutterstock.com

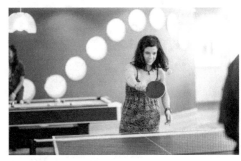

© Winthrop University

Did you know . . .

Courtesy of Shelley Hamill

According to the CDC:

There are all kinds of tests in college—beyond those you take for a grade. Examples include:

- Social and sexual pressures.
- The temptation of readily available alcohol, drugs, and unhealthy food.
- The challenge of getting enough sleep.
- Stress from trying to balance classes, friends, homework, jobs, athletics, and leadership positions (CDC, 2015)

Through wellness, an individual manages a wide range of lifestyle choices. How a person chooses to behave and the decisions they make in each of the eight dimensions of wellness will determine their overall quality of life. Making an active effort to combine and try to balance each of the eight dimensions is key to a long and fulfilling life.

The leading causes of death for all age groups are listed in figure 1.2 (CDC). While unintentional injury is clearly a significant concern for ages 1-44, it is also important to note the changes that begin to occur in leading causes of death starting with age 45. Many of these health issues are related to lifelong health risk behaviors.

10 Leading Causes of Death by Age Group, United States – 2014

Rank	<1	1-4	5-9	10-14	15-24	25-34	35-44	45-54	55-64	65+	Total
1	Congenital Anomalies 4,746	Unintentional Injury 1,216	Unintentional Injury 730	Unintentional Injury 750	Unintentional Injury 11,836	Unintentional Injury 17,357	Unintentional Injury 16,048	Malignant Neoplasms 44,834	Malignant Neoplasms 115,282	Heart Disease 489,722	Heart Disease 614,348
2	Short Gestation 4,173	Congenital Anomalies 399	Malignant Neoplasms 436	Suicide 425	Suicide 5,079	Suicide 6,569	Malignant Neoplasms 11,267	Heart Disease 34,791	Heart Disease 74,473	Malignant Neoplasms 413,885	Malignant Neoplasms 591,699
3	Maternal Pregnancy Comp. 1,574	Homicide 364	Congenital Anomalies 192	Malignant Neoplasms 416	Homicide 4,144	Homicide 4,159	Heart Disease 10,368	Unintentional Injury 20,610	Unintentional Injury 18,030	Chronic Low. Respiratory Disease 124,693	Chronic Low. Respiratory Disease 147,101
4	SIDS 1,545	Malignant Neoplasms 321	Homicide 123	Congenital Anomalies 156	Malignant Neoplasms 1,569	Malignant Neoplasms 3,624	Suicide 6,706	Suicide 8,767	Chronic Low. Respiratory Disease 16,492	Cerebro-vascular 113,308	Unintentional Injury 136,053
5	Unintentional Injury 1,161	Heart Disease 149	Heart Disease 69	Homicide 156	Heart Disease 953	Heart Disease 3,341	Homicide 2,588	Liver Disease 8,627	Diabetes Mellitus 13,342	Alzheimer's Disease 92,604	Cerebro-vascular 133,103
6	Placenta Cord. Membranes 965	Influenza & Pneumonia 109	Chronic Low. Respiratory Disease 68	Heart Disease 122	Congenital Anomalies 377	Liver Disease 725	Liver Disease 2,582	Diabetes Mellitus 6,062	Liver Disease 12,792	Diabetes Mellitus 54,161	Alzheimer's Disease 93,541
7	Bacterial Sepsis 544	Chronic Low Respiratory Disease 53	Influenza & Pneumonia 57	Chronic Low Respiratory Disease 71	Influenza & Pneumonia 199	Diabetes Mellitus 709	Diabetes Mellitus 1,999	Cerebro-vascular 5,349	Cerebro-vascular 11,727	Unintentional Injury 48,295	Diabetes Mellitus 76,488
8	Respiratory Distress 460	Septicemia 53	Cerebro-vascular 45	Cerebro-vascular 43	Diabetes Mellitus 181	HIV 583	Cerebro-vascular 1,745	Chronic Low. Respiratory Disease 4,402	Suicide 7,527	Influenza & Pneumonia 44,836	Influenza & Pneumonia 55,227
9	Circulatory System Disease 444	Benign Neoplasms 38	Benign Neoplasms 36	Influenza & Pneumonia 41	Chronic Low Respiratory Disease 178	Cerebro-vascular 579	HIV 1,174	Influenza & Pneumonia 2,731	Septicemia 5,709	Nephritis 39,957	Nephritis 48,146
10	Neonatal Hemorrhage 441	Perinatal Period 38	Septicemia 33	Benign Neoplasms 38	Cerebro-vascular 177	Influenza & Pneumonia 549	Influenza & Pneumonia 1,125	Septicemia 2,514	Influenza & Pneumonia 5,390	Septicemia 29,124	Suicide 42,773

Data Source: National Vital Statistics System, National Center for Health Statistics, CDC.
Produced by: National Center for Injury Prevention and Control, CDC using WISQARS™.

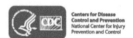

Centers for Disease Control and Prevention
National Center for Injury Prevention and Control

Figure 1.2 Courtesy of the CDC

Factors That Influence Health and Wellness

Lifestyle choices, including dietary behaviors, activity levels, tobacco use and alcohol consumption, all play a role in our overall health. While you may not see an immediate impact unless you have an acute reaction to something, you will see the consequences long term as you age. The following chart identifies the leading causes of death, but note what the contributing factors actually are. Additionally, pay attention to some of the things you can do to help reduce the risks for preventable diseases. Some of these involve things you can do on a daily basis.

Top 5 Leading Causes of Death:	Ways to Prevent Leading Causes of Death
Cancer 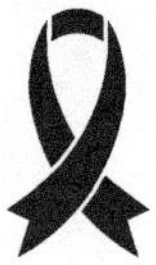	• Screenings and vaccines • Getting Tested for Hepatitis C • Avoid tobacco use • Protect your skin from sun exposure • Maintaining a healthy weight
Heart disease 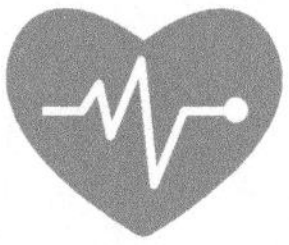	• Eating a healthy diet • Maintaining a healthy weight • Getting enough physical activity • Not smoking or using other forms of tobacco • Limiting alcohol use

Stroke 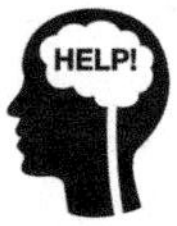	• Eating a healthy diet
	• Maintaining healthy weight
	• Not smoking or using other forms of tobacco
	• Control Medical Conditions:
	  ○ Check Cholesterol, Blood Pressure and Diabetes
	  ○ Treat your heart disease and take your medication

Chronic lower respiratory diseases (CLRD) 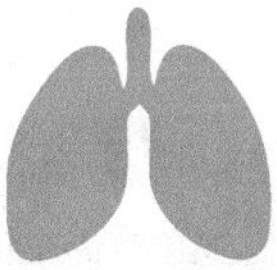	• Avoiding exposure to tobacco smoke • Avoid home and workplace air pollutants • Avoid respiratory infections by washing your hands regularly with soap and water ○ It is estimated that hands spread 80 percent of common infectious respiratory diseases like colds and flu.

Unintentional Injuries 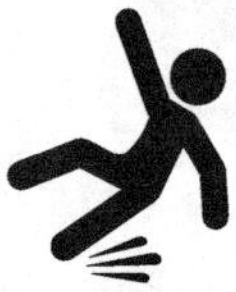	• Depending on the setting be mindful of:
	  ○ Distractions
	  ○ Your surroundings
	  ○ The people around you

Courtesy of Caylee King. Copyright © Kendall Hunt Publishing Company.

Another way to look at our dietary decisions can be seen in Figure 1.3 identifying complications from obesity. Our food choices matter long term as does our activity level or lack thereof.

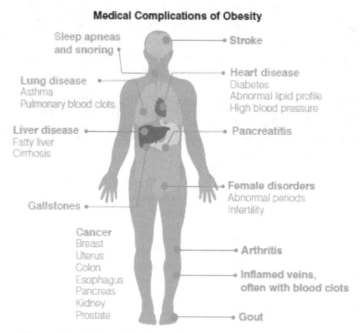

Figure 1.3 Adapted from Yale University Rudd Center for Food Policy and Obesity.

A WELLNESS PROFILE

"Living well requires constant evaluation and effort on our part. We must be aware of what we are doing, what habits we are developing, and how are they impacting our overall wellness. The following list includes important behaviors and habits to include in your daily life:

- Be responsible for your own health and wellness. Take an active role in your life and well-being.
- Learn how to recognize and manage stress effectively.
- Eat nutritious meals, exercise regularly, and maintain a healthy weight.
- Work towards healthy relationships with friends, family, and significant others.
- Avoid tobacco and other drugs; use alcohol responsibly, if at all.

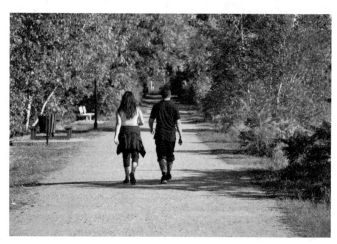

© Lester Balajadia/Shutterstock.com

- Know the facts about cardiovascular disease, cancer, infections, sexually transmitted infections, and injuries. Utilize this knowledge to protect yourself.

- Understand how the environment affects your health and take appropriate measures to improve it (adapted from Insel & Roth, 2009)."[1]

The Stages of Change

There are many models that discuss why we act or behave as we do and what occurs when we are looking to change a particular behavior. The following behavior models are examples and may be be applied across a wide range of behaviors.

"The Stages of Change Model (SCM) was originally developed in the late 1970s and early 1980s by James Prochaska and Carlo DiClemente when they were studying how smokers were able to quit smoking. The SCM model has been applied to many different behavior changes including weight loss, injury prevention, alcohol use, drug abuse, and others. The SCM consists of five stages of change: precontemplation, contemplation, preparation, action, and maintenance. The idea behind the SCM is that behavior change does not usually happen all at one time. People tend to progress through the stages until they achieve a successful behavior change or relapse. The progression through each of these stages is different depending upon the individual and the particular behavior being changed. Each person must decide when a stage is complete and when it is time to move on to the next stage."[1]

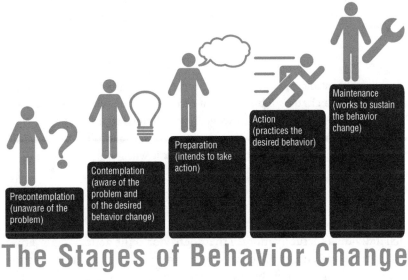

Precontemplation (unaware of the problem)

Contemplation (aware of the problem and of the desired behavior change)

Preparation (intends to take action)

Action (practices the desired behavior)

Maintenance (works to sustain the behavior change)

The Stages of Behavior Change

© Kendall Hunt Publishing Company

Precontemplation

"Precontemplation is the stage at which there is no intention to change a specific behavior in the foreseeable future. Many individuals in this stage are unaware of their unhealthy behavior. They are not thinking about change and are not interested in any help. People in this stage tend to defend their current behavior and do not feel it is a problem. They may resent efforts to help them change."[1]

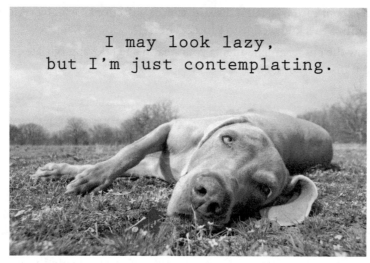

© Sari ONeal/Shutterstock.com

Contemplation

"Contemplation is the stage at which people are more aware of the consequences of their unhealthy behavior and have spent time thinking about the behavior but have not yet made a commitment to take action. They consider the possibility of changing, but tend to be ambivalent about change. In this stage, people straddle the fence, weighing the pros and cons of changing or modifying their behavior."[1]

Preparation

"The stage that combines intention and behavioral criteria is called preparation. In this stage, people have made a commitment to make a change. This can be a research phase where people are taking small steps toward change. They gather information about what they will need to do to change their behavior. Sometimes, people skip this stage and try to move directly from contemplation to action. Many times, this can result in failure because they did not research or accept what it was going to take to make a major lifestyle change."[1]

Action

"The stage at which individuals actually modify their behavior is the action stage. This requires a considerable commitment of time and energy. The amount of time people spend in the action stage varies. On average, it generally lasts about six months. In this stage, unhealthy people depend on their own willpower. They are making efforts to change the unhealthy behavior and are at greatest risk for relapse. During this stage, support from friends and family can be very helpful.

"Along the way to a permanent behavior change, most people experience a relapse. In fact, it is much more common to have at least one setback than not. Relapse is often accompanied by feelings of discouragement. While relapse can be frustrating, the majority of people who successfully change their behavior do not follow a straight path to a lifetime free of unwanted behaviors. Rather, they cycle through the five stages several times before achieving a consistent behavior change. Therefore, the SCM considers relapse to be normal. Relapses can be important opportunities for learning and becoming stronger. This is where a behavior change journal and weekly reflections can help an individual see how much progress has been made, as well as what may trigger relapses. The main thing to remember is that the goal is getting closer. Do not get upset by life or setbacks, but keep moving forward and get closer to the end goal."[1]

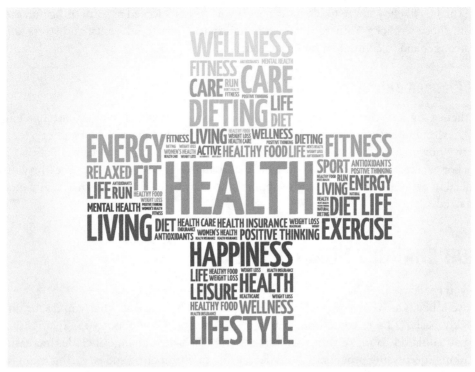

© dizain/Shutterstock.com

Maintenance

"Maintenance is the stage in which people work to prevent relapse and focus on the gains attained during the action stage. Maintenance involves being able to successfully avoid temptations to return to the previous behavior. The goal of the maintenance stage is to continue the new behavior or lack thereof without relapse. People are more able to successfully anticipate situations in which a relapse could occur and prepare coping or avoidance strategies in advance."[1]

Cognitive Dissonance

"Cognitive Dissonance refers to situations involving conflicting attitudes, beliefs or behaviors" (Simply-psychology). In 1957, Leon Festinger proposed cognitive dissonance theory, which states that a powerful motive to maintain cognitive consistency can give rise to irrational behavior. He focused on the principle of cognitive consistency, which means we want consistency in our beliefs and want to avoid disharmony.

For example, a person who smokes knows that smoking causes lung cancer. There is an underlying dissonance if they do not change that behavior. If we want to reduce dissonance, we either change our behavior, acquire new information about the behavior, (research is inconclusive about lung cancer and tobacco), or we reduce the importance of that behavior (live for today).

Another way to look at this is that as humans, we see ourselves as we want to be, our ideal selves. If there is a difference in who we really are and our ideal, there is dissonance. By utilizing the same step mentioned above, we can work towards that goal and reduce our dissonance.

Self-Efficacy

Self-efficacy centers the belief in your ability to reach goals and complete tasks. If you have a strong sense of self, and believe you can succeed, you are more likely to challenge yourself. The higher your sense of self-efficacy, the less likely you are to blame others if you do not succeed at something and are quicker to rebound from those setbacks. Your resiliency, the ability to adapt to adversity and stress, allows you to come back stronger and to continue moving forward.

Theory of Planned Behavior

Lastly, this theory suggests that your attitude about a behavior may affect your intention to engage in that behavior. Behavioral intention is generally established by attitude towards the behavior, (either good or bad), subjective norms (social pressures), and perceived behavioral control (perception of ease or difficulty to perform). For example, the likelihood you would start an exercise program is guided by your belief that you really need to get in shape, your friends support, and your belief that you can actually motivate yourself to get started.

BEHAVIOR CHANGE AND GOAL SETTING

So, how do you get started? What is the first step towards changing a behavior?

"Choose a behavior that you are really invested in. Think about what you do, or don't do, on a daily or weekly basis. Is there something you want to change? How about your relationships? Is there something you could do to make things better? Ideas for behavior change include: increasing exercise, quitting smoking, decreasing procrastination, decreasing or eliminating sodas, eating more fruits and/or vegetables, getting more sleep, drinking more water, every day, stretching, and so on.

"Only change one behavior at a time. After reviewing your habits or behaviors you would like to change, select one to focus on. People tend to get excited and want to change several different behaviors. Even if the behaviors are related, it is best to choose only one to focus on at a time. After a specific behavior has become a habit (at least six months in the maintenance stage) you can consider working on another behavior.

Once you have identified the behavior you wish to change, you need to set a goal. Your goal should be specific, **measurable**, **attainable**, **relevant** or **realistic**, and **time-bound**, otherwise known as a **SMART** goal. There are two other parts that have been added to the model and they are **evaluate** (see if your plan is working) and **revise** (if needed). Hence your goal will actually be **SMARTER**.

"The goal should be specific and measurable. The more specific the goal and the plan to achieve this goal are, the more likely the behavior change will be successful. If you want to increase fitness, it would be best to be very specific about the short- and long-term goals. For example, you should consider your baseline (where you are right now). If you are not exercising at all, you should not begin working out five times per week the following week. During the first week you may want to exercise two times for fifteen minutes each exercise session. The following week the goal could be three times at twenty minutes each exercise session. The final goal may be five days per week for thirty minutes each time. This particular goal should take at least a month or two to achieve. The Behavior Change and Goal Setting notebook activity at the end of the chapter can help outline a plan of change.

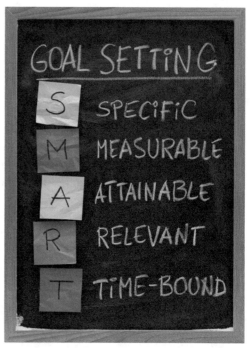

© marekuliasz/Shutterstock.com

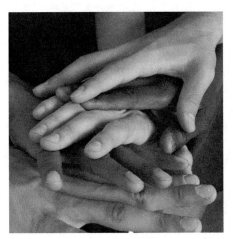

© Martin Allinger/Shutterstock.com

"**Any behavior change target should be realistic.** Often, behavior change goals include weight loss. To increase the long-term success rate, the most a person should lose is two pounds per week. One pound is equal to 3,500 calories. In order to lose two pounds per week the caloric deficit would need to be 7,000 calories. This translates to a deficit of 1,000 calories per day, which is not easy to achieve. The best way to achieve this caloric deficit is to include both exercise and limit caloric consumption. For example, you could expend part of the needed caloric deficit with exercise (approximately 500 calories per day) as well as consume fewer (approximately 500) calories per day for a total daily caloric deficit of 1,000. Remember, this is the most a person should lose per week.

"**Have a reward system.** It is nice to have short- and long-term goals that have a small reward when a goal is reached. These rewards should never be counterproductive. For example, if you are trying to lose weight, the worst type of reward would be to have a dessert. Some constructive reward ideas could be to go to a movie, go for a specific hike, buy a little something you have been wanting or just give yourself time to hang out with friends.

"**Keep a journal.** Recording notes on a regular basis is a great way to keep you focused on the behavior you are trying to change. It also creates a method to track progress and setbacks. A lot can be learned from looking at what worked and what did not in previous weeks. It is best to journal a minimum of three days per week and include a weekly reflection statement summarizing how the week progressed. This can give you critical insight that you may not have had without the journaling process.

"**Have a support group.** Tell friends and family members who will be supportive about a particular behavior change. The more people who know about the behavior change, the more likely the change will be successful. By regularly evaluating your lifestyle and making small changes, you can maintain a healthy lifestyle. There are significant benefits to choosing healthy behaviors early on. The earlier these healthy behaviors are achieved, the more graceful aging will be. In Figure 1.2 the number one cause of death is unintentional injury until the age of 44. After age 44, the leading causes of death are cancer and heart disease. The chart demonstrates how critical it is that healthy behavior choices are made now rather than waiting until an injury or disease has occurred.

Prevention

Part of the reason for changing unhealthy behaviors is to avoid short term or long term health consequences. "The best way to avoid injuries and disease is through prevention. There are three types of prevention: primary, secondary, and tertiary. **Primary prevention** utilizes behaviors to avoid the development of disease. This can include getting immunizations, exercising regularly, eating healthy meals, limiting exposure to sunlight, using sunscreen, having safe drinking water, and guarding against accidents. The focus of this textbook will be primary prevention to help individuals choose behaviors that will prevent disease and premature death.

"**Secondary prevention** is aimed at early detection of disease. This can include blood pressure screenings, mammograms, and annual pap tests to identify and detect disease in its earliest stages. This is before noticeable symptoms develop, when the disease is most

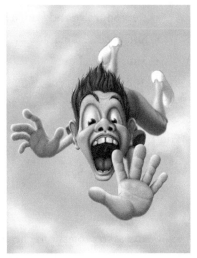

© Aidar/Shutterstock.com

likely to be treated successfully. With early detection and diagnosis, it may be possible to cure a disease, slow its progression, prevent or minimize complications, and limit disability. Another goal of secondary prevention is to prevent the spread of communicable diseases. In the community, early identification and treatment of people with communicable diseases, such as sexually transmitted infections, not only provides secondary prevention for those who are infected but also primary prevention for people who come in contact with infected individuals.

"**Tertiary prevention** works to improve the quality of life for individuals with various diseases by limiting complications and disabilities, restoring function, and slowing or stopping the progression of a disease. Tertiary prevention plays a key role for individuals with arthritis, asthma, heart disease, and diabetes."[1]

HEALTHY PEOPLE 2020: IMPROVING THE HEALTH OF AMERICANS

While we have been focused on individual goals for behavior change, there are agencies and organizations that look at goals and objectives for behavior changes for society as a whole. Not only do these goals address specific deficits in policy or access to care, but they also identify behaviors that need to be encouraged or discouraged. Additionally, there are many **health disparities** within our society. Whether associated through race, ethnicity, gender, age, sexual identity or other variables, social determinants play a significant role in the health status of individuals. As such, agencies look at how to reduce or eliminate those disparities.

Healthy People 2020 is a 10-year agenda developed with the help of numerous agencies and individuals to improve the health of the Nation. "There are twelve major public health areas, including leading health indicators. They are:

- Access to health services
- Clinical preventive services
- Environmental quality
- Injury and violence
- Maternal, infant, and child health
- Mental health
- Nutrition, physical activity, and obesity
- Oral health
- Reproductive and sexual health
- Social determinants
- Substance abuse
- Tobacco

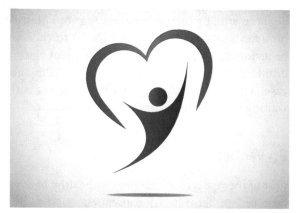

© Harish Marnad/Shutterstock.com

www.healthypeople.gov/2020/LHI.default.aspx

"There are four major factors that influence personal health:

1. personal behavior
2. heredity
3. environment
4. access to professional health care personnel

"The importance of prevention is made clear in *Healthy People 2020*. *Healthy People* was first developed in 1979 as a *Surgeon General's Report*. It has been reformulated since 1979 as *Healthy People 1990: Promoting Health/Preventing Disease, Healthy People 2000: National Health Promotion and Disease Prevention and Healthy People 2010; Objectives for Improving Health*. The original efforts of these programs were to establish national health objectives and to serve as a base of knowledge for the development of both state-level and community-level plans and programs to improve the nation's overall health. Much like the programs *Healthy People 2020* is based on, it was developed through broad consultation programs and the best and most current scientific knowledge in the public and private sectors. It is also designed in a way that will allow communities to measure the success rates, over time, of the programs they choose to implement.

"*Healthy People 2020* has four overarching goals. The first goal is to attain high quality, longer lives free of preventable disease, disability, injury, and premature death. The second goal is to achieve health equity, eliminate disparities, and improve the health of all groups. The third goal is to create social and physical environments that promote good health for all. One last goal is to promote quality of life, healthy development, and healthy behaviors across all life stages. In an attempt to meet these overarching goals, *Healthy People 2020* has forty-two topic areas—each with a concise goal statement that is designed to frame the overall purpose of each of the forty-two topic areas."[1]

Healthy Campus 2020 is a companion to Healthy People and focuses on specific issues that affect college students, faculty and staff. The intent is to provide a framework to help institutions identity priorities and develop action plans to meet individual campus needs.

Are you a healthy consumer?

We have identified many things in this chapter about wellness, health behaviors, behavior change and national health objectives. So what are you doing to foster a better health outcome? What are you, as a consumer, doing to contribute to not only your health, but the community as well? We discussed what it means to be health literate at the beginning of the chapter. What are you doing to build your health literacy and be a wise consumer? Things to think about as we continue this course.

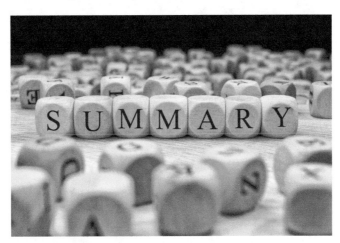

© Fabrik Bilder/Shutterstock.com

"Health is 'a state of complete physical, mental, and social well-being and not merely the absence of disease or infirmity,' according to the World Health Organization. By definition, health is a universal trait. Due to the fact that personal behaviors are one of the four major factors that influence a person's lifespan and quality of life, health also takes on a very individual and unique quality.

"The idea of wellness is an individual-based approach to health. Wellness is grounded in behavior modification strategies that result in the adoption of low-risk, health-enhancing behaviors. By balancing the seven components of wellness—emotional, intellectual, social, spiritual, physical, occupational, and environmental—a person can, to some degree, prevent disease and premature death.

"Changing behaviors and setting goals to achieve healthy change are major steps to wellness. Using the SCM can be helpful in making behavior changes. The SCM consists of precontemplation, contemplation, preparation, action, and maintenance stages. These stages are very important to recognize when preparing for a behavior change project. The key elements in a successful behavior change include planning, research, and individual willpower. Healthy behaviors chosen early in life affect an individual's wellness now and in the years to come."[1]

Prevention is a fundamental factor in promoting wellness. The three types of prevention include primary, secondary, and tertiary. Primary prevention utilizes behaviors to avoid injuries, the development of diseases, and premature death. Secondary prevention focuses on early detection of disease and tertiary prevention works to improve the quality of life for individuals with various disease processes.

Healthy People 2020 and Healthy Campus 2020 are designed to provide a plan for improving the health of our Nation. They each address specific concerns across broad areas and identify areas of disparity within various settings.

Personal Reflections . . . so, what have you learned?

1. In your own words, describe the concept of the "dimensions of wellness". How is it related to holistic health? Why is it important?

2. In which dimension would you consider yourself the most developed and why? Which one needs the most work and why?

3. Identify a behavior you might want to change. Select one of the models for behavior change and list the steps needed to make that change occur based on the model. Do not forget to make the goal "SMARTER".

4. Select one healthy objective from Healthy People 2020 and one from Healthy Campus 2020 (you will need to look these up online) that you think are the most important and explain why.

NOTES

RESOURCES ON CAMPUS FOR YOU!

Every campus has health and counseling services available to students. Identify what services are available to you and be sure to utilize their services as needed.

STUDENT LIFE

The Division of Student Life's mission is providing opportunities and services to foster student development along cognitive, personal, and interpersonal dimensions. As educators, we work with our faculty colleagues to nurture and stimulate student learning and success within a pluralistic campus community. We accomplish this by delivering primary services that provide for the out-of-classroom caring for students, the foundation upon which classroom growth occurs. We enhance the quality of campus life, establish a sense of community and school spirit, and foster students' overall maturation and ethical development.

RECREATIONAL SERVICES

Recreational Services, offers spirited and competitive activities involving intramural and extramural sports, fitness activities, special events, and aquatics.

The Office of Recreational Services is a valuable resource for students, faculty and staff who wish to pursue a healthy lifestyle. Through participation in various programs, participants can gain a multitude of personal benefits including improved levels of physical fitness and wellness, opportunities for social interaction, time management skills, engagement in a group dynamic setting, a healthy means of stress relief, as well as the creation of a sense of ownership and belonging between students and the community.

REFERENCES

Center for Disease Control, College *Health and Safety*. Retrieved from http://www.cdc.gov/family/college/. Retrieved 2016.

Corbin, C. B., Welk, G. J., Corbin, W. R. and Welk, K. A. (2010). *Concepts of Physical Fitness* (16th ed). McBrown.

Evans, R. & Sims, S. (2016). Health and Physical Education for Elementary Teachers: An integrated approach. Human Kinetics.

Floyd, P., Mims, S., and Yelding-Howard, C. (2007). *Personal Health: Perspectives and Lifestyles* (4th ed). Morton Publishing Co.

hrsa.gov/publichealth/healthliteracy

http://ahha.org http://wellness.ndsu.nodak.edu/education/dimensions.shtml

http://who.int/aboutwho/en/definition.html

https://www.cdc.gov/cancer/dcpc/prevention/index.htm

https://www.cdc.gov/cancer/dcpc/prevention/other.htm

https://www.cdc.gov/healthcommunication/toolstemplates/entertainmented/tips/chronicrespiratorydisease.html

https://www.cdc.gov/heartdisease/healthy_living.htm

http://www.cdc.gov/nchs/data/hp2k99.pdf

https://www.cdc.gov/nchs/fastats/adolescent-health.htm

https://www.cdc.gov/stroke/healthy_living.htm

https://www.cdc.gov/stroke/medical_conditions.htm

http://www.healthypeople.gov/2020/default.aspx

http://www.m-w.com/dictionary.htm

http://www.wellnesswise.com/dimensions.htm

Hyman, B., Oden, G., Bacharach, D., and Collins, R. (2006). *Fitness for living* (3rd ed). Kendall Hunt Publishing Company.

Insel, P. M. and Roth, W. T. *Core Concepts in Health* (12th ed). McGraw-Hill Publishing. 2009.

Payne, W. A., Hahn, D. B., and Lucas, E. B. (2008). *Understanding Your Health* (10th ed). McGraw-Hill Publishing.

Pruitt, B.E. and Stein, J. (1999). *Health Styles*. Allyn & Bacon.

www.simplypsychology.org/cognitive-dissonance.html

CREDITS

1. From *Health and Fitness: A Guide to a Healthy Lifestyle*, 5/e by Laura Bounds, Gayden Darnell, Kristin Brekken Shea, Dottiede Agnore. Copyright © 2012 by Kendall Hunt Publishing Company. Reprinted by permission.

NOTES

Chapter 2 +━━━━━━━━━━━━━━━━━━

Stress Management

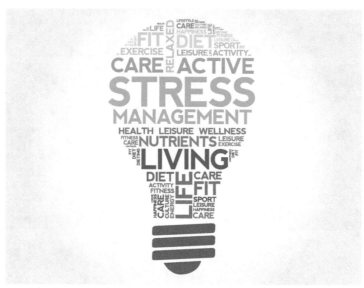

© dizain/Shutterstock.com

OBJECTIVES:

"Students will be able to:

- Define and identify the different types of stress.
- Identify different causes of stress.
- Describe the negative health complications that can result from unmanaged stress.
- Establish a link between unmanaged stress and its detrimental effect on health.
- Show the links between stress, depression, and suicidal behaviors.
- Introduce general tips to help individuals positively cope with stress.
- List characteristics of good stress managers.
- Introduce the concept of self-talk and explain the effects positive and negative self-talk can have on an individual's stress level and its impact on the person's psychological health.
- Describe the role of sleep and recommendations for effective stress management.
- Recognize and identify your universities' resources for stress management coping."[1]

"ARE YOU UNDER STRESS?

I am physically tired.	Yes	No
I am emotionally tired.	Yes	No
I have headaches.	Yes	No
I have an upset stomach.	Yes	No
I have trouble sleeping.	Yes	No
I am irritable.	Yes	No
I am too tense.	Yes	No
I am angry.	Yes	No
I get into verbal/physical fights.	Yes	No
I have a hard time concentrating.	Yes	No
I am nervous.	Yes	No
I am worried.	Yes	No

Three or more 'yes' answers can indicate a high stress level."[7]

Critical Thinking . . .

What do you think are major causes of stress in your life?

Would you consider your stress as good stress or bad stress?

Do you think you have healthy, effective, stress-coping strategies?

How does your stress level affect physical activity, sleep, nutrition, or consumer behaviors?

TYPES OF STRESS

"Stress, both positive and negative forms, has always been a part of life. One cannot hope to live and thrive without facing stressful situations daily. Most Americans live a fast-paced, over-booked lifestyle each day in an attempt to make the most of their time and talents. Due to the fact that 'working under the gun' has become the rule rather than the exception, stress has become one of the most common detriments to the overall health and well-being of Americans.

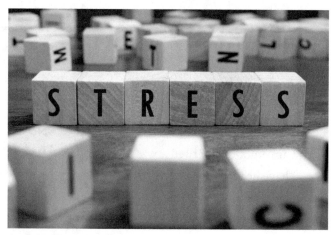

© schatzie/Shutterstock.com

"**Stress** was defined by Hans Selye as the nonspecific response to demands placed on the body. 'Nonspecific response' alludes to the production of the same physiological reaction by the body regardless of the type of stress placed on the body. Physiologically, when an individual is confronted with a stressor, they will experience a surge of adrenaline that causes the discharge of cortisol and the release of endorphins. This, in turn, will increase the person's blood pressure and heart rate, preparing him or her to take immediate action. While the physiological way in which all people react to stress is the same, the way a person physically, emotionally, or behaviorally reacts to a specific stressor can vary greatly. This is due in part to the fact that when facing the exact same event or circumstance it might be perceived as highly stressful and draining to one person but simply stimulating and exciting to someone else. The ways in which people outwardly react to stressful situations are a personal physical and emotional response to the stimuli. These responses can be either positive or negative.

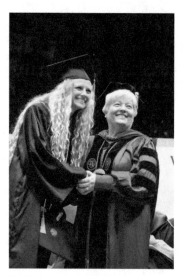

© Winthrop University

"**Eustress** is a positive stress that produces a sense of well-being. It is a healthy component of daily life. It can be harnessed to improve health and performance. Examples of activities or events that might initiate a positive stress response include competitive sports, graduation from school, dating, marriage, the birth of a baby, or a long-awaited vacation. Eustress can have positive effects on health and overall well-being. Research has shown that individuals who are experiencing eustress had more positive social behavior and improved memory (von Dawans, Fischbacher, Kirschbaum, Fehr, Heinrichs, 2012; Stauble, Thompson, Morgan, 2013). Other research has shown that long-term eustress may improve immune system function and may help individuals recover faster from injuries and illnesses (Dhabhar, Malarkey, Neri, & McEwen, 2012). It is also possible that eustress can enhance creativity and increase alertness (St. Lifer, 2013). Generally, you should look to embrace the events in your life that create a positive stress, or excitement.

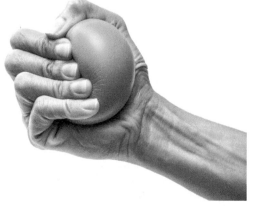

© Chutima Chaochaiya/Shutterstock.com

"**Distress** is negative stress. It is a physically and mentally damaging response to the demands placed upon the body. Distress is generally associated with changes that interrupt the natural flow of a person's life. Excessive schoolwork, loss of a job, breaking up with a significant other, or illness or death of a loved one are examples of activities or situations that may produce a negative stress response from an individual. When distress occurs, it is typical to see deterioration in the affected individual's health and performance."[1]

"Another concept related to stress is known as burnout, a complete overwhelming of stress, which causes one to shut down both personally and professionally. This term started to become mainstream in the late 60s and early 70s and was often found within professionals whose jobs included being first responders (firefighters, paramedics, police officers). During the course of their daily work lives, these people saw horrors at accident scenes, murders, fires, and violence, and when they were done with that incident, they went to the next call. By the end of their shift, the end of the week, month, year, career, they had seen so many horrible or violent things that negatively impacted their spirit, their emotions, their joy within their jobs, they were massively stressed. If you ever thought about entering one of those noble careers, when asked why, you would probably answer that you want to make a difference, you want to help individuals. You would not be ready emotionally, physically, or mentally to experience this and handle the physiological responses the first couple of times (hundreds of times) that you experienced such trauma while at work. Because these professionals were severely impacted, many left the profession due to all that they had seen and experienced. Today, we know that when people see a horrific accident or crime scene, they may need to be referred to counseling to help them work through what they saw and how it impacted them. They will talk and share the experience with a trained professional who will help them."[6]

SOURCES AND CAUSES OF STRESS

There are many individual sources and causes of stress, but we can generally categorize them into environmental, physiological, or psychosocial stressors. A **stressor** is any real or perceived event that pressures us to cope (Donatelle, 2014).

Environmental Stressors

Environmental stressors are situations or events that create stress within our environment. They can include our most immediate environment of day-to-day hassles and daily life complexities. Examples of daily situations that can create stress include: weather, noise, distractions, traffic, and even crowds. Environmental stressors can also originate from major external events, such as war, flood, or disaster.

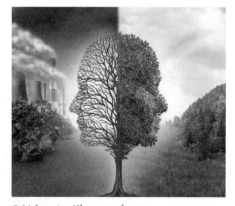

© Lightspring/Shutterstock.com

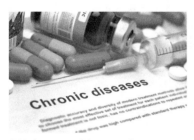

© Tashatuvango/Shutterstock.com

Physiological Stressors

Physiological stressors can be very damaging to our overall health if they persist for a long period of time, or coping strategies are ineffective. These stressors tend to be more chronic in nature, such as a long term illness or a difficult disability. Other sources might be an outcome that was very traumatic, such as the death of a loved one or a life-altering change. One physiological stressor can affect many members of a family.

Psychosocial Stressors

Psychosocial stressors include the wide variety of stressors that we encounter in our day-to-day life. Sources of psychosocial stress include the ebbs and flows of relationships with those closest to you and the range of feelings and emotions regarding these situations. Other examples can include situations such as: losing your job, breaking up with someone you loved, ending a friendship, an unplanned pregnancy, a speeding ticket, car accident, missing class, or failing an exam.

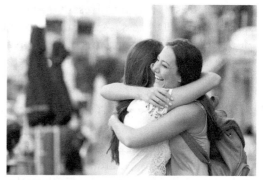

© Antonio Guillem/Shutterstock.com

STRESS IN COLLEGE – WHAT ARE STRESSORS OF COLLEGE STUDENTS?

"College can be exciting and overwhelming at the same time. New responsibilities, freedom, and relationships can challenge your ability to maintain homeostasis through a healthy lifestyle. Do you agree with the following stressors, as reported by college students?"[1]

Academic	Time	Money	Self	Social
• competition • schoolwork • grades & exams • poor resources • professors	• deadlines • procrastination • late for appointments • no time to exercise	• not enough • bills/overspending • job responsibilities • no job	• behavior • appearance • poor health • weight • self-esteem	• obligations • not dating • roommate problems • STD concerns

Think about how these stressors affect your behaviors and overall health. What can you do to effectively cope with these stressors?

The Body's Response to Stress

"The classic, automatic response to stress is known as the fight or flight response. In reality, the fight or flight response started back with our prehistoric ancestors who, when confronted by a woolly mammoth

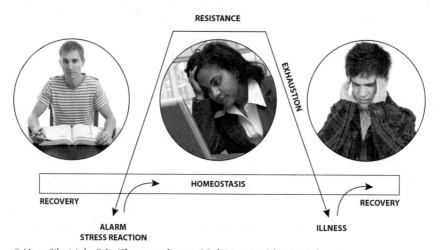

© Hugo Silveirinha Felix/Shutterstock.com, ©Rob Marmion/Shutterstock.com,
© Rui Vale de Sousa/Shutterstock.com

or saber-toothed cat, had to either fight the animal as a food source or become its food source, or decide that this battle was not in their favor and flee (the flight response). In today's version, we still have a fight or flight response, but the stakes are different, although the physiological outcomes are still similar. When discussing the fight of flight response to stress, we need to look further at the physiological response the body has to the stressor. The **General Adaptation Syndrome (GAS)**, was originally developed by Hans Selye (considered to be the father of stress research) to describe a three-stage response to stress he was investigating. This response involves both the nervous system and hormonal systems of the human body. Following is a brief overview of the GAS.

"**Stage 1.** The **alarm stage** is the immediate response to the stressor. This stage is the preparation for the fight or flight response we earlier discussed. The body releases cortisol and adrenaline, which provide the energy to deal with the stressor.

"**Stage 2.** In the **resistance stage**, also known as the adaptation stage, the body reacts to the stressor. Especially if the stressor continues, the body begins to make changes to lessen the impact of the stressor. If the stressor lessens, the body struggles to return to homeostasis (a physiological balance) and recovers from the stressor. If the stressor remains for a longer period of time, then the body moves into the last stage.

"**Stage 3.** The **exhaustion stage** occurs when the body's response to the stressor is weakening. The longer the duration of the stressor, the more likely this response will be impacted. As indicated by the name, the stressor has lasted a length of time and the body is at an overload or truly fatigued. The indication is that the body's immune system is weakened and making the individual more likely to become ill. When the individual reaches the exhaustion stage, this is where the serious health consequences from stress impact us."[6]

"There are typically four ways in which stress can surface in our lives:"[1]

Emotionally	Behaviorally
• Do you always feel rushed?	• Has your appetite changed so that you have gained or lost significant amounts of weight?
• Do you find it difficult to relax?	
• Are you irritable and moody, or easily angered?	• Are you neglecting yourself/your appearance?
• Do you want to cry for no apparent reason?	• Have you curtailed social activities?
• Is it difficult for you to listen or pay attention?	• Have you taken to substance abuse, such as cigarette smoking, drug use, or excessive alcohol or coffee intakes?
• Is it hard for you to fall or stay asleep?	
Physically	**Mentally**
• Do you have an increased heart rate or blood pressure?	• Are you indecisive in many areas of your life?
• Do you feel out of breath or have tightness in your chest?	• Is it difficult for you to concentrate?
• Do you suffer from frequent headaches or muscle aches?	• Do you regularly have bad dreams or nightmares?
• Is it difficult for you to digest food—leading to nausea or diarrhea?	• Do you have negative thoughts, including suicidal thoughts?"[1]
• Do you suffer from frequent attacks of infections?	

THE IMPACT OF STRESS ON THE BODY AND HEALTH

Symptoms of Stress

"The way each person chooses to manage the stressors that occur in life will, to a large degree, determine overall physical and emotional well-being. An individual's body naturally attempts to maintain a state of homeostasis, or balance, so that it can continue to function in an effective manner. When a stressful situation presents itself, an 'alarm' is triggered. Either the person deals with the situation and the body recovers and returns to a state of homeostasis, or the attempts to avoid or resist the stressor eventually result in exhaustion or illness. Stress is not the cause of illness, but when it goes on for long periods of time or is particularly irritating, it can become harmful by weakening an individual's immune system. This increases that person's risk of getting sick. Uncontrolled or unmanaged stress can lead to a variety of negative health consequences such as coronary heart disease, high blood pressure, ulcers, irritable bowel syndrome, migraine headaches, and insomnia. Certain forms of stress are not only normal but necessary in everyday life. However, the results of continual or inappropriately managed stress can cause disruptions that can be serious or severe to an individual's emotional, intellectual, social, spiritual, physical, occupational, and/or environmental health. It is extremely important for an individual to determine how he or she handles or reacts to stressors, especially if the stress is ongoing. The way stress manifests or 'shows itself' is going to vary depending on an individual's personality and past experiences."[1]

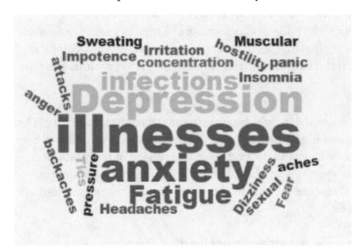

Courtesy of Joni Boyd

STRESS AND DISEASE

"**Heart Disease & Cancer** — In one study of 1,300 graduates of the Johns Hopkins Medical School, depression was found to be an important predictor of heart disease. In England, people who experienced chronic mild anxiety and depression were more likely to develop heart disease than those who did not. In a study of 10,000 Israeli men, anxiety over problems and conflicts about finances, family, and relationships with co-workers was associated with 2 to 3 times the risk of developing heart disease. In a 17-year study of 2,000 middle-aged men, depression has been associated with twice the risk of death from cancer. Dr. Donald Girard from the Oregon Health Sciences University has

The activation of the stress system

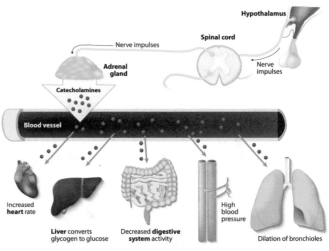

© Designua/Shutterstock.com

reviewed the literature on this subject and concluded that repressed feelings of loss, denial, depression, inflexibility, conformity, lack of social ties, high levels of anxiety and dissatisfaction, and an over-abundance of life-change events are associated with increased cancers, heart disease, and infection.

"**Colds & Flu** — A one-year study of 100 people found that flus and colds were four times as prevalent following stressful life events. An Australian study found that stressed people had twice as many days when they had flu and cold symptoms. National surveys suggest that marital happiness contributes far more to happiness in societies throughout the world than any other variable, including satisfaction with work and friendships. Divorced and separated people have poorer mental and physical health than those who remain married, or are widowed or single. Marital disruption has been found to be the single most powerful predictor of stress-related physical illness; separated partners have about 30 percent more acute illnesses and physician visits than those who remain married. It has been concluded that depression of immune function is associated with marital discord.

"**Mortality** — A number of other studies have found bereavement and a lack of social and community ties to be associated with an overall increase in mortality. A study of 95,647 widows found more than double the normal mortality rate during the first week following widowhood, primarily from cardiovascular disease, violent causes, and suicides. Dr. Ruberman of New York has reported that highly stressed and socially isolated heart disease patients (few contacts with friends, relatives, and church or club groups) had more than four times the risk of dying from heart disease of men with two levels of isolation and stress."[6]

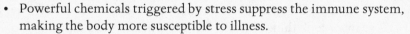

Did you know . . .

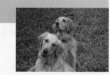

Courtesy of Shelley Hamill

"Stress and the Immune System

- Powerful chemicals triggered by stress suppress the immune system, making the body more susceptible to illness.
- Stress interferes with the body's ability to heal.
- The pituitary gland increases production of andrenocorticotropic hormone (ACTH), which in turn stimulates the release of cortisone and cortisol hormones. These hormonal releases may inhibit the functioning of disease-fighting white blood cells and suppress the immune system's response."[7]

STRESS AND ITS IMPACT ON MENTAL HEALTH

"While stress in general, and specifically unmanaged stress, can have a negative impact on a person's physical health, the impact it can have on mental health can be equally devastating. There are many types of mental health disorders. Schizophrenia, depression, general anxiety disorders, bipolar disorders, and panic disorders are just a few of the mental health disorders that can cause havoc in a person's life. These disorders typically include chronic or occasional dysfunctional feelings and/or a lost sense of self-worth that may often limit the extent to which an individual participates in life's daily activities. The many

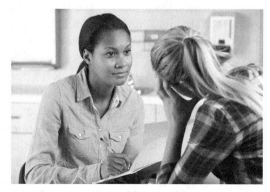

© Monkey Business Images/Shutterstock.com

different types of mental health disorders affect 90 million people. Mental health disorders are far reaching. They affect not only the individual with the disorder but also the people who have intimate and social relationships with them."[1]

Depression and Stress

"Depression is a mental health disorder that is prevalent among college populations. One of the reasons college students are particularly vulnerable to depression is that, for many students, they face large amounts of unresolved stress. College is a time filled with challenging, new, different, and stressful situations. It is important to realize that unmanaged stress and depression can quickly become a vicious cycle. The more depressed an individual is, the less day-to-day stress and the fewer activities can be coped with and the more depressed the person becomes. More information on depression is covered within the Psychological Health chapter."[1]

Suicidal Behavior and Stress

"Another area in which stress can affect an individual's mental health is thoughts of or attempts at suicide. College students are particularly vulnerable to this problem. Nationwide each year, approximately one in 10,000 college students commits suicide; many more college students have suicidal thoughts. More information on suicide is covered within the Psychological Health chapter."[1]

Eating Disorders and Stress

"Eating disorders are medically identifiable, potentially life-threatening mental health conditions related to obsessive eating patterns. Eating disorders are not new—descriptions of self-starvation have been found as far back as medieval times. Even though more young men are succumbing to eating disorders each year, the mental health condition is typically thought of as a woman's disease. Unfortunately, even grade school girls can feel pressure to 'fit in' or look thin. This can be very troubling and disruptive to young girls struggling to build a positive body image. Eating disorders are often accompanied by other psychiatric disorders, such as depression, substance abuse, or anxiety disorders. More information on eating disorders is covered within the Psychological Health chapter."[1]

EFFECTIVE STRESS COPING STRATEGIES

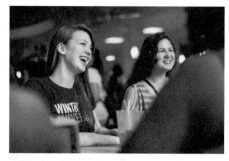

© Winthrop University

"Recognizing how stress affects their lives allows individuals to recognize stressful situations and to immediately deal with, or cope with, something that has the potential to compromise their overall well-being. While uncontrolled or unmanaged stress can lead to negative health consequences, there are a number of ways to control stress. What works for one person will not necessarily be helpful to someone else. It is important to recognize the stressor and determine the most effective way(s) to relieve, reduce, or eliminate that particular stressor. Another key to successfully managing stressors is to use a strategy that produces positive results, rather than a strategy that creates additional stress. Also, to be successful with stress management, give a particular stressor only the amount of energy it warrants—do not give a '10 cent' stressor $10 worth of time or energy. The following are general tips that can help maintain a healthy lifestyle and can prepare an individual to cope with many of the stressors found in everyday life.

1. *"Deal with the cause:* Finish the task, talk to the person, fix the tire, write the letter, make the call—do what needs to be done to deal with the situation. The longer a situation gets put off, the more stress it can create.

2. *"Put the situation into perspective:* How important is it really? How important will this be tomorrow, in six months? Most situations that tax physical/mental energies will soon be inconsequential and forgotten. Determine if anything can be done about the situation, or if it is a situation that calls for acceptance.

3. *"Pace yourself:* No one can be in 'high gear' all the time. Too often individuals stop to 'smell the roses' only after the first accident or heart attack. Set short and intermediate goals—reward yourself upon reaching these goals."[1]

Spotlight on . . .

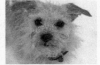

Pets & Stress

Research shows that, unless you're someone who really dislikes animals or is absolutely too busy to care for one properly, pets can provide excellent social support, stress relief and other health benefits—perhaps more than people! The following are more health benefits of pets

- Pets can improve your mood. Think how happy they are to see you and how playful they can be!
- Control blood pressure better than drugs. In a study on pets and blood pressure, groups of hypertensive New York stockbrokers who got dogs or cats were found to have lower blood pressure and heart rates than those who didn't get pets.
- Encourage you to exercise. They need to be walked and played with, right?
- Stave off loneliness and provide unconditional love. Pets can be there for you in ways that people can't. They can offer love and companionship, and can also enjoy comfortable silences, keep secrets and are excellent snugglers (Scott, 2015).

Courtesy of Shelley Hamill

4. *"Laugh at life and at yourself:* Humor is a wonderful tool. Laughing is internal jogging! She or he who laughs . . . lasts! See the humor in people and the absurdity of situations. Read the 'funny pages.'

5. *"Develop quality relationships:* Seek social and emotional support systems—individuals who care, love, and will listen to you. Express feelings constructively. Be there for others and allow others to be there for you in the good times and in the bad times.

6. *"Time management needs to be life management:* Look at goals and responsibilities from a bigger perspective; this can help

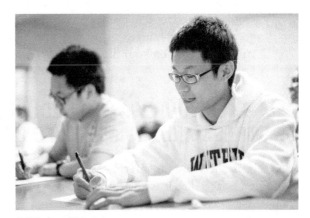

© Winthrop University

with decision making. Streamline activities by breaking big, imposing jobs into small components and list each activity in a daily planner. Seek assistance when it is needed; don't try to do everything yourself—delegate! Avoid common 'time killers'."[1]

Spotlight on . . .

Academic Success

It's understandable that academic pressures of college can be a substantial source of different stressors of college students. Class times, professors, assignments, exams, and grades can be a challenge in achieving academic success. When these stressors are coupled with the many other demands and expectations of college life, many students can feel overwhelmed. When you might feel this way, it is important to remember the priority of why you are here, which is to graduate! Putting your priorities in perspective is critical for stress management, and ultimately success in college and throughout life. Your university has several resources available for you to manage stress, from counseling and meditation sessions to exercise classes and theatrical productions. The best and most efficient means of coping with stress is an individual task for each person. What works well for your friends may not work well for you! Check the information at the end of this chapter for more on resources.

7. *"Look at situations and people in a different light—try an attitude adjustment:* Is your perception of the situation, event, or person correct? Is there another way to handle things, or is there another possible way to answer the problem? Take care of the things you can; don't worry about the things that are beyond your control.

8. *"Balance fun and responsibility:* Family, society, and community encourage and command constant work and responsibility. It is important to contribute and to meet responsibilities, but it is also important to find enjoyment and fun in life as well. Do something you find enjoyable on a regular basis and don't feel guilty!

9. *"Exercise and eat sensibly:* Exercise is one of the best stress-busters. Schedule exercise into your life. Walk, bike, swim, stretch, and recreate. Good food in proper proportions is also essential to good health and is an excellent way to reduce the negative effects stress may have on your life."[1]

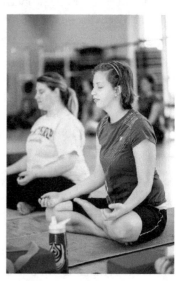
© Winthrop University

SELF-TALK YOUR WAY TO REDUCED LEVELS OF STRESS AND AN IMPROVED LIFE

"Self-talk is the constant interpretation of the different situations that individuals find themselves in throughout each day. It is that 'inner voice' that determines one's perception of a situation. Conscious thoughts, as well as subconscious thoughts, are part of a person's inner voice. Negative or positive self-talk begins early in most individuals' lives and can determine the impact stress has on each person's life.

"Negative self-talk, such as 'I am going to fail my test' or 'there is no way I can run that far or fast or perform that move' is self-defeating. Negative interpretation of a situation will often make that situation more stressful than it needs to be. Replacing negative thoughts or self-talk with positive thoughts can decrease stress levels and improve a person's productivity and overall outlook. There is a line between thinking something and feeling it! People changing the way they think can allow them to change the way they feel. Thinking positively is a habit. Like any other habit, it will take time and practice to master—but health benefits such as decreased negative stress, reduced risk of coronary heart disease, and improved coping skills make it time well spent."[1]

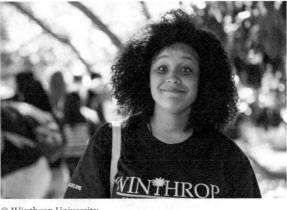
© Winthrop University

"Good Stress Managers

- are physically active, eat a healthy diet, and get adequate rest every day.
- believe they have control over events in their life (have an internal locus of control).
- understand their own feelings and accept their limitations.
- recognize, anticipate, monitor, and regulate stressors within their capabilities.
- control emotional and physical responses when distressed.
- use appropriate stress management techniques when confronted with stressors.
- recognize warning signs and symptoms of excessive stress.
- schedule daily time to unwind, relax, and evaluate the day's activities.
- control stress when called upon to perform.
- enjoy life despite occasional disappointments and frustrations.
- look success and failure squarely in the face and keep moving along a predetermined course.
- move ahead with optimism and energy and do not spend time and talent worrying about failure.
- learn from previous mistakes and use them as building blocks to prevent similar setbacks in the future.
- give of themselves freely to others.
- have a deep meaning in life."[1]

THE IMPACT OF SLEEP ON STRESS

Sleep and stress level are closely related. If we do not get enough sleep, then the energy to handle the day-to-day stressors can become overwhelming. Conversely, when stress levels rise for many people, sleep quantity and quality are often adversely affected. Many Americans suffer from some kind of sleep problems, and the college-aged population is no different. The American College Health Association's (ACHA) research on college students' health showed that less than 12% of college students reported feeling well rested from their sleep patterns. Most (60%) reported that they feel sleepy, tired, or dragged out (ACHA, 2013). Other studies have shown that most college students that average between 6–6.9 hours of sleep per night feel sad, tired, and stressed. The National Sleep Foundation (NSF) recommends college students aim for 7–8 hours of sleep each night (NSF, 2015).

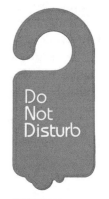
© Natapong Paopijit/ Shutterstock.com

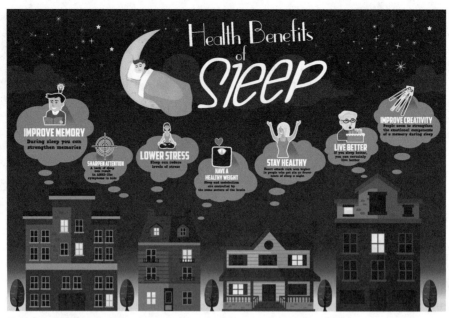

© Artisticco/Shutterstock.com

"Lack of sleep leads to problems completing a task, concentrating, making decisions, working with and getting along with other people, and unsafe actions. Sleep duration is related to length of life, with death risk increased in those sleeping less than six hours a night. Sleep deprivation is linked to approximately 100,000 vehicle crashes and 1,500 deaths each year. Insomnia early in adult life is a risk factor for the development of clinical depression and mental health disorders. Characteristics of **insomnia** (inadequate or poor sleep quality) include:

- difficulty falling or staying asleep
- non-refreshing sleep
- daytime tiredness, lack of energy, difficulty concentrating, and irritability"[3]

What happens during sleep?

"A night's sleep consists of four or five cycles, each of which progresses through several stages. During each night a person alternates between non-rapid eye movement (NREM) sleep and rapid eye movement (REM) sleep. The entire cycle of NREM and REM sleep takes about 90 minutes. The average adult sleeps 7.5 hours (five full cycles), with 25 percent of that in REM. In NREM sleep, brain activity, heart rate, respiration, blood pressure, and metabolism (vital signs) slow down, and body temperature falls, as a deep, restful state is reached. Slow wave sleep usually terminates with the sleeper's changing position. The brain waves now reverse their course as the sleeper heads for the active REM stage."[3]

"Getting a good night's sleep has proven to be a difficult goal for many people in this modern era. The National Sleep Foundation has published several guidelines for better sleep.

Here are ten guidelines for better sleep:

- Maintain a regular bed and wake time schedule, including weekends.
- Establish a regular, relaxing bedtime routine such as soaking in a hot bath or hot tub and then reading a book or listening to soothing music.
- Create a sleep-conducive environment that is dark, quiet, comfortable and cool.
- Sleep on a comfortable mattress and pillows.
- Use your bedroom only for sleep and sex. It is best to take work materials, computers, and televisions out of the sleeping environment.
- Finish eating at least two to three hours before your regular bedtime.
- Avoid nicotine (e.g., cigarettes, tobacco products). Used close to bedtime, it can lead to poor sleep.
- Avoid caffeine (e.g., coffee, tea, soft drinks, chocolate) close to bedtime. It can keep you awake.
- Avoid alcohol close to bedtime. It can lead to disrupted sleep later in the night.
- Exercise regularly."[3]

Are you a healthy consumer?

Now that you know how stress can impact certain areas of your health, let us consider how it can impact another specific area: consumerism. How does stress affect your consumer behaviors? Research has identified four basic ways in which stress can influence consumer behaviors, according to Durante and Laran (2016).

1. Stress can lead to beneficial or impulsive consumer behaviors.
2. Stress can lead to increased spending on items we deem to be necessary.
3. Stress can lead to increased saving if we perceive low income could be possible.
4. Ultimately, stress pushes us to allocate our resources so that we feel we are in control. We have identified many things in this chapter about stress, causes of stress, and impact of stress. If stress pushes you to be a healthy consumer, then you intake healthy consumption of coping strategies. Healthy foods, healthy activities, tools to relieve stress in a positive way. Impulsive behavior under stress might push you to consumer more negative coping strategies, and increase long-term stress. Tobacco, unhealthy food, risky behaviors, or just relying on a quick gratification of material things can be impulsive consumer behavior. Thinking about how stress affects your consumer behaviors, answer the following questions:

Do you believe stress influences your consumer behavior? Does your response to stress create a positive, healthy, nurturing environment? Would you consider your response to stress one that elicits impulsiveness, and enables a more stressful, negative environment?

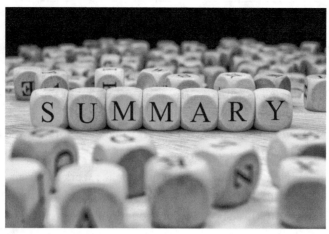

© Fabrik Bilder/Shutterstock.com

In this chapter, we have defined stress, identified stressors, and categorized stress as both positive and negative. We have compared the effects of both short-term and long-term stress, and how they affect overall health. It is also critical to understand how coping strategies also influence health. Unhealthy coping strategies essentially "double" the negative impact of stress, since they add additional health concerns to your body. Identifying unhealthy coping strategies and working to change your behavior can better reduce stress, create a positive environment, and improve overall health.

Personal Reflections . . . so, what have you learned?

1. Based on the questions from the beginning of the chapter, do you have a high stress level? What are your main sources of stress, and how much of your stress is eustress or distress?

2. What are three ways stress negatively affects your life or your health? What are three ways stress positively affects your life or your health?

3. What are three healthy coping strategies that you turn to in times of stress? What is at least one unhealthy coping strategy that you use to deal with stress?

4. How is sleep and stress related? How does our bodies use sleep to cope with stress? Does your sleep environment allow for restful, restorative sleep?

5. How can you turn any negative impulsive behavior into positive, healthy consumerism?

6. In your opinion, how does health literacy impact health consumerism, during times of eustress and distress?

NOTES

RESOURCES ON CAMPUS FOR YOU!

Academic Services

Colleges and universities offer many different types of academic support for students. Examples include:

- One-on-one consultations;
- Interim grade consultations;
- Individual and group study spaces;
- Referrals to other university support services;
- Personal assistance with academic questions or concerns;
- Individual and group tutoring opportunities;
- Academic skill development - time management, study skills, organization, etc.;
- Development of academic action plans and success contracts;
- Specialized services for students on academic probation and students with incompletes.

Workshops/Seminars

Academic success workshops are offered on many college campuses. These sessions can be facilitated for classes, residence halls, organizations, or other events. Workshop topics include the following:

- Notemaking;
- Study strategies;
- Time and stress management;
- Test taking;
- Textbook reading;
- Tutee seminars.

Tutoring

PEER TUTORS are available at all colleges and universities through academic support. Student tutors are hired each semester to assist students in developing the skills to become independent learners. Check your universities academic services centers for more information.

REFERENCES

American College Health Association. (2012) *American College Health Association- National College Health Assessment II: Reference Group Data Report Fall 2011.* Baltimore, MD: American College Health Association

Bounds. L, Gayden. D, Brekken Shea. K, Dottiede. A. (2012) *Health and fitness: A guide to a healthy lifestyle.* Dubuque, IA: Kendall Hunt Publishing Company.

Dhabhar, F.S., Malarkey, W.B., Neri, E., & McEwen, B.S. (2012). Stress-induced redistribution of immune cells–from barracks to boulevards to battlefields: A tale of three hormones. *Psychoneuroendocrinology, 37*(9) 1345–1368.

Donatelle, Rebecca J. (2014) *Access to health* (12th ed). San Francisco, California: Benjamin Cummings.

Durante, K.M. & Laran, J. (2016). The effect of stress on consumer saving and spending. *Journal of Marketing Research, 53*(5), 814–828.

National Sleep Foundation. (2015). Retrieved 2016 from https://sleepfoundation.org/.

Nieman. D. (2015) *Fitness and your health* (7th ed) Kendall Hunt Publishing Company.

Rand. C. (2012) *Stress Management: A guide to a healthier life.* Kendall Hunt Publishing Company.

Scott, E. (2015). How Owning a Dog or Cat Can Reduce Stress. Retrieved 2016 from http://stress.about .com/od/lowstresslifestyle/a/petsandstress.htm.

Stauble, M.R., Thompson, L.A., & Morgan G. (2013). Increases in cortisol are positively associated with gains in encoding and maintenance working memory performance in young men. *Stress, 16*(4), 402–410.

St. Lifer, H. (2013). 7 reasons (a little) stress can be good for you. Retrieved online at: http://www .goodhousekeeping.com/health/wellness/advice/a18528/stress/

von Dawans, B., Fischbacher, U., Kirschbaum, C., Fehr, E., & Heinrichs, M. (2012) The social dimension of stress reactivity: acute stress increases prosocial behavior in humans. *Psychological Science, 23*(6) 651–660.

Zinger. L. (2014) *Healthy happy long life* (2nd ed). Kendall Hunt Publishing Company.

CREDITS

NOTES

Chapter 3 +

Psychological Health

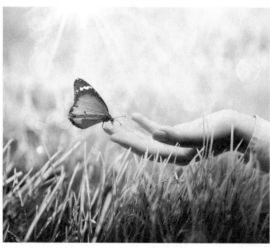

© Romolo Tavani/Shutterstock.com

OBJECTIVES:

- To identify the dimensions of psychological health.
- To define social health and the characteristics of those who are socially healthy.
- To describe how self-esteem, self-efficacy, and resiliency can affect several dimensions of psychological health.
- To describe emotional health and the characteristics of emotionally healthy individuals.
- To identify four abilities associated with emotional intelligence.
- To describe intellectual health, and individual intellectual strengths.
- To identify the discovery, process, and application disciplines associated with intellectual strengths.
- To realize and define your own preferred learning style.
- To define spiritual health and the characteristics of spiritually health individuals.
- To differentiate between religion and spirituality.
- To explore individual spirituality and what impact it has in your life.
- To identify several mental health disorders and their impact on life.
- To differentiate between depression, anxiety, panic attacks, and obsessive compulsive disorder.
- To describe the services on your college for psychological health resources.

"Are you Psychologically Healthy?   1 = Never   2 = Sometimes   3 = Always

1.	I sleep too much or too little, or I wake up constantly.	1	2	3
2.	My mood swings from depression to happiness for no reason.	1	2	3
3.	I east more than I should.	1	2	3
4.	I enjoy time playing video games more than I enjoy anything else.	1	2	3
5.	People sometimes think that I'm unstable or unreliable.	1	2	3
6.	I have poor self-esteem.	1	2	3
7.	I feel that I don't play any useful part in life.	1	2	3
8.	I have thought about ending my life.	1	2	3
9.	I am overwhelmed by thoughts I can't seem to control.	1	2	3
10.	I have disturbing dreams or recollections about my past.	1	2	3
11.	I hate the way I look.	1	2	3
12.	I cry or get very angry at times.	1	2	3
13.	My feelings are interfering with work, school, and friendships.	1	2	3
14.	I feel unhappy, sad, or worthless.	1	2	3
15.	I feel out of control.	1	2	3
16.	I feel empty or that my life has little meaning.	1	2	3
17.	I find it difficult to cope with things.	1	2	3
18.	I avoid making new friends.	1	2	3
19.	I have trouble concentrating at work or school.	1	2	3

Sum your answers for a score. Scores range between 19–57, with high scores indicating higher levels of stress. Self-reflect on your score.

Critical Thinking . . .

How does your psychological health impact your overall health?

What are the different components of psychological health and how strong are you in each?

How do your behaviors impact your psychological health and overall well-being?

Introduction to Psychological Health

Psychological health is the day-to-day combination of our feelings, thoughts, and relationships as they exist in our lives, and includes the emotional, social, intellectual (or mental) and spiritual dimensions of health (Donatelle, 2014).

SOCIAL HEALTH

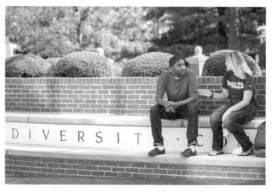

© Winthrop University

"When we begin to look at our social health, we have to reflect on where we are today in relationship to our family, our friends, our community involvement, our world involvement, and ourselves. As you begin this reflection, where you currently are is not a limit, as many of us could use more social interaction and social support in our lives. Many of you may already have a world connection through social media forums. Each of these components will impact our social health either positively or negatively. We have to consider what our personal needs are and what we are able to provide our friends and families as we grow and nurture our social health. So the beginning discussion of social health will examine where you are with each of these.

"In a discussion of our social health, we must introduce the following words: self-esteem, resiliency, self-efficacy, helplessness, depression, and happiness. Each of these words will help us to better understand our perspective of our social health and can help us grow to the next version of ourselves.

"**Self-esteem** is a feeling of self-worth, how you view yourself, happiness within your spirit, and the ability to meet life's challenges each day.

"**Resiliency** is having the ability to bounce back from obstacles and adversity within our daily lives by having the ability to cope with the life stressors we face.

"**Self-efficacy** is having the confidence in yourself to make things happen and believing in your ability to succeed in all or most of the situations that you face in your life. When we have self-efficacy, we have an innate ability to bounce back from failures, set-backs, and disappointments that arise within our life. We face the challenges given to us and believe we will overcome and be stronger for the experience. You will often see self-efficacy discussed within positive psychology and health and wellness concepts.[6]

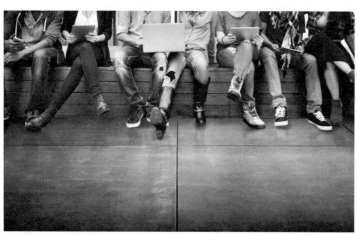

© Rawpixel.com/Shutterstock.com

Of course, we will face difficult times of adversity, failure, and even loss. It is important to not allow these moments in life define who we are mentally, spiritually, and emotionally. "Failure is only a failure if we take nothing away that can help us the next time we face the same or a similar situation. **Learned helplessness** is the anticipation or action that the individual has no control over a situation and can see no positive outcome, so they flounder with whatever occurs."[6]

Support from Family and Friends

"A discussion of our social health has to include all of the connections we have made during our lifetimes. Perhaps the most important social connections we can consistently count on are the emotional support, friendship, patience, love, understanding of our families, and being there to pick us up when we are down. Family and friends have grown up with us; they know us, can read our emotional responses, understand our mood swings, and love us unconditionally when we screw up. Yes, we all screw up during our lifetimes, and those screw-ups are actually life lessons that help us develop into who we become. As you reflect on your past life lessons, who were the people there supporting you, helping you pick up the pieces, and move forward to the next chapter in your life story?"[6]

Introvert vs. Extrovert . . . and the Impact on Health

An **introvert** is defined as someone who mentally "turns in," especially in certain environments. Most commonly, introverts tend to shy away from large crowds or awkward social interactions. They may also find energy in time spent alone, or with one or two very close friends. An **extrovert** is generally defined as the opposite, or someone who tends to find energy from interactions and time spent with others.

Research has shown both positive and negative outcomes of both introversion and extroversion. The introvert tends to form stronger bonds, have better sleep outcomes, engage in less risky behaviors, and are not stressed by the "fear of missing out" on something. However, introverts may also be less happy, have a slower reaction time when driving, and hesitate to talk to their doctor about health concerns. Extroverts tend to report higher levels of happiness, have stronger immune systems, and are more proactive about health concerns with their physician. Negative impacts of extroverts are higher levels of social-based stress, poorer sleep outcomes, and higher rates of risky behavior.

What can we do to bridge the gap between introverts and extroverts? While the college life tends to reward extroverts and their typical behavior, it is important to understand that both can acceptable and healthy, and should be embraced. Introverts can try to better understand why they may feel awkward or uncomfortable in certain situations, and incorporate strategies to effectively and healthfully deal with their emotions. Extroverts can work to engage introverts in a respectful manner, and learn to appreciate their comfort boundaries. Working together, we can understand, appreciate, and value the diversity of everyone, including personalities!

Spotlight on . . .

Body Image

"A person's body image is how a person sees him or herself in his or her mind. Body image is affected by a person's attitudes and beliefs, as well as by outside influences such as family, social pressures, and the media. It is important to have good perspective. If you are an 'apple' and naturally carry excess fat in your abdominal area, when you gain weight you will become a larger 'apple' or you may lose weight and become a smaller 'apple.' The same is true for 'pear' shaped individuals who carry their excess fat in their hips and buttocks. You cannot become a different shape, nor can you diet down to a thin waif. Accept yourself for who you are; then work on behavior changes to become healthier. The fringe benefit to becoming healthier is that you will most likely fit better in your jeans. You will also feel better while you reduce your risk of heart disease and diabetes."[1]

Commitment to Our Community, to the World

"The question as we begin this section is, how would you rank your involvement and commitment to making your community better? As you look around any college in this country, you will obviously see a wide spectrum of students who have different levels of social engagement. Your university has courses that provide service learning where you take materials related to your college courses and engage in experiential activities to immerse yourself in the learning. Most college campuses have a plethora of clubs and organizations; many are geared to provide leadership opportunities; others are created to have like-interested people who share the same passions, and others are geared as service clubs whose goals are to make a difference within the college or local community. These types of activities are the foundation for making the world around you a better place. Whether it is within the classroom experiences or from actually volunteering somewhere in your community, giving back can make a wonderful change in your attitude and increase your self-worth."[6]

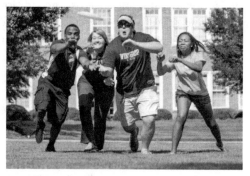

© Winthrop University

To ensure the holistic balance of health that we have and will discuss throughout the semester, social involvement is critical. Being involved on campus and within the community can engage your social health and expectations of the world. We have many opportunities for service and volunteering, both within the your college community, and the community at large.

Happiness and Joy

"How do you know when you are happy? Is there a feeling you have inside, or is it a feeling that exudes from your soul, your personality? Can we tell you're happy by your smile, your body language, how you treat others around you? What are your indicators that you are happy? Would your friends and family describe you as a happy person? Happiness and joy are often interchanged to mean the same idea. Many think that happiness and joy are similar, but view joy as a more intense experience that is of a shorter duration, and happiness is a sense of positive well-being, excitement, and contentment with your life at that moment."[6]

Joy can explain the excitement you feel when you are finally offered a job or career that you have desired. Happiness explains the emotion that you feel when going to work every day doing what you love. This is why retirement is harder for some than they thought it would be.

"Find ways to add joy and happiness into your life. Whether it is with your family, friends, or your career, joy and happiness are strong words that make life more enjoyable. When you have joy and happiness within your life, it will be easier to adjust to the life's speed bumps which we all face."[6]

INTELLECTUAL HEALTH

Intellectual, or **mental** health, refers to the dimension of "thinking" or "being rational." Those who are intellectually health are able to learn and apply new information, and often strive to do so. An intellectually healthy person can problem solve, adapt to surroundings, and develop effective strategies as they carry out responsibilities (Donatelle, 2014).

One key component of intellectual health is cognition. By definition, **cognition** refers to our processes of perception, learning, and reasoning and problem solving.

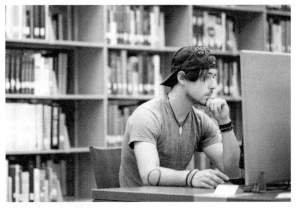

© Winthrop University

- **Perception** refers to interpreting data that you sense (hear, see, smell, feel, taste, etc.)

- **Learning** refers to the process of taking the cues that you perceived and applying them to previous ones to store as memory

- **Reasoning** and **problem solving** refer to the ability to rationalize a plan to solve a problem.

Cognition is also a link between the intellectual and emotional dimensions of the brain and can often drive our behavior about a situation. Emotions can be heightened in response to the cognitive analysis of situation or experience, and that emotional response can determine the behavior on how we choose to deal with it (Edlin & Golanty, 2014).

Intellectual Health & Learning

"Throughout recent history, intellectual capacity has been correlated to what has been termed the intelligence quotient, better known as IQ. This is determined by measuring an individual's ability to respond to visual imagery, to respond to verbal input, and to apply skills in both areas to the solution of problems. For the most part, when people talk about intellectual strengths, they are referring primarily to IQ. As a result of this, we end up with a culture where people think they are smart when they really aren't. This confusion often leads to feelings of inferiority and self-doubt related to IQ and causes uncertainty in the search for a life purpose. More recent studies have shown this to be too narrow a focus on the intellect. Howard Gardner has proposed the idea of multiple intelligences (1983). In other words, people might be 'intelligent' or 'smart' in different ways."[6] Understanding components of learning styles and learning atmosphere and how to apply those can maximize your ability to learn. Additionally, having the disciplines to allow the cognition process to run its course is key to learning and intellect."[6]

Learning Styles

"One of the primary reasons that the intellect needs to be looked at with a broader perspective is that people learn in different ways or styles. One simplified approach to learning styles divides people into three primary groups of visual, auditory, or kinesthetic/tactile learners.

- Visual learning occurs primarily through looking at images, such as pictures, diagrams, demonstrations, and body language.
- Auditory learning occurs primarily through hearing words- both spoken and written.
- Kinesthetic/tactile learning occurs through hands-on doing and interacting.

"People rarely, if ever, learn only in one style. The reality is much more a preference in learning styles. However, it is important to understand what style you prefer. This can help you approach classes and studying in a more effective manner."[6]

Learning Atmosphere

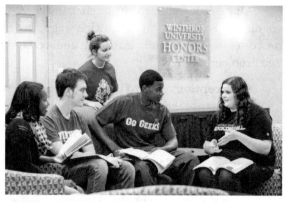

© Winthrop University

"Another approach to learning that shows our distinctiveness as individuals was developed around our preferred atmosphere or setting for learning. This concept suggests that each person has unique strengths and preferences across a full spectrum of physiological, sociological, psychological, emotional, and environmental elements. The interaction of these elements occurs differently in everyone and will affect the way they concentrate on, process, absorb, and retain new and difficult information (Dunn & Dunn, 1992, 1998, 1999).

"From our discussion we see that your true intellectual strengths are affected by your learning style and your preferred learning atmosphere. Further, we found that intellectual strengths are made up of disciplines that encompass a far greater spectrum than just IQ. This complexity, as with the other strengths, makes it harder to see when we have these strengths. Again, one of the most effective ways is listening to what others who know us well say about us."[6]

Remember, each of the psychological health dimensions provides a bridge to the other dimensions. "Intellectual health provide 'the bridge of information,' among the other strengths. What do we mean by this? It is through our intellect that we learn about what is going on with the other strengths. This adds the knowledge and understanding required to live our lives."[6]

Learning Disciplines

"**Curiosity.** A strong desire to learn more about something. People who are curious have an excitement for knowledge and eagerness to search for truth.

Persistence. A firm and steadfast continual search for knowledge and truth. People who are persistent keep on pursuing truth despite obstacles, warnings, or setbacks.

Humility. People who have intellectual humility always see themselves as a learner and are always willing to be taught by others.

Teachable spirit. A willingness and eagerness to learn. These people are open to diverse views and forms of knowledge."[6]

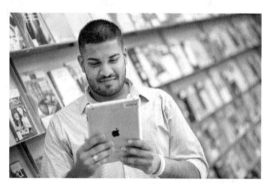

© Winthrop University

Process Disciplines

"**Integrity.** The quality or condition of interpreting information collected with honesty.

Critical thinking. The mental process of actively and skillfully conceptualizing, applying, analyzing, synthesizing, and evaluating information to reach an answer or conclusion.

Patience. The capability of calmly awaiting an outcome or result even in the face of obstacles or challenges.

Humility. Process humility is a modest view of one's own importance pertaining to the possession of understanding."[6]

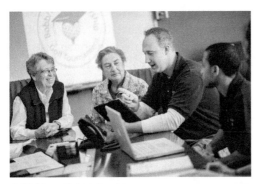

© Winthrop University

EMOTIONAL HEALTH

"What are the most important and significant experiences you will have during this school year? If you start to list them in your mind, you will find that they will likely be full of emotion. You may go to your first class and feel both excitement and apprehension. You may get your first 'A' in college and feel pride and satisfaction. You may make a new friend and gain a real sense of belonging. You may give your first speech or class presentation and feel nervous. You may try out for the varsity basketball team, and if you don't make the cut, you may feel depressed or angry at what you see as rejection. Whether they are positive, negative, or neutral, **emotions** play an important role in our lives because they alert us to something important in ourselves or our environment.

"Successfully navigating your college experience will likely call into play your ability to effectively work with your emotions, and this takes us to the concept of emotional strengths. We defined the emotional strengths domain as the capacity in our lives that enables us to experience feelings. What do we mean by these terms? When we talk about our **feelings**, we are describing an experiential state that builds within us in response to sensations, sentiments, or desires we encounter. **Sensibility** refers to our responsiveness toward other things or persons, such as the feelings of another person or changes in the environment.

"If we were to collect all the words in the English language that express our emotions, they would probably number in the hundreds. The paradox, however, is that with all those words, we still have great difficulty describing our emotional experiences to others. Why is that? Perhaps it stems from the view of emotions throughout the history of Western civilization. Emotions, for the most part, have been seen as a disruption to rational thinking and a hindrance to making good decisions. But now that view is changing.

"John Mayer, a psychologist at the University of New Hampshire, and Peter Salovey, a psychologist at Yale University (currently Dean of Yale College), proposed the concept of **emotional intelligence**, defining it as 'the ability to monitor one's own and others' feelings and emotions, to discriminate among them, and to use this information to guide one's thinking and action' (Mayer & Salovey, 1993; Salovey & Mayer, 1990). Mayer and Salovey have been joined by another psychologist, David Caruso,

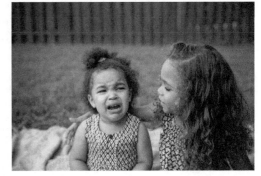

Photo by Danielle Flake.

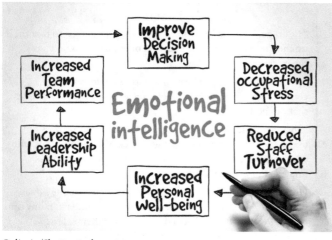

© dizain/Shutterstock.com

in systematizing the study of emotional intelligence and developing a credible tool for measuring it (Mayer-SaloveyCaruso Emotional Intelligence Test, or MSCEIT, 2002). Daniel Goleman, a journalist specializing in the area of the brain and psychology, worked from the writings of Mayer and Salovey to popularize the concept of emotional intelligence in his international bestseller, *Emotional Intelligence* (Goleman, 1995).

"Rather than seeing emotions as some sort of a primitive aberration in people that leads them to make mistakes and experience regrets, instead the findings show 'that emotion is not just important but absolutely necessary for us to make good decisions, take optimal action to solve problems, cope with change, and succeed' (Caruso & Salovey, 2004). It is not hard to see, then, that emotional strengths play an important part in the discovery of a life purpose.

"The basis for emotional intelligence is made up of four skills or strengths:

1. **Identify and express emotions.** This is the fundamental ability to recognize feelings and emotions by (a) being aware of emotional clues in yourself and in people around you, (b) being able to discern between different types of emotion, (c) being able to identify the level of intensity to which the emotion is present, and (d) being able to identify what these emotional clues mean. People with strength in this ability are better pilots of their lives because they have a surer sense of how they really feel about personal decisions from whom to marry to what job to take. They are also tuned in to the emotions of others and as a result have healthier and stronger relationships.

2. **Use or generate emotions.** This is the ability to know which emotions or moods are best for different situations and to get yourself into the 'right mood.' People with strength in this ability employ their feelings to enhance their thinking and endeavors. They realize that emotions, when rightly used, can help them solve problems, make better decisions, reason out situations, and be more creative. They will be more self-motivated and will prioritize their thinking process based on emotional input.

3. **Understand emotions.** This is the ability to recognize and grasp emotional information. This starts by gaining an emotional vocabulary—knowledge of simple and complex emotional terms. It then adds emotional comprehension—understanding how emotions combine to form another emotion, progress or intensify, or transition from one emotion to another. Finally, emotional analysis occurs—being able to understand possible causes of emotions and predict what kind of emotions people will have in different situations. People with strength in this ability have a solid grasp of emotional intelligence. They will tend to be more accurate in their interpretation of moods and emotional situations, and as a result will be more likely to deal correctly with such situations.

4. **Manage emotions.** This is the ability to regulate emotions in yourself and in other people. This involves monitoring, observing and distinguishing differences, and accurately labeling

emotions as they are encountered. This ability is based on the belief that feelings and moods can be improved or modified, with strategies being developed to accomplish this. This does not mean, however, the denial or suppression of your emotions or the emotions of others. People with strength in this ability can bounce back quickly from life's setbacks and upsets. They are also able to assess the effectiveness of how they recognize and handle emotions in various situations.

"Ironically, emotional strengths may be confused in our modern society with weakness, and society responds by not placing as great a value on this strength domain. As a result, we end up with a culture where relationships are confused and people try to hide from each other. This inner turmoil often leads to feelings of inferiority and self-doubt and causes confusion in the search for a life purpose. Emotional strengths are harder to detect than physical strengths. Once again, one of the most effective ways is listening to what others who know us well say about us. Another way is to complete exercises and assessments of our emotional strengths. Remember, each of the strength dimensions provides a bridge among the other dimensions. Emotional strengths provide the bridge of feelings among the other strengths. What do we mean by this? It is through our emotions that we actually sense and feel what is going on with the other strengths. This adds color and vitality to our lives."[6]

SPIRITUAL HEALTH

"Many people assume that religion and spirituality are the same. They can be connected, even intertwined, but they can be very different."[6] **Spiritual health** refers to the state of harmony within yourself and with others, focusing on a balance of self needs and world demands (Edin & Golanty, 2014).

Religion is defined as a specific system of beliefs, practices, rituals, and symbols for a purpose (Marr, 2015). "All religions have similarities. The followers of the religion know that when they go to church, temple, mosque, synagogue, monastery, or meeting house, they will be surrounded by others with the same beliefs, who share the sacred place housed within the building. Religious ceremonies will be consistent each time they practice them. They will listen to a religious leader or lay person, whose words will be spoken with reverence from a book, tablet, scrolls, or whatever contains the written word of their God. Each action of a ceremony will have symbolism to the followers. The service is a holy ceremony that provides comfort, faith, and support from the group who is practicing its beliefs. The ceremonies within each religious group will have their own customs, readings, and prayers. Participants will feel at home and welcomed by those of the same faith. The world's religions, of which there are many, have some very common themes, but each has its own specific beliefs and practices. If you review history, you will see many of the wars have been about religion with one culture or country trying to have another country practice its religion. If you think about it, the United States was founded on the pretense of escaping religious persecution in England."[6]

"**Spirituality** is similar and yet different. Instead of following an **organized religion**, spirituality can be based on your personal beliefs and following your inner path, still maintaining a

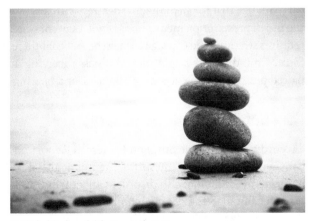

© Michal Bednarek/Shutterstock.com

belief in something larger"[6]. Realistically, one can be spiritual without following a specific religion. "When we discuss spirituality, thoughts, and feelings, we all have some concept of what we feel connected to. Usually, many people say that their spiritual makeup occurs when they are within the natural world. Others may find comfort in being surrounded by people on a busy street, and the energy that exists there helps them feel connected and ready to face the day's challenges."[6]

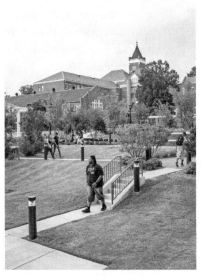

© Winthrop University

Spirituality is a combination of three integral components: healthy relationships, personal values, and a meaningful purpose in life. Although we cover healthy relationships in much more detail in a different chapter, it's important to see how it relates to spiritual health. Healthy relationships help to foster our own inner wisdom, and encourages treatment of respect, honesty, integrity, and love toward ourselves and toward others. Personal values, or principles we hold dear, help to guide our behavior in life situations. Distinguishing personal values is a type of individual spiritual journey, as they will define what we stand for and how we conduct our lives. Spiritually healthy people feel that it is their life goal to live out the purpose they were intended for. They are able to identify a meaningful purpose and work towards fulfilling that mission (Donatelle, 2014). **Spiritual intelligence** refers to an ability to access higher meanings values, abiding purposes, and unconscious aspects of the self (Zohar, 2014).

"Your spirituality should be about finding yourself, demonstrating compassion to your fellowman, and becoming a better person. What does spirituality mean to you? There are magazines, books, videos, websites, and self-help books that all discuss how, when, and where to find your spirituality. The questions we may ask are directly related to something we cannot hold, touch, or visibly see."[6]

MENTAL HEALTH DISORDERS

"There are many types of mental health disorders. Schizophrenia, depression, general anxiety disorders, bipolar disorders, and panic disorders are just a few of the mental health disorders that can cause havoc in a person's life. These disorders typically include chronic or occasional dysfunctional feelings and/or a lost sense of self-worth that may often limit the extent to which an individual participates in life's daily activities. It is critical to realize that for an individual dealing with any type of mental illness, therapy through counseling and/or the use of prescription medications is not a sign of weakness or personal failure. Accepting these means of help requires strength and courage to face the fact that there is a problem and to fight/prevail against a life-draining force. An individual with a mental illness receiving any type of therapy is much the same as a visually impaired person wearing glasses or contacts, or a hearing impaired individual using a hearing aid."[1]

Who Gets Mental Health Disorders?

"According to the 1996 Surgeon General's Report on Physical Activity and Health, one out of two Americans will suffer from some sort of mental health disorder at some point in their lifetime. The many different types of mental health disorders affect 90 million people. They affect not only the individual with the disorder but also the people who have intimate and social relationships with them. Mental health disorders have a far-reaching 'ripple effect.'"[1]

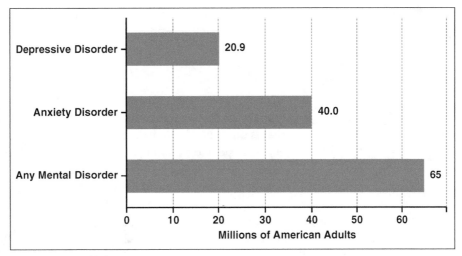

© Kendall Hunt Publishing Company

Depression

"While stress often plays a major role in depression, another type of depression also has a biological basis—endogenous depression. In this instance, a person's family mental health history can help determine if a genetic predisposition toward depression exists. This knowledge allows them to take a proactive approach

Spotlight on . . .

Exercise & Depression

"Exercise has also been shown to be effective in treating mild to moderate cases of depression. Thirty-three percent of all inactive adults consider themselves depressed. 'A recent review of more than 20 years of studies found that aerobic exercise and strength training are equally effective in treating depression, can reduce anxiety in patients with panic disorders and can be an important part of treatment for people with schizophrenia' (Payne, 2000). Recently a charity conducted a survey that found that 83 percent of those with mental health problems looked to some form of exercise to help improve their mood or reduce the amount of stress they felt they were under (news. bbc.co.uk). While exercise plays a vital role in reducing the negative impact mental health disorders have on a person's life, it should not be considered a total replacement for other treatments, and patients should always work with and under the close care of a physician."[1]

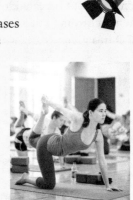

© Winthrop University

toward diagnosing and battling this mental health condition. Everyone has occasional feelings of being down or sad at some point. However, when depression results in a person crying a great deal, feeling hopeless, or being unable to take pleasure in life, professional help should be sought so that a life-threatening situation does not occur. Aside from or along with professional counseling, individual therapy or group therapy can be beneficial to an individual battling with depression. Prescription medications can be another

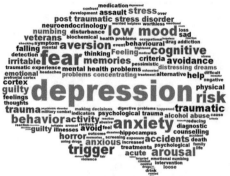

© Andrii Kondiuk/Shutterstock.com

important tool when coping with depression. They may or may not be necessary depending on each individual's situation."[1]

Anxiety Disorder

"Generalized anxiety disorder (GAD) is characterized by six months or more of chronic, exaggerated worry and tension that is unfounded or much more severe than the normal anxiety most people experience. People with this disorder usually expect the worst; they worry excessively about money, health, family, or work, even when there are no signs of trouble. They are unable to relax and often suffer from insomnia. Many people with GAD also have physical symptoms, such as fatigue, trembling, muscle tension, headaches, irritability, or hot flashes. About 2.8 percent of the U.S. population (4 million Americans) has GAD during a year's time. GAD most often strikes people in childhood or adolescence, but can begin in adulthood, too. GAD affects women more often than men. Most causes stem from stress, but individuals can be more susceptible if there is a family history."[7]

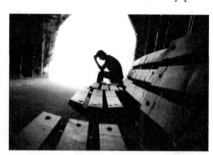

© hikrcn/Shutterstock.com

Obsessive-Compulsive Disorder (OCD)

"Individuals with OCD suffer intensely from recurrent, unwanted thoughts (obsessions) or rituals (compulsions) that they feel they cannot control. Rituals such as handwashing, counting, checking, or cleaning are often performed in hopes of preventing obsessive thoughts or making them go away. Performing these rituals, however, provides only temporary relief, and not performing them markedly increases anxiety. Left untreated, obsessions and the need to perform rituals can take over a person's life. OCD is often a chronic, relapsing illness. About 2.3 percent of the U.S. population (3.3 million Americans) has OCD in a given year. OCD affects men and women equally. OCD typically begins during adolescence or early childhood; at least one-third of the cases of adult OCD began in childhood. OCD cost the United States $8.4 billion in 1990 in social and economic losses, nearly 6 percent of the total mental health bill of $148 billion."[7]

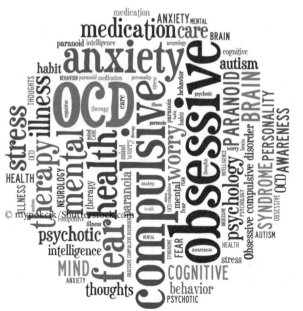

© mypokcik/Shutterstock.com

Panic Attacks

"Panic disorder is characterized by unexpected and repeated episodes of intense fear accompanied by physical symptoms that may include chest pain, heart palpitations, shortness of breath, dizziness, or abdominal distress. These sensations often mimic symptoms of a heart attack. In a given year 1.7 percent of the U.S. population (2.4 million Americans) experiences panic disorder. Women are twice as likely as men to develop panic disorder. Panic disorder typically strikes in young adulthood. Roughly

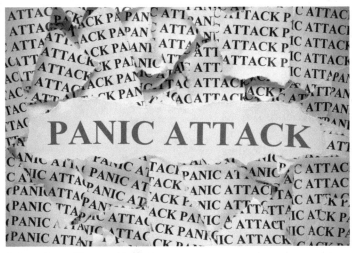

© StepanPopov/Shutterstock.com

half of all people who have panic disorder develop the condition before age 24."[7]

Suicidal Behavior

"Another area in which stress can affect an individual's mental health is thoughts of or attempts at suicide. College students are particularly vulnerable to this problem. Nationwide each year, approximately one in 10,000 college students commits suicide; many more college students have suicidal thoughts. Most people who contemplate or actually do commit suicide want something in their 'world' to change. It may be one thing that will greatly impact their life if it changes or goes away, or it may be a lot of the 'little things' that have added up. Often, a suicidal individual does not really want to die; it is just that the person has run out of ways or ideas on how to make that needed change occur. Intense pressure or stress, along with feelings of depression, alcohol misuse, drug abuse, or a personal loss such as a breakup or lack of academic success, are common causative factors in suicides. Anyone expressing suicidal thoughts should be taken seriously. Friends, roommates, or whoever should seek out help for a suicidal individual immediately."[1]

"Typical signs that an individual is contemplating suicide could include:

- skipping classes,
- giving away personal possessions,
- withdrawing from friends,
- withdrawing from 'normal' activities,
- engaging in risky behaviors not normal for that person."[1]

"An effective tool for helping someone get past suicidal thoughts or desires is counseling to help change the way he or she is thinking and coping. Medications can also be very effective in the prevention of suicidal behaviors. Hospitalization may be needed as well, in order to prevent suicide. The key to helping a suicidal or potentially suicidal individual is for those around them to be aware and actively involved in seeking out help for the person who is at risk."[1]

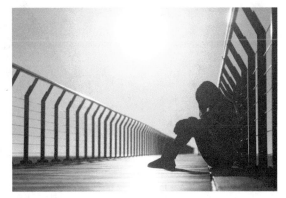

© Antonio Guillem/Shutterstock.com

EATING DISORDERS

"Typically, a person with an eating disorder seeks perfection and control over their life. Both anorexics and bulimics tend to suffer from low self-esteem and depression. They often have a conflict between a desire for perfection and feelings of personal inadequacy. Such persons typically have a distorted view of themselves, in that when they look into a mirror, they see themselves differently than others see them. Narcissism, or excessive vanity, can be linked to both anorexia and bulimia. Eating disorders are often accompanied by other psychiatric disorders, such as depression, substance abuse, or anxiety disorders. Eating disorders are very serious and may be life-threatening due to the fact that individuals suffering from these diseases can experience serious heart conditions and/or kidney failure—both of which can result in death. Therefore, it is critically important that eating disorders are recognized as real and treatable diseases."[1]

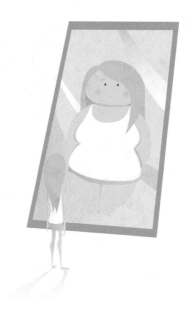

© stefanolunardi/Shutterstock.com

Anorexia Nervosa

"Anorexia nervosa is a state of starvation and emaciation, usually resulting from severe dieting and excessive exercise. An anorexic will literally stop eating in an effort to control body size. Most, if not all, anorexic individuals suffer from an extremely distorted body image. People with this disease look in a mirror and see themselves as overweight or fat even when they have become dangerously thin. Major weight loss is the most visible and the most common symptom of anorexia. Anorexic individuals often develop unusual eating habits, such as avoiding food or meals, picking out a few 'acceptable' foods and eating them in small quantities, or carefully weighing and portioning foods. Other common symptoms of this disease include absent menstruation, dry skin, excessive hair on the skin, and thinning of scalp hair. Gastrointestinal problems and orthopedic problems resulting from excessive exercise are also specific to this illness. Anorexic individuals can lose between 15 and 60 percent of their normal body weight, putting their body and their health in severe jeopardy. The medical problems associated with anorexia are numerous and serious. Starvation damages bones, organs, muscles, the immune system, the digestive system, and the nervous system."[1]

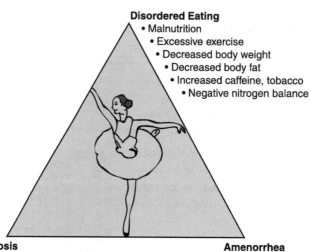

Disordered Eating
• Malnutrition
• Excessive exercise
• Decreased body weight
• Decreased body fat
• Increased caffeine, tobacco
• Negative nitrogen balance

Osteoporosis
• Inadequate calcium intake
• Excessive stress
• Low estrogen
• Decreased bone mineral content
• Injury
• Depression

Amenorrhea
• Decreased production of estrogen

© Kendall Hunt Publishing Company

Bulimia Nervosa

"Bulimia nervosa is a process of bingeing and purging. This disorder is more common than anorexia nervosa. The purging is an attempt to control body weight, though bulimics seldom starve themselves as anorexics do. They have an intense fear of becoming overweight, and usually have episodes of secretive binge eating, followed by purging, frequent weight variations, and the inability to stop eating voluntarily. Bulimics often feel hunger, overeat, and then purge to rid themselves of the guilt of overeating. Bulimic individuals are often secretive and discreet and are, therefore, often hard to identify. Typically, they have a preoccupation with food, fluctuating between fantasies of food and guilt due to overeating. Symptoms of bulimia can include cuts and calluses on the finger joints from a person sticking their fingers or hand down their throat to induce vomiting, broken blood vessels around the eyes from the strain of vomiting, and damage to tooth enamel from stomach acid."[1]

Binge-Eating Disorder

"People with binge-eating disorder typically experience frequent (at least two days a week) episodes of out-of-control eating. Binge-eating episodes are associated with at least three of the following characteristics: eating much more rapidly than normal; eating until an individual is uncomfortably full; eating large quantities of food even when not hungry; eating alone to hide the quantity of food being ingested; feeling disgusted, depressed, or guilty after overeating. Not purging their bodies of the excessive calories they have consumed is the characteristic that separates individuals with binge-eating disorder from those with bulimia. Therefore, individuals suffering from this disease are typically overweight for their height and weight."[1]

Are you a healthy consumer?

Psychological health is deeply connected to both eustress and distress, so the impact of psychological health can greatly influence your consumer behavior mentioned in chapter 2. Understanding health literacy and consumerism as they relate to psychological health is critical for proactive behaviors. Those that have less health literacy are more likely to hesitate to seek credible information regarding their health. So much of the psychological health information is confounded by miscommunication and misunderstanding of research, and can be influenced by family and friends. Where do you turn for answers to psychological health questions? If you perceive your feelings to be unhealthy or alarming, or you just have general health questions, you should turn to a physician for answers. While the internet, family, and friends can be informative, they can also provide misleading information. Be a healthy consumer!

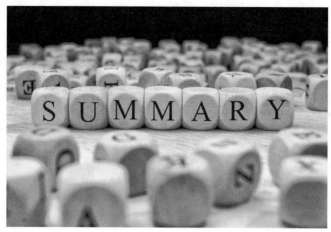

© Fabrik Bilder/Shutterstock.com

In this chapter, we learned about psychological health, and how it affects our lifestyle and overall health. Social health, intellectual health, spiritual health, and emotional health are different, yet related to the impact of our behaviors and genetic predisposition on health. Learning about our psychological health and the different components allow us to take a closer look at our stress coping behaviors, and better understand them. Additionally, we can learn to value our strengths, and work to improve the areas of psychological health that are not as strong or make us uncomfortable in non-threatening environments. After reading this chapter, you should be able to connect the information from chapters 1 and 2 to this one, and visualize how stress, behaviors, and psychological health are related.

Personal Reflections . . . so, what have you learned?

1. In your own words, describe the difference between self-esteem, resiliency, and self-efficacy. Provide an example of each as they relate to you in health related situations.

2. Reflect on how body image is related to a person's psychological health. Do you think social media is positive or negative for a person's body image?

3. Describe what the term "emotional intelligence" means to you. Provide examples to back up your theory. Do you think teenagers and college students have high emotional intelligence?

4. In your own words, what is the difference between and introvert and an extrovert? Based on your answer, how do you see yourself? How can this affect your health, both positively and negatively?

5. How is psychological health and stress related? For you, how does your stress impact your social, spiritual, intellectual, and emotional health? How do your stress coping strategies affect each of those components?

NOTES

RESOURCES ON CAMPUS FOR YOU!

Colleges and universities offer counseling and other mental health services. Many services are free or at a reduced charge from professional services. Check the services offered at your college or university!

REFERENCES

Bounds. L, Gayden. D, Brekken Shea. K, Dottiede. A. (2012). *Health and fitness: A guide to a healthy lifestyle.* Dubuque, IA: Kendall Hunt Publishing Company.

Caruso, D., & Salovey, P. (2004). *The emotionally intelligent manager: How to develop and use the four key emotional skills of leadership.* San Francisco: Jossey-Bass.

Donatelle, Rebecca J. (2014). *Access to Health* (12th ed). San Francisco, California.

Dunn, R. S., & Dunn, K. J. (1999). *The complete guide to the learning styles inservice system.* Boston: Allyn and Bacon.

Edlin G. & Golanty E. (2014). *Health and Wellness* (11th ed). Burlington, MA: Jones and Bartlett.

Goleman, D. (1995). *Emotional intelligence: Why it can matter more than IQ.* New York: Bantam Books.

Marr. J, Wilcox. S. (2015). Self-efficacy and social support mediate the relationship between internal health locus of control and health behaviors in college students. *American Journal of Health Education,* 46, 122-131.

Mayer, J. D., & Salovey, P. (1993). The intelligence of emotional intelligence. *Intelligence.* 17, 433–442.

Payne, W. A., Hahn, D. B. *Understanding Your Health* (6th ed). St. Louis, MO: Mosby. 2000

Rand. C. (2012). Stress Management: *A guide to a healthier life.* Kendall Hunt Publishing Company.

Salovey, P., & Mayer, J. D. (1990). Emotional intelligence. *Imagination, Cognition, and Personality,* 9, 185–211.

Zinger. L. (2014). *Healthy happy long life* (2nd ed). Kendall Hunt Publishing Company.

Zohar, D. (1998). *ReWiring the corporate brain: Using the new science to rethink how we structure and lead organizations.* San Francisco: Bartlett Koehler.

CREDITS

Chapter 4 +

Physical Activity & Fitness

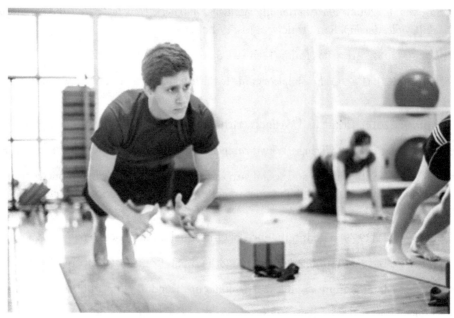

© Winthrop University

OBJECTIVES:

Students will be able to:

- Explain the benefits of regular physical activity.
- Define key terms related to cardiovascular fitness, muscular fitness, and flexibility.
- Explain the relationship between physical activity and chronic disease.
- Identify the FITT formula components.
- Identify the benefits of aerobic and anaerobic exercise.
- Identify the benefits of resistance training.
- Identify the benefits of flexibility.
- Identify the components of a workout and the importance of each component.

http://eparmedx.com/

> ### *Critical Thinking . . .*
>
> How do your physical activity habits affect your current health status?
>
> Why do you think the majority of people do not engage in regular physical activity or exercise?
>
> What is one physical activity in which you would like to participate?

WHY IS PHYSICAL ACTIVITY IMPORTANT?

"Regular physical activity decreases cardiovascular risk. Clinical, scientific, and epidemiological studies indicate that physical activity has a positive effect on the delay in development of cardiovascular disease (ACSM, 2012). In a landmark report in 1996, the Surgeon General recommended that all Americans accumulate thirty minutes of activity on most, if not all, days of the week. Recent recommendations state that thirty minutes might not be enough. The 2010 dietary guidelines recommend most Americans should bump activity time to sixty minutes daily and up to ninety minutes if a recent significant weight loss is to be maintained."[1]

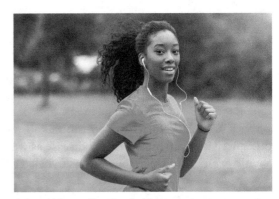

© Samuel Borges Photography/Shutterstock.com

Moderate vs. Vigorous Activities

"How do we define moderate or vigorous activities? Examples of each follow. **Moderate activities** (You can still speak while doing them) are activities like line dancing, biking with no hills, gardening, tennis (doubles), manual wheelchair wheeling, walking briskly, and water aerobics. **Vigorous activities** are aerobic dance or step aerobics, biking hills or going faster than ten miles per hour, dancing vigorously, hiking uphill, jumping rope, martial arts, race-walking, jogging or running, sports with continuous running such as basketball, soccer and hockey, swimming laps, and singles tennis. With vigorous activities it would be difficult to carry on a conversation due to the intensity of the exercise."[1]

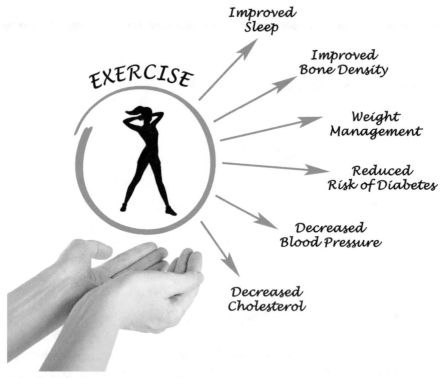

EXERCISE

Improved Sleep

Improved Bone Density

Weight Management

Reduced Risk of Diabetes

Decreased Blood Pressure

Decreased Cholesterol

© arka38/Shutterstock.com

"Try to do all of these activities for a minimum of ten minutes at a time. It is important to recognize that moderate activity is beneficial to everyone, while vigorous activity may not be appropriate for everyone. Regardless of recommendations, children and adults alike benefit from regular, consistent physical activity. Choosing to seek opportunities to move such as walking, biking, swimming, gardening, and other activities can impact risk of disease as well as quality of life. In this chapter, we will discuss why you should exercise and give suggestions to help ensure your success."[1]

The Effect of Physical Activity on Stress

As discussed in chapter 2, stress can have both positive and negative effects on health. Additionally, the way you choose to cope with stress that can have a positive or negative effect on health. Physical activity or exercise is a positive strategy for coping with both acute (short-term) and chronic (long-term) stress. Research has shown that regular participation in exercise can decrease overall levels of tension, elevate and stabilize mood, improve sleep, and improve self-esteem. It doesn't take a long bout of exercise to be effective, as even five minutes of aerobic activity has shown a reduction in anxiety and related symptoms (ADAA, 2016). As you will see throughout this chapter, the benefits of physical activity are incredibly valuable to your overall health.

The Effect of Physical Activity on Chronic Disease

"There are many benefits associated with aerobic exercise. When one is aerobically fit, there is an overall reduction in the risk of coronary artery disease, i.e., stroke, blood vessel diseases, and heart diseases. Related to this reduction, there is a decrease in resting heart rate due to the improved efficiency of the heart. There is also an increase in **stroke volume**, which is the amount of blood pumped from the heart with each heartbeat. A decrease in **systolic blood pressure**, which is the highest arterial blood pressure attained during the heart cycle, and a decrease in **diastolic blood pressure**, or lowest arterial pressure attained during the heart cycle, also occurs. There is also an increase in collateral circulation, which refers to the number of functioning capillaries both in the heart and throughout the body. Increased capillarization is an adaptation to regular aerobic activity. Delivery of oxygen to the working muscles and removal of metabolic wastes is more efficient with increased collateral circulation. In addition to the specific physiological changes just listed, other benefits of a mental, emotional, and physical nature will increase with regular aerobic exercise."[1]

Did you know . . .

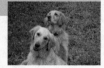

Courtesy of Shelley Hamill

"Some of the potential benefits that have been documented when aerobic fitness levels increase are:

- a decrease in percent body fat,
- an increase in strength of connective tissues,
- a reduction in mental anxiety and depression,
- improved sleep patterns,
- a decrease in the speed of the aging process,
- an improvement in stress management,
- an increase in cognitive abilities."[1]

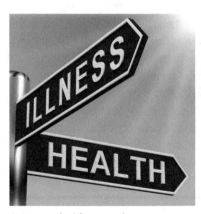

© Stuart Miles/Shutterstock.com

"Heart rate becomes elevated during exercise because of the increase in demand for oxygen in the muscle tissues. The heart is a muscle, and like other muscles, it becomes stronger due to the stress of exercise. Through regular exercise, the heart will increase slightly in size and significantly in strength, which results in an increased stroke volume. As a result of exercise, blood plasma volume increases, which allows stroke volume to increase. These two factors will cause resting heart rate to decrease, exercising heart rate will become more efficient, and there will be a quicker recovery to a resting heart rate after exercise ceases.

"Lack of exercise can contribute to many cardiovascular diseases and conditions, including **myocardial infarction**, or heart attack; **angina pectoris**, a condition caused by insufficient blood flow to the heart muscle that results in severe chest pain; and **atherosclerosis**, a build-up of fatty deposits causing blockage within the blood vessel.

"Closely associated with the function and efficiency of the heart is the function and efficiency of the **circulatory system**. As a result of aerobic exercise, blood flow to the skeletal muscles improves due to an increase in stroke volume, an increase in the number of capillaries, and an increase in the function of existing capillaries. This provides more efficient circulation both during exercise and during daily activities. Blood flow to the heart muscle is provided by two coronary arteries that branch off from the aorta and form a series of smaller vessels. With regular aerobic activity, the size of the coronary blood vessels increase and collateral circulation improves. These small blood vessels can supply oxygen to the cardiac muscle tissue when a sudden block occurs in a major vessel, such as during a heart attack. Often the degree of developed collateral circulation determines one's ability to survive a myocardial infarction, or heart attack. It appears that a regular exerciser might survive a heart attack due to collateral circulation within the heart, as the smaller collateral vessels take over when the primary artery becomes occluded, or blocked."[1]

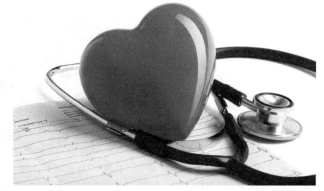

© S_L/Shutterstock.com

Types of Fitness

"**Cardiovascular fitness** refers to the ability of the heart, lungs, circulatory system, and energy supply system to perform at optimum levels for extended periods of time. **Cardiovascular endurance** is defined as the ability of the body to perform prolonged, large-muscle, dynamic exercise at moderate to high levels of intensity. The word **aerobic** means 'in the presence of oxygen' and is used synonymously with cardiovascular as well as cardiorespiratory when describing a type of exercise.

"**Complete fitness** is comprised of health-related fitness and skill-related fitness. **Health-related**

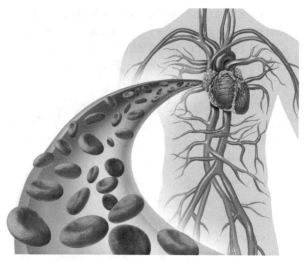

© Lightspring/Shutterstock.com

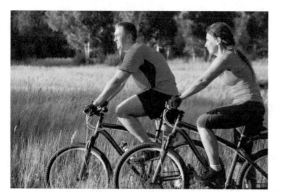

© YanLev/Shutterstock.com

fitness consists of cardiovascular fitness, muscular strength, muscular endurance, flexibility, and optimal body composition. The components of health-related fitness affect the body's ability to function efficiently and effectively. Optimal health-related fitness is not possible without regular physical activity. Most health clubs and fitness classes focus primarily on the health-related fitness components. **Skill-related fitness** includes agility, balance, coordination, reaction time, speed, and power. These attributes are critical for competitive athletes. Skill-related fitness is not essential in order to have cardiovascular fitness, nor will it necessarily make a person healthier. Balance is, however, important for seniors. Staying active helps seniors maintain strength and balance, which can be critical in avoiding injuries."[1]

Health Related Fitness
- Cardiovascular Fitness
- Muscular Strength
- Muscular Endurance
- Flexibility
- Optimal body composition

Skill-Related Fitness
- Agility
- Balance
- Coordination
- Reaction time
- Speed
- Power

Courtesy of Joni Boyd

"Cardiovascular fitness is often referred to as the most important aspect of physical fitness because of its relevance to good health and optimal performance. **Muscular fitness** is important because of its effect on efficiency of human movement and basal metabolic rate. **Flexibility** is important for everyone, athletes and non-athletes alike, especially as a person ages. Knowing how to exercise correctly for effectiveness and reduced risk of injury is also important.

The Impact of Physical Activity on Body Composition, Weight Management, and Overall Health

Physically active individuals show improvements in glucose regulation, blood pressure, blood cholesterol, bone density, and body weight. Even small amount of physical activity can have big impacts on body composition and weight management. Participation in regular physical activity is the one of the best preventive strategies against undesired weight gain. Regular physical activity can significantly affect body weight and body composition for those that are overweight or obese. A loss of 5 to 10 percent of body weight can dramatically change body composition and overall health risk. Your biggest risk is to stay sedentary, which increases your chance of obesity, disease, and preventable death.

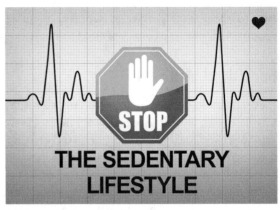

© Hriana/Shutterstock.com

How important is participation in physical activity in achieving and maintaining good health? Since 1992, the American Heart Association has considered inactivity as important a risk factor for heart disease as high blood cholesterol,high blood pressure, and cigarette smoking."[1]

Aerobic and Anaerobic Exercise

"**Aerobic exercise** is activity that requires the body to supply oxygen to support performance over a period of time. Aerobic exercise is characterized by the use

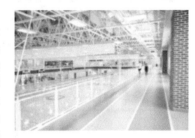

© Winthrop University

of the large muscle groups in a rhythmic mode with an increase in respiration and heart rate. Aerobic literally means 'with oxygen.' Walking, the most common form of exercise in the United States, is an aerobic activity. Other aerobic exercises include running, swimming, biking, cardio kickboxing, rowing, jump-roping, and any activity that fits the above criteria. As with most exercise, the rate of energy expenditure varies with an individual's skill level and intensity of exercise. Aerobic activities of low intensity are ideal for the beginning or sedentary exerciser because they can be maintained for a longer period of time and have been shown to be effective in promoting weight loss and enhancing cardiovascular health. Many activities are too intense to be maintained more than a few minutes; these activities are considered anaerobic.

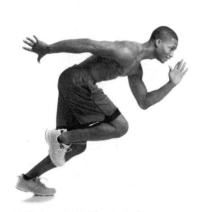

© Flashon Studio/Shutterstock.com

"Anaerobic literally means 'in the absence of oxygen.' **Anaerobic exercise** is exercise performed at intensity levels so great that the body's demand for oxygen exceeds its ability to supply it. Examples of anaerobic activities include strength training, sprinting, and interval training. Sprinting requires so much energy that the intensity of the activity cannot be maintained for a long period of time. Anaerobic training can enhance the body's ability to cope with the effects of fatigue, thus promoting greater anaerobic fitness."[1]

Muscular Fitness

"Muscular fitness includes two specific components: muscular strength and muscular endurance. Muscular strength is the force or tension a muscle or muscle group can exert against a resistance in one maximal effort. Muscular endurance is the ability or capacity of a muscle group to perform repeated contractions against a load, or to sustain a contraction for an extended period of time. In February 2002, ACSM released a new position stand regarding resistance training progression. The position stand reported that everyone would benefit from resistance training two to three days per week, working eight to ten muscle groups with one to two sets of eight to twelve repetitions."[1]

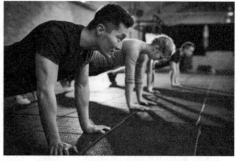

© Uber Images/Shutterstock.com

Benefits of Muscular Fitness

"Several physiological adaptations occur as a result of resistance training. Strength gains can be seen within the first six weeks, with little or no change in muscle size, and are attributed to neural changes. As strength training activities continue, hypertrophy, or an increase in the size of the muscle fibers, can occur. Another result from training is an increase in the amount of energy available for contraction. Carbohydrates are stored in the form of glycogen in the muscle and can be used as the primary energy source for contraction. These muscle glycogen stores increase as a result of training. Bone and connective tissue also undergo changes with resistance training, including an increase in bone matrix, an increase in bone mineral density, and an increase in mass and tensile strength of ligaments and tendons. These increases help prevent injury and decrease the chance of development of osteoporosis after middle age.

Did you know . . .

ACSM Resistance Training Guidelines:

- 2–3 non-consecutive days per week
- 8–10 total exercises
- 2–4 sets of each exercise
- 8–12 repetitions of each set

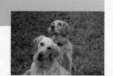

Courtesy of Shelley Hamill

Benefits of muscular fitness include:

an increase in muscular strength, power and endurance

a higher percent of muscle mass

increased strength of tendons & ligaments

increased bone mass

increased metabolic rate

increased resistance to fatigue

improved posture

improved movement

decreased risk of low back pain or other injuries

increased energy & vitality

weight loss

higher self-esteem

improved well-being

Courtesy of Joni Boyd

"More muscle mass increases an individual's basal metabolic rate, which is why weight training is excellent for those wanting to reduce their percentage of body fat. 'An increase in one pound of muscle elevates basal metabolic rate by approximately 2–3 percent' (Powers and Dodd, 2009). Along with the physiological adaptations previously discussed come benefits that improve the quality of one's life."[1]

Spotlight on . . .

"**Interval training** has been used for years. The concept is simple: work for a shorter amount of time, but work harder. Working with a coach or personal trainer is recommended so that you also work smarter. Interval training involves high intensity cardiovascular exercise alternating between short rest and active rest periods. People who tend to get bored just running for 40 minutes often enjoy the variety and change in routine. The increased challenge of a 40-minute interval workout means increased energy expenditure. The basic variables manipulated when designing an interval training program include:

1. Duration (time/distance) of intervals
2. Duration of rest/recovery phase
3. Number of repetitions of intervals
4. Intensity (speed) of intervals
5. Frequency of interval workout sessions"[1]

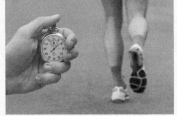

© Leszek Bogdewicz/Shutterstock.com

Training for the Best Results

Understand that your body type, your experience and fitness levels, as well as your motivation should dictate the type of training that would be best for you. Not every program works at the same rate for every individual person. A few rules to remember can ensure that you do not make the typical mistake of doing too much too soon.

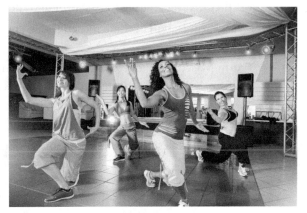

© Val Thoermer/Shutterstock.com

1. **Always warm-up.** A short 5–10 minute warm-up of light, full-body movement is your best protection against injury.

2. **Start light.** Don't jump in too quickly. Give your body time to adjust to the demands you place on it.

3. **Stay consistent.** It's going to take time to see changes! You will see changes as long as you stay consistent with SOME type of activity.

Trying to do a fitness or exercise program that is not well designed for you increases your chance of burnout, injury, and giving up. "As with any type of training program, watch for signs of **over-training**, which can lead to burning out. With muscular fitness training, these indicators include a decrease in physical performance and weight loss, increase in muscle soreness, increase in resting heart rate, sleeplessness, nausea after a workout, constant fatigue, and decreased interest in exercise."[1]

"**True or False? Weight Training Myths**

1. Myth: Weight training causes one to lose flexibility.

   Truth: Resistance training will increase muscle size, but it does not necessarily make one less flexible. In fact, proper strength training can actually increase flexibility when a full range of motion is used.

2. Myth: Resistance training or 'spot reducing' is beneficial in reducing deposits of fat from specific areas on the body, such as in the hips, thighs, and waist.

   Truth: Resistance training focuses on the muscles used. Fat is not removed from one area of the body by working the muscles in that area. Creating a caloric deficit consistently, through diet, exercise, or a combination of both, loses fat. The location of fat deposits is determined genetically.

3. Myth: Fat will be converted to muscle with resistance training.

   Truth: Fat is not converted to muscle with exercise, nor is muscle converted to fat through disuse. Muscle cells and fat cells are different entities. The size of muscle cells can be increased with resistance training. Fat cell size is increased with sedentary living combined with a poor diet.

4. Myth: Dietary supplements will make one bigger and stronger.

   Truth: A balanced diet and hard work in the weight room will increase muscle size and strength. Most dietary supplements will only cause the manufacturer's wallet to become bigger. Often when a person spends money on a supplement believing that supplement to work, the placebo effect might result in some apparent short-term improvement.

5. Myth: Performance-enhancing drugs such as steroids, growth hormones, diuretics, and metabolism boosters will help make one fit.

   Truth: These drugs are extremely dangerous and potentially fatal. They can contribute to aesthetic changes, but can also have a negative impact on health. Some fitness enthusiasts have lost their lives searching for a short-cut to health by using supplements.

6. Myth: Women will become masculine in appearance by participating in resistance training activities.

   Truth: Masculinity and femininity are determined through hormones, not through resistance training. Resistance training will cause an increase in muscle tone, which is perceived to increase the attractiveness of both males and females.

7. Myth: Kids should not weight train.

   Truth: Pre-adolescent children can and should use their body as resistance. Swinging on the monkey bars or climbing a tree are good examples of using one's body as resistance; push-ups, sit-ups, and tumbling activities are also great."[1]

Spotlight on . . .

WOMEN AND STRENGTH TRAINING

Women considering strength training are sometimes concerned that strength exercises will make them appear less feminine. The fear is that training will produce large, unsightly, bulging muscles. In the past few years, research has disputed this myth. Women have the same muscle properties as men, but because of endocrinological differences, they respond to a training stimulus in different ways. The result is that men develop a greater quantity of muscle tissue and respond with a greater gain of muscle mass when they engage in a strength program. In most cases, women will not gain a large amount of muscle mass when training, but they will obtain increased strength, which will enable them to better perform daily activities. There is no physiological reason for women not to engage in a strength training program and no need to suggest different training programs on the basis of sex. Both women and men can experience the same general benefits; it is only the degree of gain in muscle tissue that will differ. (Allsen, 2009)

Flexibility

"Can you touch your toes? Think of how much your flexibility has changed in the last ten years. How much more will it change in the next ten years? Truly, if you don't stretch or if you are not active, flexibility will be lost. Why is this a concern? Loss of flexibility with age or injury can greatly affect a person's quality of life. Simple activities such as putting on your socks or bending to lift a toddler can be painful or even impossible. Individuals who are active tend to be more flexible simply because they tend to use a full

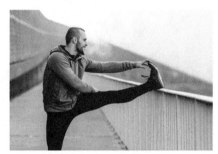

© baranq/Shutterstock.com

range of motion in their activity. Active individuals are also more likely to engage in health enhancing behaviors. Several factors can have an impact on the amount of flexibility a person can achieve, including gender, age, genetic composition, activity level, muscle core temperature, and previous or current injury. Old injuries often hamper flexibility for adults later in life, therefore affecting future activity.

"Flexibility and balance are a concern for the aging population. Non-impact activities such as tai chi and yoga are gaining in popularity with all ages, both of which are appropriate to the aging population. Flexibility is defined as the range of motion around a joint. **Flexibility** is also specific to individual joints. For instance, an individual may have complete range of motion in the wrist but be very limited or stiff in the shoulder. An individual could be very flexible on the right side of the body, and inflexible on the left side.

"Flexibility exercises should be included in all exercise programs regardless of the objectives. The benefits of maintaining flexibility include having the ability to perform daily activities without developing muscle strains or tears and being able to participate in sports with enhanced performance. A swimmer who increases shoulder flexibility is able to reach further and pull more water, and thus swims faster. "Stretching exercises are identified through three specific categories: ballistic, static, and PNF."[1]

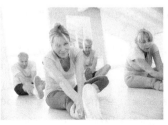

© goodluz/Shutterstock.com

"Yoga is gaining in popularity in the United States. Most forms of yoga encourage the buildup of heat within the body to facilitate movement and internal focus. Relaxation is a common goal of most yoga participants, yet most experience enhanced flexibility and increased strength as a fringe benefit. One style of yoga, Bikram yoga, advocates practicing yoga in rooms with temperatures as high as 105 degrees. The premise is that the heat will allow the tendons, ligaments, and muscles to loosen up more and stretch further. A common yoga truism is that even steel, when hot enough, will bend."[1]

Types of Stretches

Ballistic stretching involves rapid movements, or "bouncing." Ballistic stretching is not recommended for the general population as a means to improve flexibility. An exception is athletes who have ballistic movement in their sport.

© d13/Shutterstock.com

Static stretching involves a held stretch to the point of mild discomfort and maintaining that angle for 15–60 seconds before allowing the muscle to relax. The entire procedure should be repeated several times for maximum benefit.

© lzf/Shutterstock.com

Proprioceptive neuromuscular facilitation or PNF requires a partner. The basic formula for this activity is to isometrically resist against a partner using the muscle groups surrounding a particular joint, causing contraction, and then relaxing the same muscle group.

© fizkes/Shutterstock.com

COMPONENTS OF AN EXERCISE SESSION

Warm-Up

"A good cardiovascular workout follows a specific sequence of events. First and foremost, to prepare the body and increase the comfort level for a cardiovascular workout, a warm-up is crucial. The purpose of the warm-up is to prepare the body, especially the heart, for the more vigorous work to come. The warmup should increase body temperature, increase heart rate, increase blood flow to the muscles that will be used during the workout, and include some rhythmic movement to loosen muscles that may be cold and/or tight. A warm-up should raise the pulse from a resting level to a rate somewhere near the low end of the recommended heart rate training zone. Beginning vigorous exercise without some kind of warm-up is not only difficult physically and mentally, but it can also contribute to musculoskeletal injuries."[1]

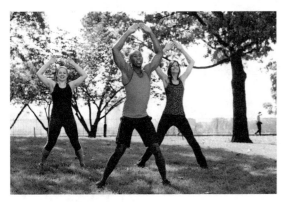

© Tyler Olson/Shutterstock.com

Pre-Stretch

"It is important to warm up the muscles that will be used during the workout. Use caution when stretching prior to the workout, holding the stretches for a brief time and not stretching with much intensity. Stretching prior to the workout is optional. Many athletes choose to go through rhythmic limbering, with dynamic movements focusing on functional movement patterns that will be used in the race, sport, or fitness class rather than holding a static stretch."[1]

Cooldown and Stretch

"After an exercise session, heart rate should be lowered gradually by slowly reducing the intensity of the exercise. Sudden stops are not recommended and can lead to muscle cramps, dizziness, and blood pooling in the legs. After a gradual cooldown such as walking, static stretching of the muscle groups is needed and highly recommended. When muscle core and body core temperature are elevated, it is an optimal time to stretch for increased flexibility. Warmer muscle core temperature increases the pliability of the muscle, allowing it to lengthen."[1]

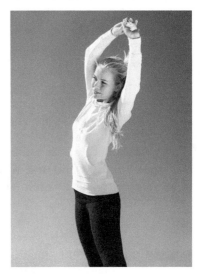

© Syda Productions/Shutterstock.com

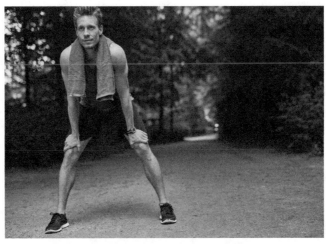

© Uber Images/Shutterstock.com

PRINCIPLES OF FITNESS TRAINING — THE RULES

"There are specific principles that can be applied to any exercise program. Understanding these exercise principles will increase a person's chance of success with his/her exercise program."[1]

Overload and Adaptation

OVERLOAD

"The principle of overload and adaptation states that in order for a body system to become more efficient or stronger, it must be stressed beyond its normal working level. In other words, it must be overloaded. When this overload occurs, the system will respond by gradually adapting to this new load and increasing its work efficiency until another plateau is reached. The cardiovascular system can be overloaded in more than one way. In terms of weight training, any time a person adds more weight to the bench press or increases the number of repetitions, that person is using the principle of overload. **In order for improvements to be realized, overload must occur.** The principle of overload and adaptation applies to muscular strength, cardiovascular and muscular endurance, and flexibility training."[1]

Specificity

SPECIFICITY

"The principle of specificity refers to training specifically for an activity, or isolating a specific muscle group and/or movement pattern one would like to improve. For example, a 200-m sprinter would not train by running long, slow distances. Likewise, a racewalker would not train for competition by swimming. Workouts must be specific to one's goal with respect to the type of exercise, intensity, and duration. The warm-up should also be specific to a particular activity."[1]

Individual Differences

INDIVIDUAL

"The principle of individual differences reminds us that individuals will respond differently to the same training protocol. Some individuals may be what are called 'low responders' to an exercise stimulus. It is not clear why individuals vary in response to exercise, but initial fitness level, age, gender, genetic composition, and previous history will also cause individual responses to specific activities to differ. Coaches, athletic trainers, and personal trainers should be especially aware of this principle when designing workouts in order to achieve maximum performance levels. It is also critical that individuals realize that body type is genetically determined. Body fat distribution and metabolism are individual. Lifestyle and activity can affect one's physique; however, a large-framed person will never be a small-framed person and vice versa. Focusing more on enhanced health rather than trying to change one's body type is prudent."[1]

Reversibility

REVERSIBILITY

"The inevitable process of losing cardiovascular benefits with cessation of aerobic activity is known as the reversibility principle. The old adage 'if you don't use it you lose it' applies here. Physiological changes will occur within the first two weeks of detraining and will continue for several months. Bed rest causes this detraining process to greatly accelerate. Consider the muscle atrophy that occurs with disuse when a cast is removed from a body part that has been immobilized for several weeks. The reversibility principle is clearly the justification for off-season programs for athletes and immediate initiation of physical rehabilitation programs for individuals with limited mobility or for those individuals recovering from injury."[1]

Exercise Prescription Using the FITT Principles

Type of Activity	Frequency	Intensity	Time	Type
Physical Activity	Most days of the week	Moderate level	at least 30 minutes	Any moderate – vigorous activity
Aerobic Exercise	3–5 days per week	30–85% HRR 12–16 RPE scale	20–60 minutes	Any full body, repetitive movement
Resistance Training	2–3 nonconsecutive days per week	Point of muscle fatigue	2–4 sets 8–12 reps	8–10 exercises for full body
Flexibility	Minimum 2–3 days per week	Hold stretch until point of discomfort	15–60 seconds Repeat	Static stretches

American College of Sports Medicine, 2013

"To improve cardiovascular fitness, one must have a well-designed regimen of cardiovascular exercise. In order for improvement to occur, specific guidelines must be adhered to when designing a personal exercise program. As will be discussed later, the following guidelines apply not only to aerobic exercise, but to other components of physical fitness, as well. The FITT acronym is easy to remember when identifying an appropriate cardiovascular exercise prescription: **frequency, intensity, time,** and **type**."[1]

Frequency

"Frequency refers to the number of exercise sessions per week. For individuals with a low level of aerobic fitness, beginning an exercise program by working out two times a week will result in an initial increase in aerobic fitness level. However, after some time, frequency and/or intensity will need to be increased for improvement to continue."[1]

Intensity

"Intensity refers to how hard one is working, and it can be measured by several techniques. These techniques include **measuring the heart rate** while exercising, **rating of perceived exertion (RPE)**, and the **talk test**. To use heart rate as a measure of intensity, one's target heart rate range needs to be calculated before exercising. **Target heart rate range** is the intensity of training necessary to achieve cardiovascular improvement. This target heart rate range indicates what an individual's heart rate should be during exercise. Calculation of target heart rate range using the Karvonen formula is done by multiplying maximum heart rate (220 minus one's age) by a designated intensity percentage. The American College of Sports Medicine guidelines for intensity recommends working between 55 and 90 percent of maximum heart rate, or between 50 and 85 percent of heart rate reserve (maximum heart

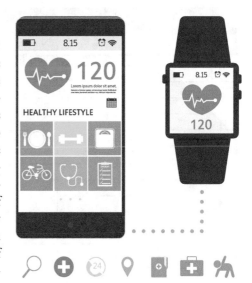

© Felicity.S/Shutterstock.com

rate minus resting heart rate). For individuals who are very unfit, the recommended range is 55 to 64 percent of maximum heart rate or 40 to 49 percent of heart rate reserve (Pollock, Gaesser, Butcher, Despres, Dishman, et al., 1998). Use of a heart rate monitor is also useful for specific heart rate and intensity feedback. Programs can be designed using heart rate to alleviate boredom and increase efficiency of the workout.

"Another technique for measuring exercise intensity is through subjective self-evaluation of how hard one is working. Gunner Borg designed the **Rating of Perceived Exertion Scale (RPE)** in the early 1950s. It is a numbered scale from 6 to 20, with the lowest numbers being 'very, very light' exercise, the highest numbers being 'maximal' exercise, and the numbers in between representing a gradual increase in exercise intensity, from low to high. Using this scale, a rating of 10 corresponds roughly to 50 percent of maximal heart rate and a rating of 16 corresponds roughly to 90 percent of maximal heart rate. A person estimates his or her exercise intensity level by taking into consideration or 'perceiving' how they feel, how much sleep they have had, whether or not they have eaten, whether or not they are ill, and so on. This scale is a useful tool for estimating exercise intensity when exact measures are not needed, and it is often used in a clinical setting as well as fitness classes and health clubs. Perceived exertion is also useful when a person is taking medication that can alter the heart rate.

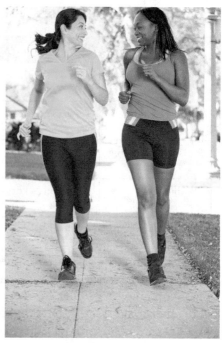

© Monkey Business Images/Shutterstock.com

"A third, and probably the easiest, technique to measure exercise intensity is the talk test. If you are exercising and must laboriously breathe rather than participate in a conversation, the exercise intensity is too high and training heart rate has probably been exceeded. Exercise at this intensity will be difficult to maintain for long periods of time. On the other hand, if you are able to sing, intensity level is probably insufficient for improvement in your fitness level."[1]

BORG RPE	Modified RPE	Breathing	% of Max HR
6	0	No effort. Very easy.	50–60%
7		Very light activity.	
8	1		
9			
10	2	Breathing is deeper, but pace can be maintained for long time.	60–70%
11			
12	3	You can talk, but holding a conversation is more difficult.	70–80%
13			
14	4	Breathing is much deeper and it is uncomfortable to talk.	80–90%
15	5		
16	6		
17	7	You do not want to talk at all. Focus is on deep, forceful breaths.	90–100%
18	8		
19	9	Very difficult to continue for any period of time	
20	10	Total Maximum Exertion	

Time

"The third factor to be considered when designing a cardiovascular exercise workout is **time**, or duration. For benefits to be accrued in the cardiovascular system, exercise duration should be a minimum of twenty minutes of continuous exercise or several intermittent exercise sessions of a minimum of ten minutes each. Some beginning exercisers may not be capable of exercising continuously for twenty minutes at a prescribed intensity. While a minimum of twenty minutes is recommended, a duration of ten minutes can certainly be beneficial to people who are at a low fitness level and just beginning an exercise program."[1]

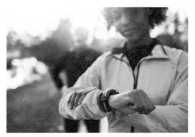
© Uber Images/Shutterstock.com

Type

"Another factor that should be considered in determining a cardiovascular exercise prescription is **type**, or mode, of exercise. The choice of exercise modality is up to each individual, but one must keep in mind the specific requirements of cardiovascular exercise: use the large muscle groups via continuous and rhythmic movement, and exercise for a duration of twenty to thirty minutes or more in the target heart rate range a minimum of three to five times per week. Common types of aerobic exercise include running, walking, swimming, step aerobics, cross-country skiing, biking, or using a machine such as a rower, stair stepper, or treadmill. However, these are certainly not the only types of exercise available."[1]

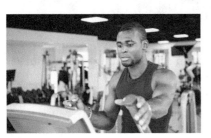
© pio3/Shutterstock.com

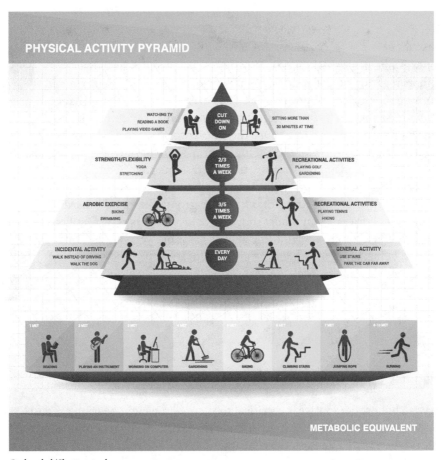
© elenabsl/Shutterstock.com

INJURIES & INJURY PREVENTION

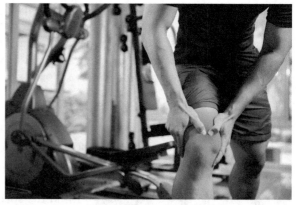

© VectorLifestylepic/Shutterstock.com

"Although injuries do occur during exercise, the benefits of regular exercise far out-weigh the risk of injury. In most cases, proper training, clothing, and equipment will prevent injuries. Avoiding injury requires common sense and moderation. One should not attempt to self-diagnose, nor try to 'train through the pain.' Pain is a signal that something is wrong, and activity should be stopped until the source of the pain is identified and a trained medical professional can advise you. Some common injuries resulting from exercise include joint sprains, muscle strains, and other musculoskeletal problems. Knowing how to treat an acute, or immediate, injury is important. **RICE** most injuries, such as a twisted ankle: Rest, Ice, Compression, and Elevation.

"Of course, using proper equipment, wearing proper clothing and shoes, and practicing correct technique are essential for injury prevention. Weight-bearing forms of exercise will obviously cause more stress on the joints, but also have benefits that non-weight-bearing activities do not have, such as increasing strength of the bones and other connective tissues."[1]

Did you know . . .

Courtesy of Shelley Hamill

"Christopher McDougall's 2009 publication Born to Run started a discourse between runners regarding what is the best way to run—wearing $160.00 state-of-the-art running shoes or running barefoot? The barefoot crowd claims that a barefoot runner has a more natural gait, striking with the mid or forefoot first. Shoes with cushioning and a high heel cause the runner to strike the ground with the heel first. Vibram's successful FiveFingers brand popularized the minimalist shoe movement in California and first-place runners in marathons have been seen wearing them. Barefoot runners using the FiveFingers shoe can "feel" the road and may run with a more natural gate and yet still have protection from irritants on the ground like small shards of glass. There are 2 categories of minimalist shoes—the FiveFingers type that fits snug on your foot, and a minimalist running shoe (a cross between a traditional running shoe and being barefoot) which has just a bit of structure and support. If you decide to try the minimalist route, progress slowly and use caution. (Ellingson, Linda, The Basics of Barefoot/Minimalist Running, Jan. 2012, REI expert advice online.)"[1]

© MawRhis/Shutterstock.com

Proper Footwear

"It may seem trivial, but proper footwear is critical to success in weight bearing exercise. Shoe technology has come a long way in the past decade. Sport specific shoes are highly recommended to avoid injury and to enhance performance. Unfortunately, the consumer pays for the research and technology, as well as the logo on the shoes. A good cross trainer shoe is the way to go if you like to do a variety of activities. Cross

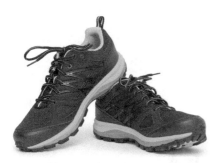

© cocoo/Shutterstock.com

trainers are not, however, recommended for aerobic dance or running. Running shoes are also not appropriate for 'studio activities' such as aerobic dance, step aerobics, BOSU activities, as well as court activities like tennis or racquetball. Running shoes have little lateral support and the higher flared heel can actually cause a person participating in step aerobics to be more prone to twisting an ankle or knee joint. Some steps also have a rubber top which can grip the waffle sole of the running shoe and increase the risk of injury. In any athletic shoe, fit and comfort are of the utmost importance. It is worth going to a store staffed by knowledgeable personnel. Often they can give you good insight into the type of shoe that is most appropriate for your foot and your gait."[1]

Environmental Conditions

"Take into consideration environmental conditions such as temperature, air pollution, wind-chill, altitude, and humidity that can affect one's health and safety. Dressing appropriately is important when exercising in extreme weather conditions. When exercising in the cold weather, layering of clothes is advised. There are new fabrics that can wick away moisture from the body better than fabrics such as wool, polypropylene, and cotton. Avoid cotton as a base layer in cold weather because if it gets wet with perspiration it will stay wet and make you colder.

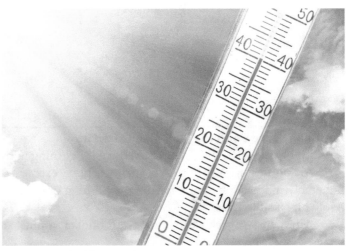

© Juergen Faelchle/Shutterstock.com

"Exercising in the heat can be a challenge. It is important to acclimate to the heat and humidity, especially when moving from an area that is cool and arid. Gradually increase duration and intensity when exercising in a new type of environment. Especially in the Southern states, heat injuries are a real concern.

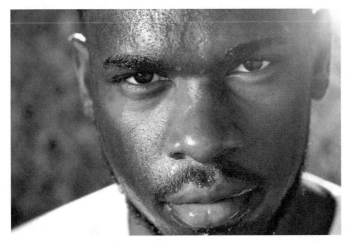

© mimagephotography/Shutterstock.com

Heat cramps, **heat exhaustion**, and **heat stroke** can all occur with prolonged exposure to the heat. Heat stroke is a life-threatening condition, and necessitates hospitalization. Heat exhaustion is more common, with individuals typically suffering from dehydration. In order for the body to effectively cool, evaporation of sweat needs to occur. In a humid environment when perspiration drips off of a person, evaporation is not occurring, and therefore cooling is not taking place. A hot and humid environment is especially risky to the very young, the old, and those with low cardiovascular fitness levels."[1]

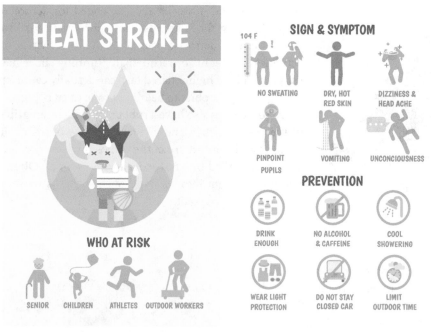

© Falara/Shutterstock.com

Common Sense Concerns for Outside Activity

Lightning—DO NOT exercise if there is lightning in the area. Stay indoors.

Air pollution—When the air quality is poor, exercise early in the morning, later in the evening, or preferably indoors, especially for those with lung or heart disease. Pay attention to air pollution alerts. Avoid high traffic areas.

Allergens—Check weather reports for pollen counts, and avoid outdoor vigorous exercise when the pollen count is high.

Night exercise—It is common for some to walk, jog, or bike on the shoulder of roads. Drivers need to use caution; sometimes the glare from oncoming traffic can obscure visibility. However, night exercisers must be responsible and make themselves more visible at night:

1. Use a flashlight.
2. Dress in white clothing—there is an amazing difference in visibility between gray and white shirts at night.
3. Wear a reflective vest or reflective arm bands.
4. Walk in a well-lit, safe area if possible.
5. Be safe and aware of your surroundings, and use common sense.
6. Don't go alone; go with friends or borrow a dog if you don't have your own.
7. Carry ID with you.
8. Do NOT let headphones distract you from traffic or safety concerns.
9. Use flashing lights that can be attached to a belt or arm band.
10. Remember when walking to face the oncoming traffic if possible.
11. Let someone know your route and expected time back.
12. Be aware that drivers may have difficulty seeing you at twilight.

Use common sense when environmental conditions are significant!"[1]

Hydration

"Heat injuries are much less likely to occur if a person is adequately hydrated. Proper hydration is necessary for the body to function properly. Water aids in controlling body temperature, contributes to the structure and form of the body, and provides the liquid environment for cell processes. When the thirst mechanism is activated, dehydration has already begun. It is important to pre-hydrate, drink before thirst occurs, and especially drink before exercising. The standard recommendation is to drink at least eight eight-ounce glasses of water a day. Exercise increases the body's

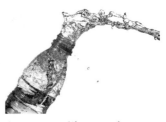

© Mariyana M/Shutterstock.com

demand for water due to an increase in metabolic rate and body temperature. Therefore, this amount should be increased. Drinking water every waking hour is a good habit for individuals who exercise on a regular basis."[1]

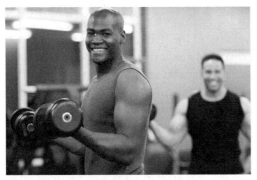

© michaeljung/Shutterstock.com

Illness

"Use common sense when ill. If you have cold symptoms with no fever, then possibly a light workout might make you feel better. If fever is present, you have a headache, extreme fatigue, muscle aches, swollen lymph glands, or if you have flu-like symptoms, then bed rest is recommended. Marathon efforts of high intensity and long duration have been shown to temporarily suppress the immune system.

The Biggest Risk to Exercise is Not Starting!"[1]

Are you a healthy consumer?

Many people would consider themselves a consumer of fitness products . . . but not necessarily of fitness itself. Millions of consumers own fitness memberships, equipment, videos, and apps of exercise, and that doesn't include the recent popularity of "wellness coaches," aka—personal trainers. While purchasing these items can be beneficial, efficient, and preferable, they are not always necessary. You don't have to spend money to be physically active, lose or gain weight, or get fit. Make sure you spend wisely when it comes to exercise, and only purchase items in which you see real value. Research products, people, and facilities, and always read the fine print before making big-ticket commitments. The only thing you need to succeed in physical activity is you!

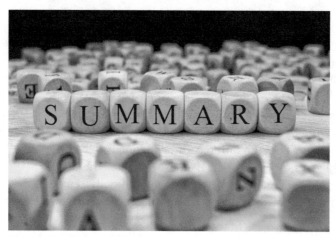

© Fabrik Bilder/Shutterstock.com

"Staying active has clearly been shown to enhance a person's quality of life. Exercise is for everyone; it is never too early or too late to start. Most people know that they would benefit from participating in an exercise program, but for many it is difficult to get started. Find an activity you enjoy. Make a plan. Write it down. Get a workout buddy. Start slowly, and listen to your body. Pain is usually a signal that something is wrong. The old adage 'no pain, no gain' can cause beginners to become frustrated. Balance activity, leisure time, and rest each week. With consistency, activity can have a positive impact on reducing risk for many conditions associated with too little activity, called hypokinetic conditions. And most importantly, you should experience increased stamina, enthusiasm, and enhanced mental well-being in your daily life."[1]

Check out your university's resources on the next page to get you started on your fitness/exercise goals!

NOTES

Personal reflection . . . so, what have you learned?

1. In your own words, summarize (in about 5 sentences) how participation in a regular physical activity program would affect you specifically. Include information from all sections that describe the impact of physical activity on any health component.

2. What are the ACSM guidelines for physical activity, aerobic exercise, resistance training, and flexibility? Provide one example of each type of activity/exercise.

3. What type of physical activities are available to you at little or no cost?

4. What is one myth about physical activity/exercise from the chapter that surprised you and why?

NOTES

RESOURCES ON CAMPUS FOR YOU!

Recreational services is a valuable resource for students, faculty and staff who wish to pursue a healthy lifestyle. Through participation in various programs, participants can gain a multitude of personal benefits including improved levels of physical fitness and wellness, opportunities for social interaction, time management skills, engagement in a group dynamic setting, a healthy means of stress relief, as well as the creation of a sense of ownership and belonging between students and your college community. Check the services offered on your campus through recreational services.

Examples of services include:

- Fitness and Wellness
- Group Fitness
- Intramural Sports
- Club Sports
- Personal Training
- Aquatics
- Aqua Tone Water Running
- Swimming Lessons

REFERENCES

Allsen, P. (2009). *Strength training: beginners, body builders, and athletes* (5th edition). Dubuque, IA: Kendall Hunt Publishing Company.

American College of Sports Medicine [ACSM]. (2012). ACSM's Health/Fitness Facility Standards and Guidelines. Human Kinetics: Champagne, IL.

American College of Sports Medicine. (2013). ACSM information on: Resistance training for health & fitness. Retrieved from www.acsm.org

American College of Sports Medicine, & American Heart Association. (2007). Exercise and acute cardiovascular events: placing risks into perspective." *Medicine and Science in Sports and Exercise*, 39, 5, 886–97.

American Heart Association, & American Stroke Association. (2012). *Heart and Stroke Statistical Update*. Dallas, TX: American Heart Association.

Anxiety and Depression Association of America [ADAA]. (2016). Physical Activity Reduces Stress. Retrieved from: https://adaa.org/understanding-anxiety/related-illnesses/other-related-conditions/stress/physical-activity-reduces-st

Canadian Society for Exercise Physiology. (2002). Physical Activity Readiness Questionnaire. Retrieved from www.csep.ca/forms

Ellingsen, Jan, & The Basics of Barefoot/Minimalist Running Jan. (2012). REI expert advice online. Retrieved from www.physicalactivityplan.org

Pollock, M. L., Gaesser, G. A., Butcher, J. D., Despres, J-P., Dishman, R. K., et al. (1998). ACSM Position Stand on the Recommended Quantity and Quality of Exercise for Developing and Maintaining Cardiorespiratory and Muscular Fitness, and Flexibility in Healthy Adults. **Medicine & Science in Sports & Exercise**, 30, 6, 975–991. 975–991.

Powers, S. K., Dodd, S. L., Jackson, E.M., & Miller, M.K. (2009). *Total fitness and wellness* (5th ed). San Francisco: Pearson/Benjamin Cummings.

CREDITS

1. From *Health and Fitness: A Guide to a Healthy Lifestyle*, 5/e by Laura Bounds, Gayden Darnell, Kristin Brekken Shea, Dottiede Agnore. Copyright © 2012 by Kendall Hunt Publishing Company. Reprinted by permission.

NOTES

NOTES

Chapter 5 ✛

Nutrition

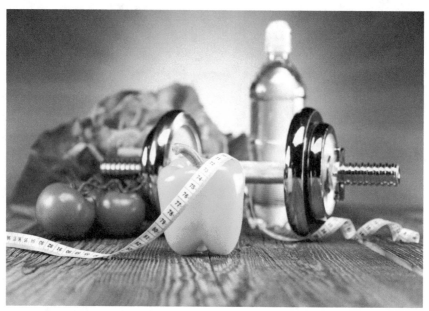

© Sebastian Duda/Shutterstock.com

OBJECTIVES:

Students will be able to:

- Identify the difference between macronutrients and micronutrients.
- Identify essential nutrients and their role in daily nurition.
- Introduce and explain the nutritional guidelines and recommendations.
- Recognize healthy sources of macro- and micronutrients, as well as the different types of food through the use of the MyPlate food groups.
- Discuss the food nutrition label and the different types of information it presents.
- Compare and contrast the four types of vegetarianism.
- Describe the value and factors of organic foods.
- Identify food safety hazards and describe prevention strategies.

Nutrition Knowledge Assessment. Circle the correct answer.

1. Which of the following is a macronutrient?

   A. carbohydrate   B. vitamin D   C. water

2. Which of the following food is considered high in fiber?

   A. chicken   B. almonds   C. eggs

3. Which of the following fats can benefit cholesterol levels?

   A. trans fat   B. saturated fat   C. unsaturated fat

4. For most adults, how much protein is recommended each day?

   A. 20–25 g   B. 45–65 g   C. 75–80 g

5. Which of the following nutrients can slow aging by suppressing cell deterioration?

   A. antioxidants   B. water   C. carbohydrates

6. Superfoods have been shown to reduce the risk of:

   A. heart disease   B. cancer   C. both A & B

7. What type of vegetarian will consume only dairy, fruit, and vegetables?

   A. semivegetarian   B. vegan   C. lactovegetarian

8. Minerals that the body needs in relatively large quantaties are called:

   A. microminerals   B. macrominerals   C. water-soluble vitamins

9. In addition to calcium, milk and dairy products are excellent sources of:

   A. vitamin B12   B. vitamin C   C. zinc

10. Protein amino acids that we must consume in our diet are called:

    A. non-essential   B. essential   C. polyunsaturated

Check your knowledge:

Answers: 1–A; 2–B; 3–C; 4–B; 5–A; 6–C; 7–C; 8–B; 9–A; 10–B

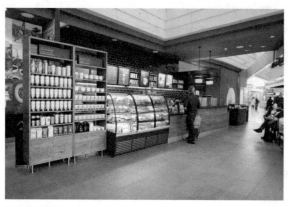

© Sorbis/Shutterstock.com

Introduction to Nutrition

"Good, sound nutritional choices are necessary for maintaining a healthy lifestyle. Making the effort to obtain the essential nutrients through daily dietary intake is not something in which most Americans are proficient. In general, Americans eat too much salt, sugar, and fat and do not consume the recommended daily allowance (RDA) of vitamins and minerals. Poor dietary habits, along with being physically inactive, are major factors that result in Americans becoming increasingly overweight and obese. Being overweight or obese is a major risk factor for chronic health problems such as hypertension, cardiovascular disease, diabetes, and certain types of cancers. With this in mind, the importance of building a knowledge base that will allow an individual to develop sound, life-long nutritional habits and practices becomes clear. Once an individual has made the effort to gather information that will allow him or her to make good nutritional choices, he or she must then make a concentrated effort to obtain the essential macronutrients and micronutrients through their daily food selections.

"**Macronutrients** provide energy in the form of calories. Carbohydrates, fats, and proteins make up the sources of macronutrients. **Micronutrients**, which include vitamins and minerals, regulate bodily functions such as metabolism, growth, and cellular development. Together, macronutrients and micronutrients are responsible for the following three tasks that are necessary for the continuance of life:

1. growth, repair, and maintenance of all tissues,
2. regulation of body processes, and
3. providing energy

"Because nutrition information is often filled with scientific terminology and unfamiliar jargon, it is many times misleading or appears to be overly complicated. Several government agencies, such as the U.S. Department of Agriculture (USDA) and the U.S. Department of Health and Human Services (DHHS), have teamed up in an effort to simplify and streamline nutritional information widely available to the general public in an effort to decrease the amount of misinformation on nutrition and increase the prevalence of practical, easy-to-apply, user-friendly information."[1]

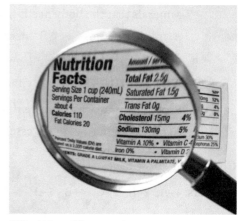

© Yossi Manor/Shutterstock.com

DIETARY GUIDELINES FOR AMERICANS

"In 1980 the Dietary Guidelines for Americans was first published as a scientifically-based health promotion that attempted to reduce an individual's risk for chronic diseases through diet and increased levels of physical activity. The USDA and the DHHS have updated and republished these Dietary Guidelines every five years since their inception in 1980."[1]

The most current version of the Dietary Guidelines was published in late 2015 (http://health.gov/dietaryguidelines/2015/guidelines/executive-summary/). The following is a list of the key recommendations of the Dietary Guidelines.

The Guidelines

1. **Follow a healthy eating pattern across the lifespan.** All food and beverage choices matter. Choose a healthy eating pattern at an appropriate calorie level to help achieve and maintain a healthy body weight, support nutrient adequacy, and reduce the risk of chronic disease.

2. **Focus on variety, nutrient density, and amount.** To meet nutrient needs within calorie limits, choose a variety of nutrient-dense foods across and within all food groups in recommended amounts.

3. **Limit calories from added sugars and saturated fats and reduce sodium intake.** Consume an eating pattern low in added sugars, saturated fats, and sodium. Cut back on foods and beverages higher in these components to amounts that fit within healthy eating patterns.

4. **Shift to healthier food and beverage choices.** Choose nutrient-dense foods and beverages across and within all food groups in place of less healthy choices. Consider cultural and personal preferences to make these shifts easier to accomplish and maintain.

5. **Support healthy eating patterns for all.** Everyone has a role in helping to create and support healthy eating patterns in multiple settings nationwide, from home to school to work to communities.

Key Recommendations

Consume a healthy eating pattern that accounts for all foods and beverages within an appropriate calorie level.

A healthy eating pattern includes:

- A variety of vegetables from all of the subgroups- dark green, red and orange, legumes (beans and peas), starchy, and other
- Fruits, especially whole fruits
- Grains, at least half of which are whole grains
- Fat-free or low-fat dairy, including milk, yogurt, cheese, and/or fortified soy beverages
- A variety of protein foods, including seafood, lean meats and poultry, eggs, legumes (beans and peas), and nuts, seeds, and soy products
- Oils

A healthy eating pattern limits:

- Saturated fats and *trans* fats, added sugars, and sodium
- Consume less than 10 percent of calories per day from added sugars
- Consume less than 10 percent of calories per day from saturated fats
- Consume less than 2,300 milligrams per day of sodium
- If alcohol is consumed, it should be consumed in moderation- up to one drink a day for women and up to two drinks per day for men- and only by adults of legal drinking age

Meet the *Physical Activity Guidelines for Americans* (See Chapter 4 Physical Activity & Exercise).

CARB, FAT AND PROTEIN DAILY RATE

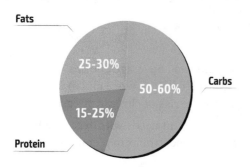

Fats 25-30%

Carbs 50-60%

Protein 15-25%

Healthy protein, carbohydrates, and fat sources

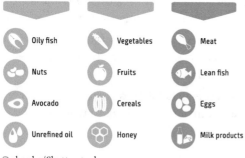

- Oily fish
- Nuts
- Avocado
- Unrefined oil
- Vegetables
- Fruits
- Cereals
- Honey
- Meat
- Lean fish
- Eggs
- Milk products

© shonka/Shutterstock.com

Macronutrients

"It is necessary for an individual to ingest more than forty different nutrients in order to maintain good health. Because no single food source contains all of these nutrients, variety in one's diet is essential. Eating a wide variety of foods will help ensure adequate intake of carbohydrates, fats, and proteins."[1]

Carbohydrates

"**Carbohydrates** should be the body's main source of fuel. Between 55 and 60 percent of an individual's diet should be composed of carbohydrates. Of this 55 to 60 percent, 45 to 50 percent of total daily caloric intake should be from complex carbohydrates, leaving simple carbohydrates to account for less than 10 percent of the daily carbohydrate intake. **Complex carbohydrates** are relatively low in calories (4 calories per gram), nutritionally dense, and are a rich source of vitamins, minerals, and water. Complex carbohydrates provide the body with a steady source of energy for hours. The best sources of complex carbohydrates are breads, cereals, pastas, and grains. Simple carbohydrates are sugars that have little nutritive value beyond their energy content. Foods high in simple sugars are sometimes dismissed as "empty calories." Examples of these foods include candy, cakes, jellies, and sodas."[1]

© Juice Team/Shutterstock.com

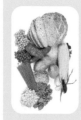

Complex Carbohydrates
- high in micronutrients (minerals & vitamins)
- high in fiber
- more filling
- sustained energy

© Robyn Mackenzie/Shutterstock.com

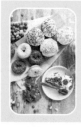

Simple Carbohydrates
- high in sugar (usually processed/refined)
- low in nutrients
- less filling
- can contribute to rapid changes in blood sugar

© Syda Productions/Shutterstock.com

Simple carbohydrates are higher in calories and sugar, and have lower amounts of vitamins, minerals and fiber. A healthy diet is one that is high in complex carbohydrates and low in simple carbohydrates.

"**Dietary fiber**, also known as roughage or bulk, is a type of complex carbohydrate that is present mainly in leaves, roots, skins, and seeds and is the part of a plant that is not digested in the small intestine. Dietary fiber helps decrease the risk of cardiovascular disease and cancer, and may lower an individual's risk of coronary heart disease. Dietary fiber is either soluble or insoluble. **Soluble fiber** dissolves in water. It helps the body excrete fats and has been shown to reduce levels of blood cholesterol

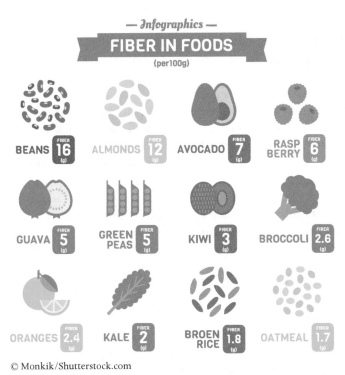

— *Infographics* —

FIBER IN FOODS

(per 100g)

BEANS **16** (g) ALMONDS **12** (g) AVOCADO **7** (g) RASP BERRY **6** (g)

GUAVA **5** (g) GREEN PEAS **5** (g) KIWI **3** (g) BROCCOLI **2.6** (g)

ORANGES **2.4** (g) KALE **2** (g) BROEN RICE **1.8** (g) OATMEAL **1.7** (g)

© Monkik/Shutterstock.com

and blood sugar, as well as helping to control diabetes. Water soluble fiber travels through the digestive tract in gel-like form, pacing the absorption of cholesterol, which helps prevent dramatic shifts in blood sugar levels. Soluble fiber is found primarily in oats, fruits, barley, and legumes.

"Insoluble fiber does not dissolve easily in water; therefore, it cannot be digested by the body. Insoluble fiber causes softer, bulkier stool that increases peristalsis. This, in turn, reduces the risk of colon cancer by allowing food residues to pass through the intestinal tract more quickly, limiting the exposure and absorption time of toxic substances within the waste materials. Primary sources of insoluble fiber include wheat, cereals, vegetables, and the skins of fruits. The recommended daily intake of fiber is 25–30 g per day. Health disorders associated with low fiber intake include constipation, diverticulitis, hemorrhoids, gall bladder disease, and obesity. Problems associated with ingesting too much fiber include losses of calcium, phosphorous, iron, and disturbances of the gastrointestinal system."[1]

Fats

"Fats are the body's primary source of energy, and supply the body with 9 calories of energy per gram ingested. While many Americans consume too many of their daily calories from fats (37 to 40 percent), dietary fat is not necessarily a 'bad' component of an individual's diet at moderate levels of consumption. At moderate amounts, between 25 and 30 percent of daily calories, fat is crucial to good nutrition.

"Fat has many essential functions: providing the body with stored energy, insulating the body to preserve body heat, contributing to cellular structure, and protecting vital organs by absorbing shock. Fat not only adds flavor and texture to foods and helps satisfy an individual's appetite because it is digested more slowly, it also supplies the body with essential fatty acids and transports fat-soluble vitamins A, E, D, and K. Fat is also necessary for normal growth and healthy skin, and is essential in the synthesis of certain hormones.

"Fats become counterproductive to good health when they are consumed in excess. Too much fat in many Americans' diets is the reason Americans lead

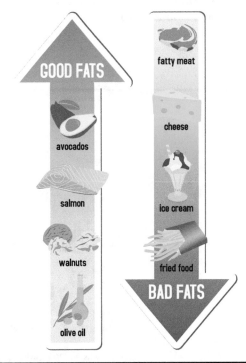

GOOD FATS

fatty meat

cheese

avocados

salmon

ice cream

walnuts

fried food

olive oil

BAD FATS

GOOD FATS vs. BAD FATS

© Elizabeta Lexa/Shutterstock.com

the world in heart disease. Excess fat intake elevates blood cholesterol levels and leads to atherosclerosis. Diets with excess fat have attributed to 30 to 40 percent of all cancers in men and 60 percent of all cancers in women, and have also been linked to cancer of the breast, colon, and prostate more frequently than any other dietary factor.

"There are different types of dietary fat. **Saturated fats** are found primarily in animal products such as meats, lard, cream, butter, cheese, and whole milk. However, coconut and palm oils are two plant sources of saturated fat. A defining characteristic of saturated fats is that they typically do not melt at room temperature (an exception being the above mentioned oils that are 'almost solid' at room temperature). Saturated fats increase low-density lipoproteins (LDL) or "bad cholesterol" levels and in turn increase an individual's risk for heart disease and colorectal cancer.

"**Unsaturated fats** are derived primarily from plant products such as vegetable oils, avocados, and most nuts, and do not raise the body's blood cholesterol. Unsaturated fats include both monounsaturated and polyunsaturated fats. **Monounsaturated fats** are found in foods such as olives, peanuts, canola oil, peanut oil, and olive oil. **Polyunsaturated fats** are found in margarine, pecans, corn oil, cottonseed oil, sunflower oil, and soybean oil.

"**Trans fat** is different from other types of fat in that it typically does not occur naturally in plant or animal products. While a small amount of trans fat is found naturally, the majority of trans fat is formed when liquid oils are made into solid fats (i.e., shortening and some margarines). Trans fat is made during hydrogenation—when hydrogen is added to vegetable oil. This process is used to increase the shelf life of foods and to help foods maintain their original flavor. Many fried foods and 'store bought' sweets and treats have high amounts of this type of fat. While most individuals consume four to five times more saturated fat than trans fat, it is important to be aware of the amount of trans fat in one's diet because it raises LDL, 'bad,' cholesterol and increases the risk of coronary heart disease. Starting January 1, 2006, the Food and Drug Administration (FDA) required all foods to list the amount of trans fat contained in the product on the Nutrition Facts panel. *The exception to this new requirement is that if the total fat in a food is less than 0.5 g per serving and no claims are made about fat, fatty acid, or cholesterol content, trans fat does not have to be listed.*"[1]

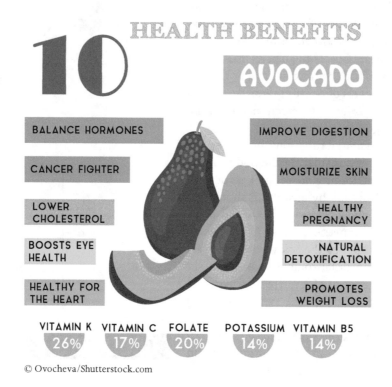

© Ovocheva/Shutterstock.com

Dietary Fat

Unsaturated Fat	Saturated Fat	Trans Fat
Food Examples	**Food Examples**	**Food Examples**
Almonds Vegetables Fish Olives Olive Oil	Beef Butter Pizza Ice Cream Lard	Cookies Donuts Cakes Fries Hydrogenated Oil
Benefits	**Benefits**	**Benefits**
Works in conjunction with saturated fats to prevent heart attacks and strokes Raises good cholesterol levels	Works in conjunction with unsaturated fats to prevent heart attacks and strokes	None

© John T Takai/Shutterstock.com

Protein

"Even though proteins should make up only 12–15 percent of total calories ingested, they are the essential 'building blocks' of the body. Proteins are needed for the growth, maintenance, and repair of all body tissues, that is, muscles, blood, bones, internal organs, skin, hair, and nails. Proteins also help maintain the normal balance of body fluids and are needed to make enzymes, hormones, and antibodies that fight infection. Proteins are made up of approximately twenty amino acids. An individual's body uses all twenty of these amino acids in the formation of different proteins. Eleven of the twenty are **non-essential amino acids**—they are manufactured in the body if food proteins in a person's diet provide enough nitrogen. Nine of the twenty are **essential amino acids**—the body cannot produce these, and thus must be supplied through an individual's diet. All amino acids must be present at the same time for particular protein synthesis to occur."[1]

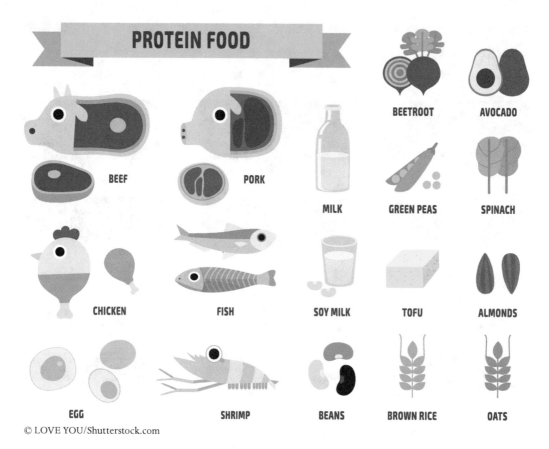

© LOVE YOU/Shutterstock.com

"The suggested RDA of protein for adults is 45 through 65 g per day (intake should not exceed 1.6 g/kg of body weight (1kg. = 2.2 lbs). A few exceptions to this rule should be noted: Overweight individuals need slightly less than the calculated 'norm,' and women who are pregnant or lactating need slightly more protein per pound of body weight than the calculation indicates."[1]

Spotlight on . . .

Protein Supplements & Shakes!

Many people believe that once they begin an exercise program, they should consume extra protein through supplements, and most commonly, protein shakes. While some individuals who train at extremely high levels may need supplementation to address protein needs, this is not the case for most of the general population. "It is inadvisable to consume more protein than the daily recommended dosage (45–65 g/day), particularly in the form of protein supplements. Excessive protein supplementation can damage the kidneys, increase calcium excretion, negatively affect bone health, inhibit muscle growth, and can be detrimental to endurance performance. Individuals who are trying to maximize muscular strength, endurance, and growth should take in the recommended 1.5 g of protein per kilogram of body weight, as well as an additional 500 calories of complex carbohydrates. The recommended protein and additional complex carbohydrates will work together to provide the extra nutrients and glucose needed for the increased muscular work load."[1]

Micronutrients

All macronutrients provide the body with calories, only the healthier sources will have higher amounts of micronutrients, which are vitamins, minerals, and water. We need these three nutrients for regulations and processes within the body.

Vitamins

"**Vitamins** are necessary for normal body metabolism, growth, and development. They do not provide the body with energy, but they do allow the energy from consumed carbohydrates, fats, and proteins to be released. Although vitamins are vital to life, they are required in minute amounts. Due primarily to adequate food supply, vitamin deficiencies in Americans are rare. However, there are some situations that may alter an individual's requirements, including pregnancy and smoking. Non-smokers need to consume 60 mg of vitamin C each day; a smoker must ingest 100 mg of vitamin C each day in order to gain the same nutritional benefits. A man or a non-pregnant woman should consume 180–200 mcg of folic acid, while a pregnant woman should consume approximately 400 mcg of folic acid per day."[1]

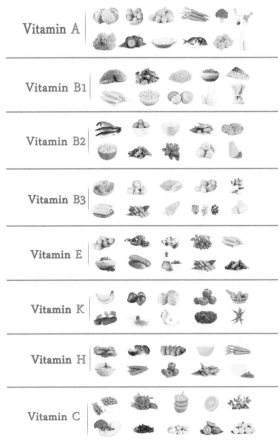

© Africa Studio/Shutterstock.com

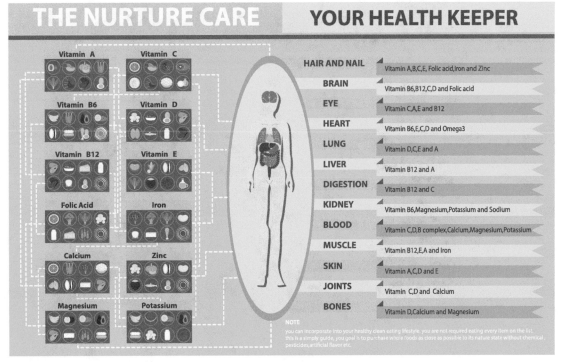

© PattyK/Shutterstock.com

"Vitamins are grouped as either fat soluble or water soluble. **Fat-soluble vitamins** are transported by the body's fat cells and by the liver. They include vitamins A, E, D, and K. Fat-soluble vitamins are not excreted in urine; therefore, they are stored in the body for relatively long periods of time (many months), and can build up to potentially toxic levels if excessive doses are consumed over time. **Water-soluble vitamins** include the B vitamins and vitamin C. These vitamins are not stored in the body for a significant amount of time, and the amounts that are consumed and not used relatively quickly by the body are excreted through urine and sweat. For this reason, water-soluble vitamins must be replaced daily."[1]

Minerals

"**Minerals** are inorganic substances that are critical to many enzyme functions in the body. Approximately twenty-five minerals have important roles in bodily functions. Minerals are contained in all cells and are concentrated in hard parts of the body—nails, teeth, and bones—and are crucial to maintaining water balance and the acid-base balance. Minerals are essential components of respiratory pigments, enzymes, and enzyme systems, while also regulating muscular and nervous tissue excitability, blood clotting, and normal heart rhythm.

"Two groups of minerals are necessary in an individual's diet: macrominerals and microminerals. **Macrominerals** are the seven minerals the body needs in relatively large quantities (100 mg or more each day). These seven minerals are: calcium, chloride, magnesium, phosphorus, potassium, sodium, and sulfur. In most cases, these minerals can be acquired by eating a variety of foods each day. While **microminerals** are essential to healthy living, they are needed in smaller quantities (less than 100 mg per day) than

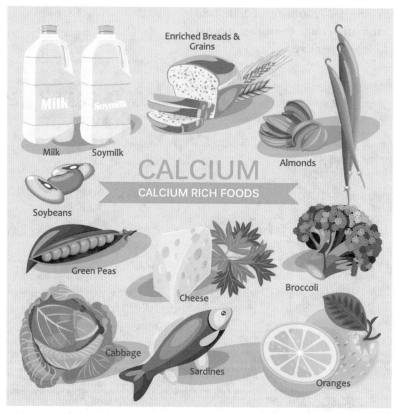

© Tatsiana Tsyhanova/Shutterstock.com

macrominerals. Examples of these minerals include chromium, cobalt, copper, fluoride, iodine, iron, manganese, molybdenum, selenium, and zinc."[1]

Antioxidants

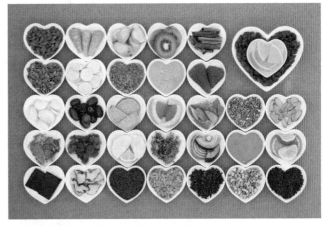

© Marilyn barbone/Shutterstock.com

"**Antioxidants** are compounds that aid each cell in the body facing an ongoing barrage of damage resulting from daily oxygen exposure, environmental pollution, chemicals and pesticides, additives in processed foods, stress hormones, and sun radiation. Studies continue to show the ability of antioxidants to suppress cell deterioration and to "slow" the aging process. Realizing the potential power of these substances should encourage Americans to take action by eating at least five servings of a wide variety of fruits and vegetables each day. There are many proven health benefits of antioxidants. Vitamin C speeds the healing process, helps prevent infection, and prevents scurvy. Vitamin E helps prevent heart disease by stopping the oxidation of low-density lipoprotein (the harmful form of cholesterol); strengthens the immune system; and may play a role in the prevention of Alzheimer's disease, cataracts, and some forms of cancer, providing further proof of the benefits of antioxidants. Adequate amounts of vitamins, minerals, and antioxidants are crucial to good overall health."[1]

Spotlight on . . .

Organic Foods

"**Organic foods** are foods that are grown without the use of pesticides. These chemical-free foods are much more difficult to grow because they are more vulnerable to disease and pests; thus, they are not 'high yield' crops. Due to the fact that they are less common and harder to grow successfully, organic foods are more expensive. Whether the expense is justified by the improved nutritional quality and overall health benefits is yet to be determined.

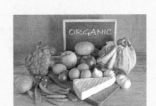

© PIxelbliss/Shutterstock.com

Functional Foods

Functional foods are foods with benefits that go above and beyond basic nutrition. A person's overall health can be greatly affected by the food choices they make. Functional benefits of foods that have been consumed for decades are being discovered and new foods are being developed for their helpful dietary components.

Water

"In many cases, **water** is the 'forgotten nutrient.' Although water does not provide energy to the body in the form of calories, it is a substance that is essential to life. Among other things, water lubricates joints,

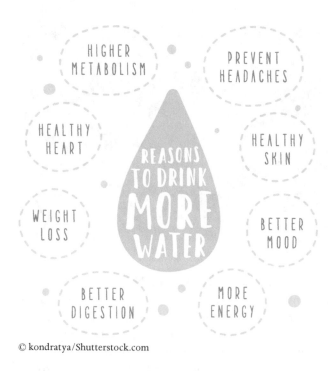

© kondratya/Shutterstock.com

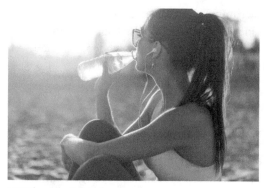

© Undrey/Shutterstock.com

absorbs shock, regulates body temperature, maintains blood volume, and transports fluids throughout the body, while comprising 60 percent of an individual's body. While it is clear that adequate hydration is crucial to proper physiological functioning, many people are in a semi-hydrated state most of the time. Whether exercising or not, hydration should be a continuous process. Prolonged periods of dehydration can result in as much as a 10 percent loss of intracellular water concentration and can result in death. Individuals more susceptible to dehydration include: persons who are overweight; deconditioned or not acclimatized to heat; very old and very young; and individuals who do not eat breakfast or drink water."[1]

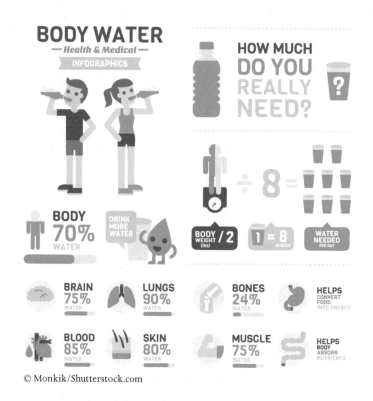

© Monkik/Shutterstock.com

"To ensure proper water balance and prevent dehydration, approximately six to eight eight-ounce glasses of water should be consumed each day an individual is not exercising. When working out, current recommendations for water intake are two to three eight-ounce cups of water before exercising, four to six ounces of cool water every fifteen minutes during the workout, and rehydrating thoroughly after the activity."[1]

BUILDING A HEALTHY PLATE

"MyPlate is an idea based on the 2010 Dietary Guidelines for Americans. The idea behind MyPlate is to simplify the concept of making better/healthier food choices. MyPlate uses the familiar place setting, using a plate 9 inches in diameter, to illustrate the five food groups and the relative proportions in which they should be consumed. When used in conjunction with the ChooseMyPlate.gov website, consumers have access to practical, easy to understand information that will enable them to easily build a healthier diet. Some select messages ChooseMyPlate uses to help consumers focus in on key behaviors include:

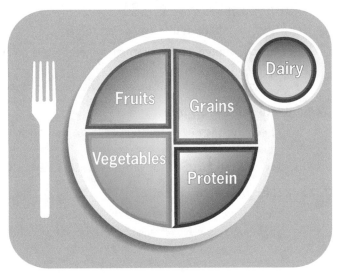

© Basheera Designs/Shutterstock.com

- **Eat the right amount of calories for you.** Everyone has a personal calorie limit. Staying within yours can help you get to or maintain a healthy weight. People who are successful at managing their weight have found ways to keep track of how much they eat in a day, even if they don't count every calorie.
- **Enjoy your food, but eat less.**
- **Cook more often at home, where you are in control of what's in your food. When eating out, choose lower calorie menu options.**
- **Write down what you eat to keep track of how much you eat. If you drink alcoholic beverages, do so sensibly—limit to 1 drink a day for women or to 2 drinks a day for men.**
- **Build a healthy plate.** Before you eat, think about what goes on your plate or in your cup or bowl. Foods like vegetables, fruits, whole grains, low-fat dairy products, and lean protein foods contain the nutrients you need without too many calories. Try some of these options.
- **Keep your food safe to eat—learn more at www.FoodSafety.gov.**
- **Cut back on foods high in solid fats, added sugars, and salt.** Many people eat foods with too much solid fats, added sugars, and salt (sodium). Added sugars and fats load foods with extra calories you don't need. Too much sodium may increase your blood pressure.
- **Choose foods and drinks with little or no added sugars.**
- **Look out for salt (sodium) in foods you buy—it all adds up.**
- **Eat fewer foods that are high in solid fats.**"[1]

Spotlight on . . .

MyPlate Food Groups

Make at least half your grains whole.

- Choose 100% whole-grain cereals, breads, crackers, rice, and pasta.
- Check the ingredients list on food packages to find whole-grain foods.

Make half your plate fruits and vegetables.

- Eat red, orange, and dark-green vegetables, such as tomatoes, sweet potatoes, and broccoli, in main and side dishes.
- Eat fruit, vegetables, or unsalted nuts as snacks—they are nature's original fast foods.

Switch to skim or 1% milk.

- They have the same amount of calcium and other essential nutrients as whole milk, but less fat and calories.
- Try calcium-fortified soy products as an alternative to dairy foods.

Vary your protein food choices.

- Twice a week, make seafood the protein on your plate.
- Eat beans, which are a natural source of fiber and protein.

Grains

"When examining options of food choices within this group it is important to not only choose a majority on one's daily calories from grains, but also to remember that it is nutritionally prudent to make half of the grains chosen whole grains. Whole grains are defined by the American Association of Cereal Chemists as 'food made from the entire grain seed, usually called the kernel, which consists of the bran, germ, and endosperm (AACC International Board of Directors, 1999). If the kernel has been cracked, crushed, or flaked, it must retain nearly the same relative proportions of bran, germ, and endosperm as the original grain.' Examples of easy-to-find whole grains include brown rice, bulgur (cracked wheat), popcorn, whole rye, wild rice, whole oats/oatmeal, whole-grain barley, and whole wheat. Selections of whole-grain products from this group will help an individual maximize their intake of dietary fiber as well as other nutrients. One serving from the grain group equals one slice of bread, half a bagel or one sixteen-inch tortilla."[1]

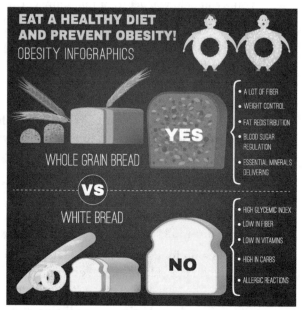

© Double Brain/Shutterstock.com

Vegetables

"Vegetables are an excellent source of natural fiber, they are low in fat, and provide the body with vitamins, especially vitamins A and C. While all vegetables are good nutritional choices, to maximize the benefits of eating vegetables, one should vary the type of vegetables eaten. It is also important when choosing vegetables to ingest not only a variety of the brightly colored vegetables such as corn, squash, and peas, but also the green and orange vegetables such as carrots, yams, and broccoli. One serving from the vegetable group equals one cup of raw, lefty greens; half cup of other chopped vegetables; or three-quarter cup of vegetable juice."[1]

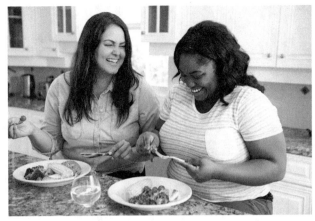

© Monkey Business Images/Shutterstock.com

Did you know . . .

Superfoods are foods that have been shown to reduce the chances of some diseases such as heart disease, cancer, and diabetes. They can also provide valuable nutrients that improve quality of life such as immune support and memory. Many whole grains, fruits, and vegetables have been shown to have superfood properties!

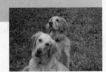

Courtesy of Shelley Hamill

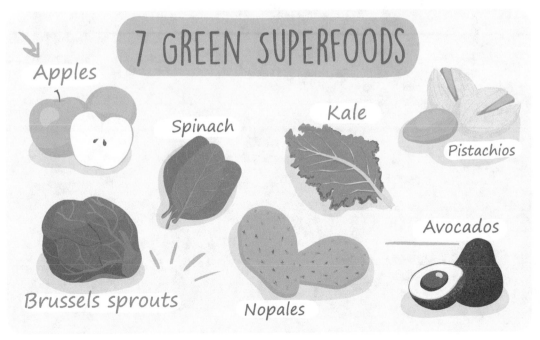

© On Theway/Shutterstock.com

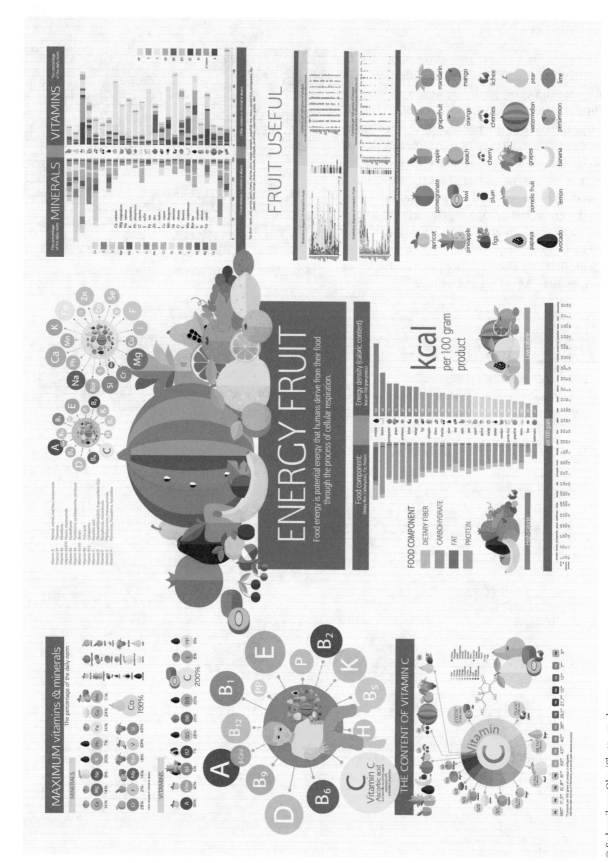

Fruits

"Fresh, canned, frozen, or dried fruits are all excellent sources of vitamins and minerals, most notably vitamin C. It is, however, important to watch for heavy, sugary syrups when selecting canned fruits. Fruits canned in lite syrups or the fruit's own natural juice allow an individual to take in the same amount of vitamins and minerals as their heavily syrup counterparts without adding unnecessary and/or unwanted sugar, fat, and calories to their diet. Fruit juices are another important part of many people's diet that should be monitored for 'hidden' sugars and calories. When possible, freshly squeezed juices are an ideal alternative. Serving equivalents for the fruit group are: one serving equals one medium apple, banana, or orange; one melon wedge; half cup of chopped berries, or three-quarter cup of fruit juice."[1]

Milk/Dairy

"Milk products are not only the body's best source of calcium, but they are also an excellent source of protein and vitamin B12. To maximize the benefits of calcium-rich foods and minimize the calories, cholesterol, fat, and saturated fat per selection, low-fat and skim alternatives should be chosen. One serving from the milk group equals one cup of milk or yogurt, or one and a half ounces of cheese."[1]

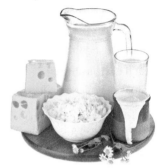

© Madlen/Shutterstock.com

Protein/Meats and Beans

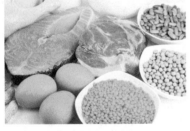

© Africa Studio/Shutterstock.com

"Meats and beans are excellent sources of protein, iron, zinc, and B vitamins. It is important to be aware of the fact that many food selections within this food group can be relatively high in fat content, especially saturated fats. Lower fat alternatives within this group that remain a rich source of vitamins and minerals include beans, fish, poultry, and lean cuts of beef. Serving equivalents for the meat and beans group are as follows: one serving equals two to three ounces of cooked lean beef, poultry, or fish; one egg; half cup of cooked beans; or two tablespoons of seeds or nuts."[1]

Oils

"As in all other areas of the pyramid, it is important to choose your source(s) of oils carefully. As a general rule, oils such as olive oil, peanut oil, and canola oil contain unsaturated fats. These oils do not raise an individual's blood cholesterol and are therefore a healthier option."[1]

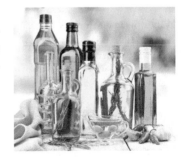

© Africa Studio/Shutterstock.com

READING AND UNDERSTANDING THE NUTRITION FACTS LABEL

"Food labels are legally required to include the number of servings per container, serving size, and the number of calories per serving. They must also list the percentage of the daily value of total fat, saturated fat, and trans fat. Nutrition Facts Labels must also list the percentage of the daily value of cholesterol, sodium, total carbohydrates (including dietary fiber and sugars), proteins, vitamins, and minerals."[1]

Food Label: Nutrition Facts

Serving Size

Is your serving the same size as the one on the label? If you eat double the serving size listed, you need to double the nutrient and calorie values. If you eat one-half the serving size shown here, cut the nutrient and calorie values in half.

Calories

Are you overweight? Cut back a little on calories! Look here to see how a serving of the food adds to your daily total. A 5'4", 138-lb. active woman needs about 2,200 calories each day. A 5'10", 174-lb. active man needs about 2,900. How about you?

Total Carbohydrate

When you cut down on fat, you can eat more carbohydrates. Carbohydrates are in foods like bread, potatoes, fruits, and vegetables. Choose these often! They give you more nutrients than sugars like soda pop and candy.

Dietary Fiber

Grandmother called it "roughage," but her advice to eat more is still up-to-date! That goes for both soluble and insoluble kinds of dietary fiber. Fruits, vegetables, whole-grain foods, beans, and peas are all good sources and can help reduce the risk of heart disease and cancer.

Protein

Most Americans get more protein than they need. Where there is animal protein, there is also fat and cholesterol. Eat small servings of lean meat, fish, and poultry. Use skim or low-fat milk, yogurt, and cheese. Try vegetable proteins like beans, grains, and cereals.

Vitamins and Minerals

Your goal here is 100 percent of each for the day. Don't count on one food to do it all. Let a combination of foods add up to a winning score.

Nutrition Facts		
Serving Size 1 cup (228g)		
Servings Per Container 2		
Amount Per Serving		
Calories 250	Calories from Fat 110	
	% Daily Value*	
Total Fat 12g		**18%**
Saturated Fat 3g		**15%**
Trans Fat 3g		
Cholesterol 30mg		**10%**
Sodium 470mg		**20%**
Total Carbohydrate 31g		**10%**
Dietary Fiber 0g		**0%**
Sugars 5g		
Protein 5g		
Vitamin A		4%
Vitamin C		2%
Calcium		20%
Iron		4%

*Percent Daily Values are based on a 2,000 calorie diet. Your Daily Values may be higher or lower depending on your calorie needs:

	Calories	2,000	2,500
Total Fat	Less than	65g	80g
Sat Fat	Less than	20g	25g
Cholesterol	Less than	300mg	300mg
Sodium	Less than	2,400mg	2,400mg
Total Carbohydrate		300g	375g
Fiber		25g	30g

Calories per gram:

Fat 9 • Carbohydrates 4 • Protein 4

More nutrients may be listed on some labels.

Total Fat

Aim low. Most people need to cut back on fat! Too much fat may contribute to heart disease and cancer. Try to limit your calories from fat. For a healthy heart, choose foods with a big difference between the total number of calories and the number of calories from fat.

Saturated Fat

A new kind of fat? No—saturated fat is part of the total fat in food. It is listed separately because it's the key player in raising blood cholesterol and your risk of heart disease. Eat less!

Cholesterol

Too much cholesterol—a second cousin to fat—can lead to heart disease. Challenge yourself to eat less than 300 mg each day.

Sodium

You call it "salt," the label calls it "sodium." Either way, it may add up to high blood pressure in some people. So, keep your sodium intake low—2,400 to 3,000 mg or less each day.*

*The AHA recommends no more than 3,000 mg sodium per day for healthy adults.

Daily Value

Feel like you're drowning in numbers? Let the Daily Value be your guide. Daily Values are listed for people who eat 2,000 or 2,500 calories each day. If you eat more, your personal daily value may be higher than what's listed on the label. If you eat less, your personal daily value may be lower.

For fat, saturated fat, cholesterol, and sodium, choose foods with a low percent Daily Value. For total carbohydrate, dietary fiber, vitamins, and minerals, your daily value goal is to reach 100 percent of each.

g = grams (About 28 g = 1 ounce)
mg = milligrams (1,000 mg = 1 g)

Did you know . . .

Percent fat of a food refers to the amount of a food that is just fat. You can determine the percent fat of a food by dividing the calories from fat by total calories. For example, for this nutrition label, calories from fat = 100 and total calories = 310.

Courtesy of Shelley Hamill

100/310 = 32% of this food's calories are from fat. Foods that are 35% or higher are considered a high-fat food. Try to limit foods that have higher percentages of fat (Bounds, 2012).

Nutrition Facts

Serving Size 5 oz. (144g)
Servings Per Container 4

Amount Per Serving

Calories 310	Calories from Fat 100

	% Daily Value*
Total Fat 15g	**21%**
Saturated Fat 2.6g	**17%**
Trans Fat 1g	
Cholesterol 118mg	**39%**
Sodium 560mg	**28%**
Total Carbohydrate 12g	**4%**
Dietary Fiber 1g	**4%**
Sugars 1g	
Protein 24g	

Vitamin A 1%	•	Vitamin C 2%
Calcium 2%	•	Iron 5%

*Percent Daily Values are based on a 2,000 calorie diet. Your daily values may be higher or lower depending on your calorie needs:

		Calories	2,000	2,500
Total Fat	Less Than		65g	80g
Saturated Fat	Less Than		20g	25g
Cholesterol	Less Than		300mg	300mg
Sodium	Less Than		2,400mg	2,400mg
Total Carbohydrate			300g	375g
Dietary Fiber			25g	30g

Calories per gram:
Fat 9 • Carbohydrate 4 • Protein 4

© Shelby Allison/Shutterstock.com

Vegetarianism

"There have always been people who, for one reason or another (religious, ethical, or philosophical), have chosen to follow a vegetarian diet. However, in recent years, a vegetarian diet has become increasingly popular. There are four different types of vegetarian diets:

"**Vegans** are considered true vegetarians. Their diets are completely void of meat, chicken, fish, eggs, or milk products. A vegan's primary sources of protein are vegetables, fruits, and grains. Because vitamin B12 is normally found only in meat products, many vegans choose to supplement their diet with this vitamin.

"**Lactovegetarians** eat dairy products, fruits, and vegetables but do not consume any other animal products (meat, poultry, fish, or eggs).

"**Ovolactovegetarians** are another type of vegetarians. They eat eggs as well as dairy products, fruits, and vegetables, but still do not consume meat, poultry, or fish.

VEGAN SOURCES OF PROTEIN

QUINOA   LEAFY GREENS   TOFU   GREEN PEAS

BROCCOLI   HEMP SEEDS   BEANS   MUSHROOMS

LENTILS   AVOCADO   CHIA SEEDS   NUTS

TEMPEH   BUCKWHEAT   SOYBEANS   CHICKPEAS

© kondratya/Shutterstock.com

"A person who eats fruits, vegetables, dairy products, eggs, and a small selection of poultry, fish, and other seafood is a partial or **semivegetarian**. These individuals do not consume any beef or pork.

"Vegetarians of all four types can meet all their daily dietary needs through the food selections available to them. However, because certain foods or groups of foods that are high in specific nutrients are forbidden, it is critical that a vegetarian is diligent in selecting his or her food combinations so that the nutritional benefits of the foods allowed are maximized. If food combinations from a wide variety of sources are not selected, nutritional deficiencies of proteins, vitamins, and minerals can rapidly occur and proper growth, development, and function may not occur."[1]

The Impact of Nutrition on Body Composition & Weight Management

Other than physical activity and exercise, nutrition intake plays the biggest role in body composition and weight management. The basis of body weight equals the amount of calories consumed versus the amount of calories burned (or used). If you are participating in higher amounts of physical activity than previously, then you are probably burning more calories that you are consuming, which would lead to weight loss. If you are eating more calories than you are burning through exercise, physical activity, or daily movements, then you have a higher caloric intake, which will lead to weight gain. If you consume the same amount of calories that you burn, then you will stay about the same body weight.

Products that claim to increase the body's metabolism may contain dangerous substances, such as ephedra, or they may just contain increased levels of caffeine, which might have adverse effects. The best weight loss plan is one of balance. Weight is controlled by many factors, including genetics and learned behaviors, but the basics of weight gain or loss is a balance between calories in and calories out. If you burn more calories than you consume, you will lose weight. The rate at which the body burns calories varies and is affected by gender and age, among other factors. The best weight loss plan is one that results in one to two pounds a week loss of weight. Programs that result in drastic weight loss in a short period of time are not easily sustained because most of the weight lost is due to dehydration (Hamilton, 2010).

If you are trying to lose weight, remember a few important points:

- Body weight and body composition are highly influenced by your genetics.
- Your ability to lose weight is dependent on the types of foods you consume, and how much physical activity you perform.
- Never starve yourself. Just consume more healthy foods that are low in calories, fat, and sugar, and are higher in nutrients.

If you are trying to gain weight, remember a few important points:

- Body weight and body composition are highly influenced by your genetics.
- Increase overall caloric intake, but still focus on healthy foods.
- Include resistance training to increase muscle mass.

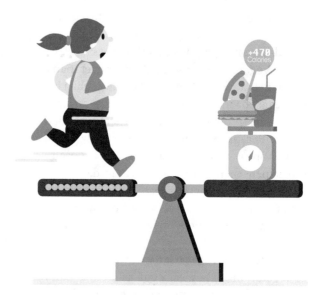

© Mangssab/Shutterstock.com

Spotlight on . . .

Diets and Diet Plans

Many Americans have a desire to lose weight. Many diet plans are marketed as quick, easy, and effective, and some of them might live up to this claim. Diets that promote eating only one food for a long period of time are not recommended. Limiting the diet to only one food source is not healthy because this limits vitamin and mineral intake. If a diet asks for the elimination of one energy source, such as carbohydrates, this is also not a healthy choice because it limits the body's source of energy and all sources play a unique role in the maintenance of total wellness.

Diets that severely limit caloric intake or require a period of fasting are never a good idea because this will put the body into starvation mode. If the body perceives that starvation is imminent, it will stop naturally burning calories by shutting down metabolism. It's very difficult to jump start the body's metabolism once it slows.

Are you a healthy consumer?

Nutrition and consumerism are strongly related. Most of us do not grow the foods we eat, so we must purchase them from a food market or restaurant. Consumer research within nutrition focuses on various types of behaviors. When do you tend to make your nutrition consumer choices? If you are waiting until you are really hungry or thirsty, you may be more likely to just choose anything, regardless if it's healthy or not. Do you use emotion when you purchase your food? If you are sad or anxious or depressed, you may purchase food that you perceive is "comforting." Realistically, most of the "comfort" foods that people gravitate to are not very healthy.

Being a healthy consumer of nutrition products includes a health literacy component. It's easier for those that have some general knowledge or education about nutrition to use tools to make healthy decisions. Understanding how to read and use the information on food labels is critical to becoming a healthy consumer of nutrition products. Beware of "fad" diets or products that make boastful claims about their effectiveness. Be smart about where you are spending your money, even as it relates to your nutrition consumer behaviors!

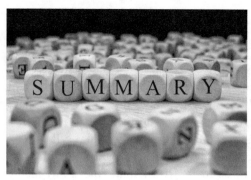

© Fabrik Bilder/Shutterstock.com

In this chapter, we defined and described basic nutrition information regarding macronutrients and micronutrients. We identified sources of both healthy and unhealthy foods, and described the current dietary guidelines by the US Department of Health and Human Services. We discussed strategies for individuals to make healthier nutrition choices. This chapter also covered the importance of reading and understanding the food nutrition labels, in order to be a more healthy consumer of nutrition products. By understanding macronutrient and micronutrient needs, functions, and sources, students can feel in control of their dietary needs, body composition, and weight management.

Personal Reflections . . . so, what have you learned?

1. Why do you think it is so difficult for most people to eat healthy?

2. In your own words of AT LEAST 5 sentences, summarize the nutrition guidelines and key recommendations for healthy Americans.

3. List the purpose of the following nutrients: carbohydrates, fats, proteins & fiber. What is at least one healthy source of each?

4. What impact does your current nutrition choices have on your overall health?

5. Identify at least one change you would like to implement in your nutrition behaviors here. How can you make the change effective?

NOTES

REFERENCES

Bounds, L., Darnell, G., Shea, K.B., & Agnore, D. (2012). *Health and fitness: A guide to a healthy lifestyle* (5th ed.). Dubuque, IA: Kendall Hunt Publishing Company.

Hamilton, A.R. (2010). *Health and the environment: Choices that lead to better health.* Dubuque, IA: Kendall Hunt Publishing Company.

U.S. Department of Agriculture. (2016). *Building a healthy eating style.* Retrieved from http://choosemyplate.gov/MyPlate

U.S. Department of Health and Human Services and U.S. Department of Agriculture. (2015). *2015–2020 dietary guidelines for Americans* (8th ed.). Retrieved from http://health.gov/dietaryguidelines/2015/guidelines/

Wing, R. & Hill, J. (2001). Successful weight loss maintenance. *Annual Review of Nutrition, 21,* 323–341.

CREDITS

1. From *Health and Fitness: A Guide to a Healthy Lifestyle,* 5/e by Laura Bounds, Gayden Darnell, Kristin Brekken Shea, Dottiede Agnore. Copyright © 2012 by Kendall Hunt Publishing Company. Reprinted by permission.

Chapter 6 ╋ ──────────────

Relationships

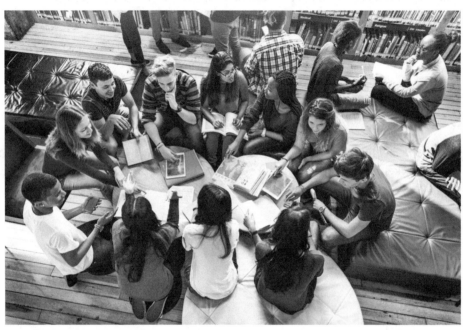

© Rawpixel.com/Shutterstock.com

OBJECTIVES:

Students will be able to:

- Identify the differences in communication patterns.
- Discuss how technology may impact communication
- "List and describe the elements of a healthy relationship.
- "List warning signs of an unhealthy relationship.
- "Identify types of abuse and describe the cycle of abuse and why it's difficult for the victim to end the relationship."[1]

RELATIONSHIP SURVEY

Think about the following questions:

1. What are the top 10 qualities you want in an intimate partner?
2. Which ones are non-negotiable, as in they must have these qualities for you to be with them?
3. Do you think you will have the same requirements in 5 years? Why or why not?
4. What would you say are your own top 10 qualities?

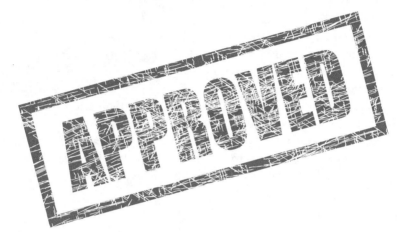

© Mahesh Patil/Shutterstock.com

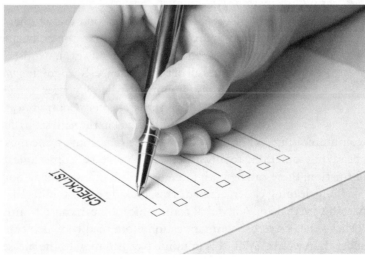

© Di Studio/Shutterstock.com

HEALTHY RELATIONSHIPS

"There are numerous types of relationships that exist. They range from casual acquaintances to life-long partners. It is important to realize the different types and stages that relationships grow into, as well as what represents a healthy relationship."[1]

Positive Self-Worth

"The first step to having a healthy relationship is developing a positive self-worth. This self-worth comes from many different sources. These may include family members, close friends, co-workers, occupation, achievements, and so on."[1] While our foundation for having a positive self-worth may come from our relationship with others, as we grow emotionally, developing and sustaining that positive image from within becomes important. If we continue to rely on others to provide that sense of worth, if they are no longer in our lives for some reason we may find ourselves losing our sense of value if those people are no longer in our lives.

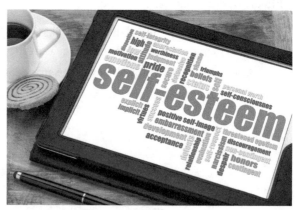

© marekuliasz/Shutterstock.com

   "A positive self-worth is represented in confidence, a healthy body, and a positive attitude about yourself and others. This is not to say that one has to be completely healthy in order to have a healthy relationship, but the closer to this goal the better relationships typically will be."[1]

Communication

According to the Oxford dictionary, communication is the "imparting or exchanging of information by speaking, writing, or using some other medium; the conveying or sharing of ideas and feelings; the means of sending or receiving ideas or information" (Oxford dictionaries).

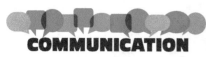

© Qvasimodo art/Shutterstock.com

Tone, pitch and intonation are another part of communication. You are paying attention to the body language, and you hear the words, but do you really **hear** the words? Sometimes the inflection makes all of the difference. Recognizing what someone is really saying is also important when it comes to **consent**, which we will talk about later in this chapter. Communication has many layers and it is important to develop the skill set to decipher the messages.

   We are always communicating. While the words we use may convey one message, our non-verbal communication may be saying something totally different. "Non-verbal communication includes unwritten and unspoken information; these can be both intentional and unintentional. Some examples include smiling, eye contact, nodding, leaning closer, crossed arms, looking off in another direction, and even rolling one's eyes. A mismatch of verbal and nonverbal communication can cause confusion. When this happens, people tend to believe the nonverbal communication more readily, which comes from the old saying, 'Actions speak louder than words.' With this in mind, pay attention to the messages you are sending nonverbally."[1]

   "There are different spatial zones that exist. Some individuals will lean closer to let a person know they are interested in them or in what is being said. There is an acceptable amount of space or a 'zone' that individuals claim as their personal space. Depending upon the circumstance, geographic location (such as a crowded city), or culture one grew up in, this zone changes. For example, this zone is larger when an individual is in a public or social environment, but typically becomes smaller when they are in a more personal or intimate setting. If your personal zone becomes too small for your comfort level, take two steps backward to increase the size of the space."[1]

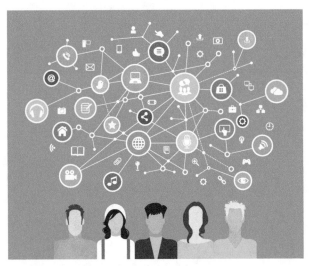

© VLADGRIN/Shutterstock.com

Communication in the Age of Technology

According to the Pew Research Center, nearly two thirds of Americans owned smart phones in 2015 (Pew Research Center). According to a the Pew Institute, the number of text messages sent monthly in the United States went from 14 billion in 2000 to 188 billion in 2010 and that number shows no signs of abating (CNN). Americans ages 18–29 send and receive an average of nearly 88 text messages per day (CNN). Of course, that does not include instant messaging, Snapchat, Twitter, and the many other electronically-assisted correspondences.

While electronic communication may be fast, it isn't always easy. How do you convey your tone or emotions when you are texting? Do you use emoticons or acronyms? We have a new language where we know what "lol" or "btw" mean. Have you ever been misunderstood in a text? There are countless articles citing how electronic communication has impacted our ability to communicate face-to-face. Think about how you communicate and how that may impact your present and future relationships.

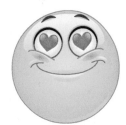

©Yayayoyo/Shutterstock.com

Open Communication

"Healthy relationships include open communication, compromise, trust, respect, caring, selflessness, as well as many other attributes. Researchers have found that 70 to 93 percent of messages sent come from nonverbal communication.

"Open communication involves actively listening, talking effectively, and body language. Minimize or alleviate other distractions in order to maximize open communication with your partner or friend. This may include removing the headphones, looking up from the iPhone, or maybe getting away from other friends and/or roommates. During a discussion truly listen to the other person. Do not interrupt or simply wait until they are finished speaking to interject your thought or advice. So much of the time people only hear the first part of a sentence or a concept because they are busy forming their thoughts and ideas of how they are going to reply. Be open to questions. Do not continuously lead the conversation. Let the other person talk and listen to what they have to say."[1]

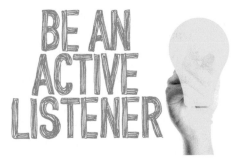

© Gustavo Frazao/Shutterstock.com

Did you know . . .

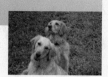
Courtesy of Shelley Hamill

According to Forbes (2016) there are 10 steps to Effective Listening:

1. Face the speaker and maintain eye contact.
2. Be attentive, but relaxed.
3. Keep an open mind
4. Listen to the words and try to picture what the speaker is saying
5. Don't interrupt and don't impose your "solutions".
6. Wait for the speaker to pause to ask clarifying questions.
7. Ask questions only to ensure understanding.
8. Try to feel what the speaker is feeling.
9. Give the speaker regular feedback
10. Pay attention to non-verbal cues,

Communication Styles

"There are numerous ways to communicate with one another. Each individual has their own style of communication. The type of communication an individual chooses to use at any given time is dependent upon the current situation, how important the concept or information is to them, and their personality. Communication styles are learned throughout one's life from parents, siblings, peers, and co-workers and are blended into a style that is preferred and compatible with one's personality.

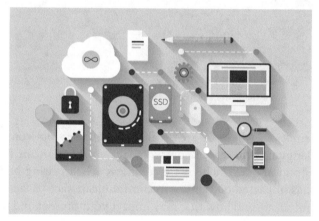
© Bloomua/Shutterstock.com

Spelling a Healthy Relationship
(adapted from Kuriansky, 2002)

Honesty—always tell the truth even if it will initially hurt.

Harmony—enrich one another's differences.

Heart—give your whole heart.

Honor—hold others in high regard.

Happy—be happy with each other.

Empathy—be able to understand what each other feel.

Equality—treat the other as your equal.

Energetic—be spontaneous, relationships take energy.

Enthusiasm—be excited about being together.

Empowerment—support each other.

Acceptance—know that you approve of each other just the way they are.

Accommodation—make adjustments for each other's needs.

Appreciation—be grateful for each other.

Adaptability—be able to make changes when necessary.

Agreements—make an agreement and hold to it.

Love—should be unconditional.

Loyalty—be devoted, never betray each other.

Listening—actively listen, it makes the other person feel important.

Laughter—have fun together.

Lust—sparks the union.

Trust—being able to relax around the other person.

Talking—communication is the key.

Time—spend time together. Nothing is more important than time.

Tenderness—treat each other with kindness.

Thoughtfulness—show consideration in thoughts and actions.

Home—create a safe haven.

Healing—work together to heal new and old wounds.

Humility—admit when you are wrong.

Hope—for a better tomorrow when things are not at their best.

Homework—relationships are not easy, they do require constant work.

YES! Say yes as often as you can.

It is helpful to recognize and understand communication styles and differences early in relationships regardless if they are personal or professional to help strengthen communication and minimize miscommunication."[1]

Left-Brain vs. Right-Brain . . . there is really no such thing

So, what does this mean? *Psychology about Health* (2015) notes that many people believe they are left brain or right brain thinkers. From books to television programs, you've probably heard the phrase mentioned numerous times or perhaps you've even taken an online test to determine which type best describes you. You've probably spotted at least a few infographics on Pinterest or Facebook claiming to reveal your dominant brain hemisphere.

People who identify as **left-brain thinkers** might feel that they have strong math and logic skills. Those who profess to be **right-brain thinkers**, on the other hand, feel that their talents are more on the creative side of things. Given the popularity of the idea of "right brained" and "left brained" thinkers, it might surprise you learn that this idea is just one of many myths about the brain. Additionally, people are said to prefer one type of thinking over the other. For example, a person who is "left-brained" is often said to be more logical, analytical,

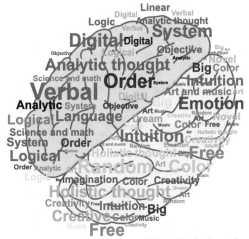

Left Brain Functions

Right Brain Functions

© Photoraidz/Shutterstock.com

and objective. A person who is "right-brained" is said to be more intuitive, thoughtful, and subjective. **The truth is both sides of the brain work together to process whatever is necessary to fulfill the task at hand.**

That said, some use this concept to note differences in communication patterns. Popular wisdom over the years has stated that men and women communicate differently and listed the specifics of what that looked like. The focus of males being more "logical" and females being more "emotional" continued to be emphasized in communication patterns. The reality is that **gender does not determine a person's communication pattern.** Not only that, a person's pattern of communication may be dependent upon the situation they are in at the time. Perhaps what is more significant is recognizing what that communication pattern is so that the exchange can be more meaningful or less frustrating.

Effective communication entails actually communicating. Some people play "guess what I am thinking" or "if you really cared you would know what I mean," but the reality is we are not mind readers! If you have something to say, say it. If you have an opinion or something is bothering you, let it be known. Making someone guess can create unnecessary stress and misunderstanding in relationships.

Compromise

Conflict is part of any relationship at some point. If you and your partner or friend reach an impasse on an issue or situation, it may be necessary to compromise. There are always at least two sides to every issue or situation. If you and your partner cannot reach an agreement, talk about the positives and negatives from your respective positions. Why do you feel something needs to happen and listen to why the other person believes differently? If you still can't reach agreement, then find some middle ground. Of course, sometimes compromise just isn't possible and one person may concede the position. That's fine as long as one person is not always conceding.

Trust

Trust is the foundation for any healthy relationship. It does not matter whether a friend or a partner, establishing trust is key for individuals that are spending time together and sharing their life experiences. Remember, trust takes time to develop and does not happen over night. Some use the "Onion Theory" of communication when describing building relationships. We share or disclose something about ourselves to another and want them to reciprocate. Nothing too deep or personal until we know we can trust them. As we continue to build trust, those layers

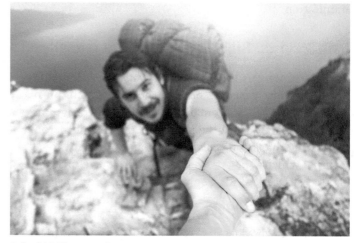

© frankie's/Shutterstock.com

of the onion are peeled back. "Be cautious and do not expose deep feelings and internal ideas too early, but at the same time give others a chance to build trust little by little. In a relationship built upon trust one can discuss issues with confidence and know that these ideas will be kept private if necessary. Another element associated with trust is that in this person's absence one can trust the friend's ideas and actions. A relationship built upon trust can have incredible rewards. With this added element each person is comfortable being themselves and the relationship can develop to a completely different level. When complete trust exists many problems such as jealousy are non-existent in the relationship."[1]

TYPES OF RELATIONSHIPS

"There are many types of relationships, which fulfill many different needs. We begin with our family relationships, parents, siblings, aunts, uncles, and so on. This is the core of our foundation. In today's society we have many different structures that represent 'family.' Some individuals are raised by both of their biological parents, or maybe just one parent, others by grandparents, and others are adopted, to name a few. These initial relationships have a huge impact upon how we relate with others. What type of relationship do you have with your parents? Is it close? What changes would you make in your relationships with family members if you had the chance? Who has impacted you the most in your family? Was this a positive or negative impact? When there is a good foundation of healthy relationships with family members this typically carries over to friendships and intimate relationships."[1]

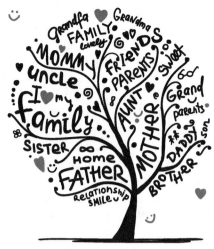

© Kudryashka/Shutterstock.com

Parental Relationship

"Similar to most relationships, the parental and child relationship has many stages in which it progresses through in an individual's life. These different stages can have easy, routine, or difficult transitions. As with most situations, open, honest, and respectful communication is one of the key elements to a successful relationship. It is helpful when both parties recognize the ever-changing dynamics of this very unique relationship. Problems can arise when one party is ready or needs to transition to the next stage, but the other half of the relationship is not ready or does not recognize the need for a change. It only takes one side of the equation to be unaware of the change in the relationship for communication problems to develop."[1]

Making the Transition to College

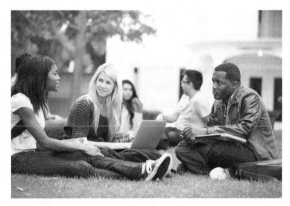

© Monkey Business Images/Shutterstock.com

While there have been many developmental changes along the way, transitioning from high school to college can be a stressful and challenging time for both students and parents. Moving from the position of child or adolescent to young adult in just a few short months after graduation can create uncertainty about roles and responsibilities. The transition from dependence to independence can create difficulties in "deciphering boundaries and expectations. This is especially true if the parents are still paying for living and college expenses. The young adult is experiencing complete independence for the first time in their life. No one is there to tell them when to be home, what and when to eat, who to hang out with, et cetera. This is refreshing and exhilarating to most students, but it can also be a significant unrecognized stressor. It is not uncommon for the new college student to feel anxiety from the new situation, but not immediately recognize its source. Many college freshmen report an internal struggle between their need for complete independence and the relative comfort of the past parent-child bond. This unfamiliar situation can result in a new form of tension when the college student returns home for winter and summer break."[1]

"It is important to remember that both the college student and the parents have gone through significant transitions in their lives. Confusion and conflict can come from two different realities. Some parents assume the past relationships will be unchanged when the student returns home and hold onto the former expectations. It is still the parent's house and their child is coming back. Many parents believe that if they are under their roof, then the parent's rules apply. The college student, however, has become accustomed to complete freedom and typically does not life the increased control in their life. On the other hand, some parents have moved on to the next stage of their lives. They become accustomed to an empty house with fewer obligations to a dependent child in the home. In this case, tension may arise when the student comes home with the expectation, or even the need, for everything to be as it was when they left. Anxiety can be inadvertently increased when the student realizes that their safety net is no longer the same place they remember. It is likely still there, it just feels or looks different.

"One way to bridge this gap of expectations is to recognize that different perspectives exist and have open dialogue with one another about each other's needs and wants prior to visiting or shortly after arriving. Try to keep emotions calm and allow everyone ample time to speak. It may be helpful for everyone involved to write down and prioritize their expectations and needs before having a discussion. By doing this, it can help identify the areas that are less important and thus can be compromised upon and the areas that cannot be compromised. If at all possible, it is best to try and meet in the middle on the majority of the differing expectations. Recognizing that everyone is in a different stage of life than they were just a year or two before can help ease this transition."[1]

Peer Relationships

College provides the opportunity to meet many new people from diverse backgrounds and experiences. It is the opportunity to expand your circle of friends and to adjust to new relationships with peers. Learning how to navigate through the any opportunities with new peers in various settings can be an important part of the college experience.

Roommates

"Another important relationship that is typically new to a college student is that of a roommate. Many people think that if they were best friends in high school, they will make perfect college roommates. There are more complicated dynamics that exist with roommates far beyond that of a traditional friendship. Making this assumption can set one up for possible roommate struggles. In some cases, the prior friendship creates barriers to living together harmoniously. Various hygiene habits, different sleep patterns, and different expectations for residence hall or apartment cleanliness can make the best of friends experience difficulty."[1] What about living with a complete stranger, which often happens during the first semester of school? How do you navigate through those expectations while still getting to know the person?

"In addition to adjusting to a new living arrangement, one must also learn to balance new-found freedom, and the responsibilities that go along with college education demands. It is helpful to recognize these

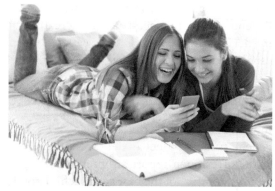

© Stock Rocket/Shutterstock.com

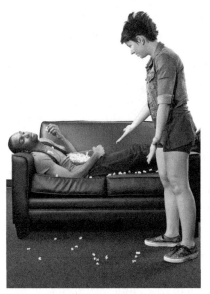

© Rommel Canlas/Shutterstock.com

adjustments and work toward a smooth transition. Any of these changes can cause stress and friction between roommates which can interrupt sleep, study time, and crate uncomfortable living arrangements."[1] As previously discussed in the section on communication, people need to talk with one another. "Interpersonal skills and open communication (talking versus social networking, e.g., texting, Facebook messages, etc.) are critical for conflict resolution should they arise. Though deciding the 'big' things like who gets which room or financial obligations if in an apartment, don't forget to include even the mundane tasks of taking out the garbage and washing the dishes as part of the discussion on responsibilities. All of the little things can add up over time and create conflict if not dealt with constructively. Some of the key elements for successful roommates are setting boundaries and expectations early in the relationship."[1]

Spotlight on . . .

"Within the first month of living together, develop a **roommate agreement**.

At a minimum, address the following questions:

1. How will we split up household duties?
2. What are the expectations of the shared space (e.g., living room)? How late can the TV be on? Is there designated 'study' or 'quiet' time? Does this space need to remain clean or is it okay to leave personal items (clothes, textbooks, dishes) in the shared space?
3. Are overnight guests (same or opposite gender) allowed?
4. Are pets allowed? If so, what type?
5. If you share a bathroom, who will clean it and how often?
6. Are you going to purchase your own food or buy together and share?
7. Are you allowed to borrow each other's clothes? What if something gets stained, torn, or ruined? Are there certain items that are off limits?
8. Other items?

Have each roommate sign the agreement and keep a copy for future reference. At a minimum, review and update the agreement once a year."[1]

"If conflict arises, address your concerns early and in a respectful and calm manner. If the concern is relatively minor, don't make too big of a deal out of it, but be sure to address it if it will bother you if the behavior continues. Remember, your roommate cannot read your mind. A simple reminder (verbal or written) may be all that is needed. If the problem persists or is more serious in nature, decide which method of communication is best based upon the personalities involved.

"Typically, class and work schedules will change from semester to semester and roommate agreements will likely need to be updated or revisited. These revisions and compromises need to benefit all parties. One person should not feel like they are always giving in to the other roommate's requests.

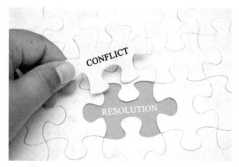

© Kendall Hunt Publishing Company

"When discussions and compromise do not resolve more serious problems, then it is time to consider consulting a third party or a new living arrangement. Most dorms have a resident assistant (RA) to help with these types of situations. Be sure that the RA is able to hear all sides of the situation so that they have a good understanding of what is actually happening. Remember, there are always two sides (or more) to every story. If you do not believe that this type of conflict resolution will be helpful to the problem, then it is probably time to consider moving to a different room or find a new roommate (adapted from http://bailey-shoemaker-richards.suite101.com /dorm-lifeconflict-resolution-strategies-a275040)."[1]

Lesbian, Gay, Bisexual, and Transgender (LGBT)

Adjusting to college is stressful enough for many students, but for some LGBT students, college may be a time when they first publically acknowledge their sexual identity or sexual orientation. While it may be a liberating experience for some, it can also be a stressful situation filled with fear of rejection from peers and/or family. Some may find their campus community is supportive and accepting, only to find that their family back home is not. While this may create some dissonance, it is important for all students to feel loved and accepted. Accessing support services, as needed, and having supportive peers is an important part of the life journey.

Types of Friendships

"There different levels of friendship: casual, close, and intimate. Each of these friendships can be very beneficial. The key ingredients to a successful friendship include steadfastness, honesty, reliability, and trust. Casual friendships are good for camaraderie, someone to see a movie with, or eat lunch. In close friendships, there is typically a greater investment of time and emotional energy. Benefits typically seen with close friendships are those that can stand the test of time. There is a connection beyond the surface and a history with this person. Typically close friends know more about you than a casual acquaintance and can be called upon more easily in a time of need."[1]

"More often people are meeting others and developing relationships over the Internet. This can be very beneficial in that you can express your opinions and thoughts anonymously and receive feedback. It can also help fill a void on a lonely Friday night. Use this method of meeting people with extreme caution and never give your full name, address, or other personal information for the entire world to see. Remember, you never know exactly to whom you are talking through the Internet."[1] Be cautious when using Facebook, Snapchat, or Tinder type apps. Posting personal information on the Internet can make it easy for those wishing to cause harm to have access to you and your information. It is relatively easy for criminals to piece together random information and figure out where you live or what your usual routine is.

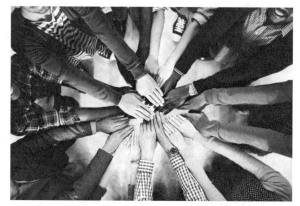

© Rawpixel.com/Shutterstock.com

Dating in the Age of Technology

"Dating is the process of getting to know other people as well as yourself while growing with and from each relationship. Typically a date is stimulated by physical attraction, which can lead to emotional and physical intimacy. One of the outcomes of this process can be finding someone with whom we can happily spend the rest of our life. This process can be incredibly exciting and frustrating all at the same time. Each new relationship exposes one to new and exciting experiences. While dating, your abilities, strengths, and interests can be maximized. As you are learning who you are and what you like, you should prioritize which characteristics are important and which are not. There is so much to be learned during the dating process. How do you relate to your partner in an intimate setting? What expectations do you have for the person with whom you want to live the rest of your life?"[1]

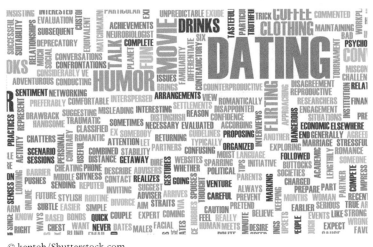

© kentoh/Shutterstock.com

But how do you find someone you want to date? While many people meet through friends or engaging in activities of mutual interest, in today's world there are many other ways to meet people you may be interested in dating. The internet is full

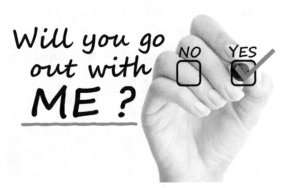

© Ai825/Shutterstock.com

of information on apps you can download to "find your perfect match for dating or hooking up". One study reports that 73% of college students report using Tinder to find a potential date. Other apps like Grindr, Scruff, and Her are designed for the Lesbian, Gay, and Bisexual (LGB) population and a new app has just been released called Thurst for LGBTQ , which includes transsexuals and queer. New apps are springing up regularly like "Friendsy" which offers students matches specific to their own college or university. However, even though there may be many more options to meet people, safety still has to be a consideration when deciding to meet someone from an app.

"As mentioned earlier, after the initial physical attraction, individuals may choose to become emotionally and/or physically intimate. There are many responsibilities that follow when taking this next step. There is more at risk—mentally, physically, and financially. A scenario to contemplate is: How long does it take the average person to decide to buy a car? Or maybe a house? How long will these items be an influence on an individual's life? How long does the average person contemplate sexual intimacy or sexual intercourse? What are some of the repercussions associated with these decisions and how long might they affect an individual's life? It is best to fully consider the consequences before proceeding. Make sure that you and your partner are ready to deal with the consequences."[1] For more information on protection against sexually transmitted infections (STIs) and pregnancy, see Chapter 7.

If you and your partner do decide to become sexually intimate, here is a quick reminder about some sexual activities and their risk for STIs and or pregnancy.

"Rating Safe Sex Activities

Safer sex activities include:

- Dry kissing

- Hugging

- Frottage (rubbing against each other)

- Massage

- Telephone sex

- Tantric sex (extended love-making techniques from the Orient that do not involve penetration)

Riskier activities include:

- Open mouth or deep tongue kissing

- Oral sex (with condoms or dental dams)

- Vaginal intercourse with a condom

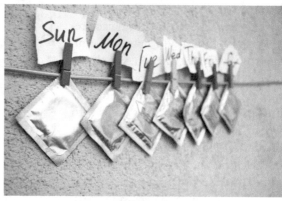

© romantitov/Shutterstock.com

Unsafe sex activities include:

- Vaginal intercourse without a condom (even if pulling out before ejaculation)

- Oral sex without a condom (even if pulling out before ejaculation)

- Oral sex or vaginal penetration without a condom during a woman's period

- Anal sex without a condom"[1]

Date Rape

Though this information is discussed in more detail in another chapter, it bears reminding people that sometimes violence can occur in dating situations. Six in ten acquaintance rapes on college campuses occur in dating relationships (New, 2014). Consent means to agree, approve, or permit. If individuals have not mutually consented to a sexual encounter in an unaltered state of mind, then the situation might be considered sexual assault. If a person is intoxicated or unconscious, they would be deemed to be in an altered state and therefore unable to give consent. Remember:

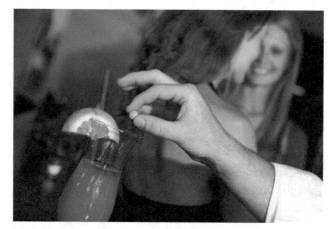

© Monkey Business Images/Shutterstock.com

- "Develop clear lines of communication with the person you are dating.

- "Communicate and clearly understand what each of you want and expect from the date.

- "Do not use psychoactive substances, including alcohol, in dating situations.

- "Do not be coerced into unwanted sexual activities."[1]

"If you are the victim of date rape, remember it is not your fault. Seek medical treatment and counseling immediately. There is information listed at the end of this chapter."[1]

What's Love Got to Do with It?

"There are probably as many different definitions of love as there are people in this world. For this reason, it makes answering 'When is it love?' very difficult. One definition of love is a strong affection or liking for someone or something. Some signs it might be love include: verbally expressing affection, such as saying 'I love you'; feeling happier or more secure when this person is present; putting the other person's interests before yours (in a healthy give and-take relationship); respecting the other person for who they are; and not minding the other person's idiosyncrasies (adapted from Yarber et al., 2009).

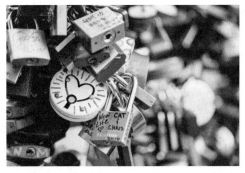

© Grisha Bruev/Shutterstock.com

"Historically, there are several different models of love. Two common ones are described below. The first is Sternberg's (1988) love triangle which includes three components: passion, intimacy, and commitment. Passion tends to occur at the beginning of relationships, peaks relatively quickly, and then reduces to a stable level. Passion generates romance, physical attraction, and sometimes intercourse. Intimacy is the feeling of closeness that exists between two people. Intimacy tends to peak slower than passion and then gradually reduces to a lower level. This level typically changes throughout a relationship. Commitment is the decision to further a loving relationship with another individual. The level of commitment typically rises slowly in the beginning, speeds up, and then gradually levels off. Sternberg describes the various types of love as a composition of different combinations of these three components. These various kinds of love change over time as the relationship matures."[1]

"John Lee (1973) describes six styles of loving:

EROS—passionate love

- Become sexually involved quickly
- Intense focus on partner and shares all of him/herself
- Quick to develop, quick to end

LUDUS—game-playing love

- Love and sex are seen only as fun, an activity, a diversion
- Move from partner to partner and often have several at a time
- Passion for the game, not the partner

STORGE—friendship love

- Long-term commitment
- Strong and secure, places less emphasis on passion

MANIA—obsessive love

- Turbulent and ambivalent
- Intense mental preoccupation, but little satisfaction
- Likely to be possessive and jealous

PRAGMA—realistic love

- Rational and practical
- Often for evolutionary and economic purposes
- Intense feelings may develop once a partner is chosen

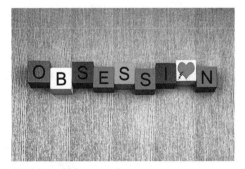

© Ed Samuel/Shutterstock.com

AGAPE—altruistic love

- Generous, unselfish giving of oneself
- Less emphasis on passion and sexuality"[1]

Taming the Green-Eyed Monster

While some people like to think jealousy is a sign of caring or love, actually "jealousy typically comes from a lack of self-esteem and/or lack of confidence. Jealousy will undermine an otherwise healthy relationship and drive potential partners away."[1] Attempting to test your partner to see if they will get jealous shows your insecurity and can damage the relationship.

If you and your partner find that jealousy is creeping in to your relationship, find a time to talk about what's going on and don't allow it to fester. Make sure you both are on the same page and there are not misunderstandings. Also remember that not only can jealousy be from insecurity, but it can also come from one individual wanting to control another. That may be a sign of an unhealthy relationship developing.

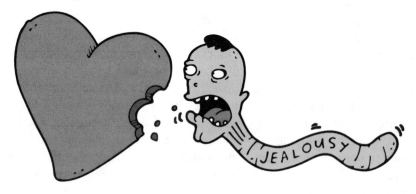

© tetsuu/Shutterstock.com

Every day may not be all sunshine and happiness in most relationships. You will disagree and probably argue from time to time but that is absolutely normal. Problems arise when you find you are disagreeing more than agreeing or when the arguments escalate because you don't actually know how to argue! The most common things couples argue about are listed below. These things, while perhaps changing in order, seem to remain constant over time.

Did you know . . .

"The most common topics couples argue about include:

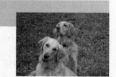

Courtesy of Shelley Hamill

- When to see each other
- How often to see each other
- Flirting with other people
- Being late
- Forgetting important dates (birthdays and anniversaries)
- Being faithful
- Who spends how much money and on what
- How you spend time (watching too much TV and going out with friends)
- The amount or type of sex you have
- Family (when and whom to visit) (Kuriansky, 2003)"[1]

When couples do find themselves to have a conflict, the following rules are helpful to go by. Remember, once you say something, you cannot take it back. Though a person may forgive you, it can be very difficult to forget.

Spotlight on . . .

"Rules for Arguing Fairly
(adapted from Godek, 1997)

1. Stay with the initial issue, do not bring up everything that is bothering you.
2. Stay in the present, do not bring up past problems and issues.
3. Say what you feel.
4. Do not generalize. ('You always . . .' You are just like your mother . . .)
5. Do not threaten (verbally or physically).
6. Absolutely, no violence. (Men: Not even the slightest touch. Women: This includes slapping his face.)
7. State your needs as specific requests for different behavior.
8. Work toward a solution. Do not add fuel to the fire."[1]

LOVING RELATIONSHIPS

"One definition of love is a passionate affection of one person for another. Another definition is 'The emotion evoked when two souls resonate or fit together naturally. It is close, but still not perfect' (Godek, 1997). There is no one exact definition that sums up all of the meanings of the word love. It is very different and personal to each individual. Different types of love exist with regard to partners, parents, children, and friends. Within a loving relationship there are five important elements:"[1]

1. Honesty
2. Loyalty
3. Thoughtfulness
4. Sharing
5. Sacrifice

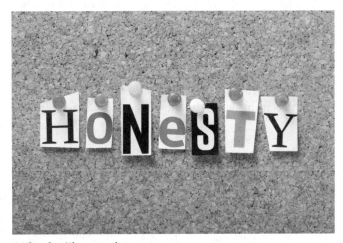

© Thinglass/Shutterstock.com

"Honesty is the foundation that relationships are formed upon. Without this one cannot deepen or enrich a relationship further. Loyalty is also incredibly important. Your partner must always realize where your loyalty lies regardless if they are present. This loyalty also builds the foundation to further enhance your relationship. Thoughtfulness is an expression of how you feel about the other person. These actions should indicate to your partner how important they are to you. Another fulfilling element of a loving relationship includes sharing. This includes sharing possessions as well as experiences. Most experiences are enhanced if accompanied by someone you love. This could include a trip, dinner, sporting activity, and the menial tasks that go along with life. Finally sacrifice, loving someone enough to do without so they may have what they desire. This is sacrificing without being a martyr, because it is freely given without strings attached."[1]

Is Marriage in the Future?

There was a time when this question only pertained to one segment of society. Now that laws have changed, those of legal age, no matter their sexual orientation, may look at their intimate relationships with the idea of marriage in mind. "There are many things to consider when contemplating marriage. Is this the person with whom you truly want to spend the rest of your life? Are we compatible? Do we have similar values? These are just a few of the questions that should be asked."[1]

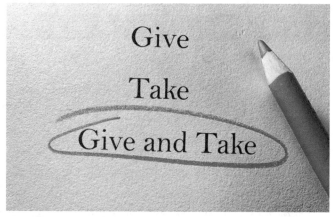

© zimmytws/Shutterstock.com

"The question of compatibility is one that takes time to answer. Some characteristics that comprise compatibility include similar interests, ways of doing things, as well as the ability to compromise when you do not see 'eye to eye.' Do you both like to participate in outdoor or indoor activities? Are your activity levels similar? Do you need structure to your life or is spontaneity more your style? Are you both outgoing or do you complement each other with some differences? What are your long-term goals and are they similar to your partner's? Do you have similar views on finances? Are you thrifty or extravagant? Do both of you want children? This is not to say that you and your ideal partner have to be identical. In fact, it is helpful to have some differences (within reason) to help complement the other's weaknesses. For example, if one of you is somewhat over reactive and the other one is more grounded, then you will probably balance one another out. Problems arise when there are so many differences that you cannot relate or the differences simply irritate one another. With this said, it is very helpful to have similar interests and ways of doing things that can carry past the initial infatuation stage.

"Values are defined as beliefs or standards. Are your values similar? For example, how you treat other people, volunteer work, religion, and child rearing. What do you hold very dear to your heart? Are there any specific lines that you would never cross and expect the same out of a life-long partner? Some examples include drug use, infidelity, or lying. What are your views of marriage? What does this word mean to you, and is it similar to the meaning your partner places on it?"[1]

Unhealthy Relationships

"It takes work to have a healthy relationship; they don't just happen. Sometimes there is a process of growing through unhealthy relationships in order to find the right one for you. Some signs of an unhealthy relationship include (Kuriansky, 2002):

- You feel insecure and weak around each other.
- You suffer from low self-esteem as a result of what happens between you.
- You are dishonest with each other.
- You spend more time feeling hurt than feeling good about how you treat each other.

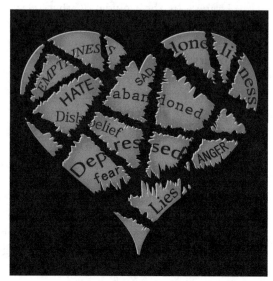

© Athanasia Nomikou/Shutterstock.com

- You find yourself complaining to others about your relationship.
- You are unable to talk about your feelings or problems with your partner, much less solve them.
- You are unable to resolve your differences together.
- You become unenthusiastic about life because of what goes on between you.
- Your trust is irrevocably broken.
- Seemingly small things erode your relationship, like trickling water that wears away at a rock over time.
- Priorities other than each other constantly present themselves.
- What goes on between you interferes with other aspects of your life."[1]

If you or your partner decide that the relationship is not in the best interests of both of you, it may be time to consider ending your time together.

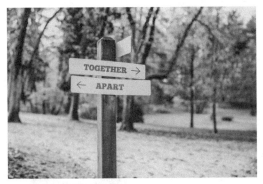

© Gajus/Shutterstock.com

Ending a Relationship

"In most cases the first individual you date will not be the person you remain with for the rest of your life. There are many reasons that exist to end a relationship. Some of these include initial misperceptions, changes in life routes, surfacing unattractive behaviors, infidelity, or even boredom. Typically only one individual sees a need for the change in the relationship, which makes ending a relationship a difficult situation."[1]

If you are the one to end a relationship always try to be as tactful as possible. Remember that at one point you were interested enough in this person to pursue a relationship. Be open and honest about the reason(s) you wish to end the relationship. Sending a text message or posting on Facebook that you are no longer in a relationship is NOT the way to let someone know you are no longer interested in being involved. It may be uncomfortable to tell someone face to face but think how you would feel if it happened to you.

If you are the one being told the relationship is over, listen carefully to what the person is saying and do not respond desperately or defensively. If this truly is the end of this relationship, realize and accept that there will be a better match for you at some point in the future.

Abusive Relationships

To be very clear, NO ONE should have to stay in an abusive relationship. Abuse may be subtle at first whether physical or emotional, but these will almost always escalate to dangerous episodes. When signs of abusive behavior appear, it is definitely time to get out of the relationship. Abuse can happen between partners of any sex, sexual orientation, or gender identity and should not be stereotyped as only occurring in certain types of relationships. One in five students report they have experienced domestic violence with a current partner while more than 30% of students say they have experienced domestic violence with a previous partner (New, 2014).

"Sometimes it is incredibly hard for the abused partner to leave because their self-esteem is so low. They honestly feel the only person that would 'put up' with them is their partner, so they feel trapped. The abusing partner typically isolates their partner from friends and family over an extended period of time. This evolves into a very controlling and abusive relationship. The abuser may threaten to harm the

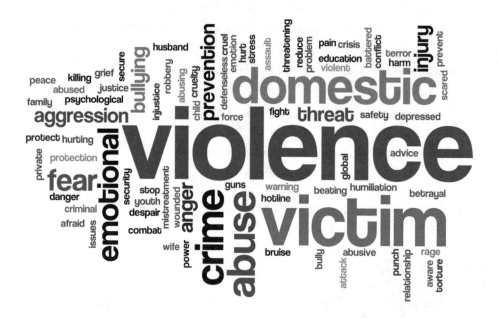

© ibreakstock/Shutterstock.com

partner, partner's family or even the family pet if they try to leave. Contact campus police to get assistance. Access counseling services for support. If this is the case, do not let your partner know you are thinking about leaving. Wait until you know your partner will be gone for an extended period of time and call someone whom your partner does not know for help.

"In some instances restraining orders are necessary to keep an individual from stalking or harassing. Be very careful in these situations because they can and have become life threatening. Remember that if you are in an abusive relationship more likely than not this individual will continue to abuse you until the relationship is over. Also, the abuse will typically escalate over time."[1]

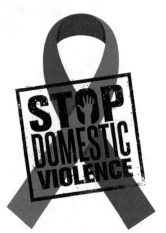

© wow.subtropica/Shutterstock
.com

Are you a wise consumer?

What are you doing to improve your communication skills? Are you really paying attention? Are you participating in your relationships or are you letting others "do all the work"? When you go out with friends in partying situations, do you look out for each other? Are you taking care of you? All of these things matter and you are an active participant.

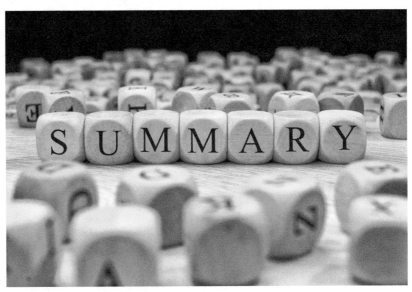

© Fabrik Bilder/Shutterstock.com

Developing and maintaining healthy relationships is a part of developing as well-rounded individuals. Self-confidence and recognizing qualities within ourselves that support our abilities to engage with others in healthy ways is important. Learning the skills necessary for good communication as well as the ability to stand up for ourselves when necessary are all part of our growth. Your campus has many resources to assist students navigate through the challenges of college life. Please make sure to access those services if and when you ever need them.

NOTES

Personal Reflections . . . so, what have you learned?

1. Answer questions 1–3 under the relationship survey at the beginning of your chapter. Answer these based on what you want not necessarily what you may currently have in a partner.

2. What would you say are your own top 10 qualities? Why do you think these are you best qualities and how will you protect the in a relationship?

3. Of the top 10 steps for being an effective listener, which three do you do well and which three might you need to work on?

4. What advice would you give to incoming freshman regarding their relationships with the following during their transition to college?
   a. Parents and siblings
   b. Living with other students (roommates)

5. What advice would you give to incoming freshman regarding their expectations with dating and intimate relationships in college?

6. Now that you have given such great advice, what do you think someone 5–10 years older than you would give you about your journey once you graduate?

NOTES

RESOURCES ON CAMPUS FOR YOU!

Victims Assistance

Find out if your institution offers any victims assistance services to survivors of sexual assault, domestic violence, dating violence, and stalking on campus. Be sure to take advantage of the educational programs to prevent these crimes from occurring.

In case of an emergency, please call your Campus Police, the local police, or the local rape crisis center in your area.

Health and Counseling Services

Believe in the dignity, integrity, growth potential, and innate worth of the individual, and offer services to foster whole-person health through prevention, education, assessment, treatment, and advocacy.

REFERENCES

Cherry K. (2015) about health. *Left brain vs right brain.* Retrieved 2016 from http://psychology.about.com /od/cognitivepsychology/a/left-brain-right-brain.htm.

dysavil (2010). *Group projects: A conflict resolution guide for students.* Retrieved 2016 from www.scribd.com /doc/26177419/Group-Projects-a-Conflict-Resolution-GuideFor

Floyd, P.A., Mimms, S. E., & Yelding-Howards, C. (2008). *Personal health: Perspectives and lifestyles* (4th ed). Belmont, Calif: Thomson Wadsworth.

Godek, G. (1997). *Love: The course they forgot to teach you in school.* Naperville, IL: Casablanca Press.

Schilling, D. (2012). 10 steps to effective listening. Retrieved 2016 http://www.forbes.com/sites /womensmedia/2012/11/09/10-steps-to-effective-listening/#1d4f230f26fb.

Kluger J. (2012) We never talk any more: the problem with text messaging. Retrieved 2016 from http://www.cnn.com/2012/08/31/tech/mobile/problem-text-messaging-oms/index.html

Kuriansky, J. (2002). *The complete idiot's guide to a healthy relationship* (2nd ed). Indianapolis, IN: Alpha

Kuriansky, J. (2003). *The complete idiot's guide to dating* (3rd ed). Indianapolis, IN: Alpha Books.

Lee, J. A. (1973). *Colours of love: an exploration of the ways of loving.* Toronto: New Press.

New, J. (2014). *Deadly dating violence.* Retrieved 2016 from https://www.insidehighered.com /news/2014/12/02/domestic-abuse-prevalent-sexual-assault-college-campuses.

Oxford Dictionaries (2016). *Communication.* Retrieved 2016 from http://www.oxforddictionaries.com /definition/english/communication

Smith, A. (2015). *U.S. Smartphone use in 2015.* Retrieved 2016 from http://www.pewinternet .org/2015/04/01/us-smartphone-use-in-2015/

Sternberg, R. J. (1998). *The triangle of love: Intimacy, passion, commitment.* New York: Basic Books.

Yarber, W., Sayad, B., & Strong, B. (2010). *Human sexuality: Diversity in contemporary America* (7th ed). McGraw-Hill.

CREDITS

NOTES

Chapter 7 +———————————

Sexual Health

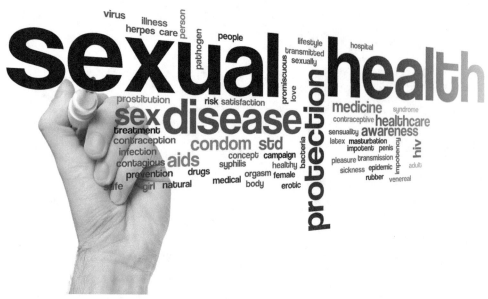

© ibreakstock/Shutterstock.com

OBJECTIVES:

"Students will be able to:

- "Identify structures of the female and male sexual anatomy
- "Describe the stages of the menstrual cycle and pregnancy."[1]
- Identify the advantages and disadvantages of various methods of contraception.
- List the most common sexually transmitted infections, their pathogens, symptoms, methods of transmission, treatment, and whether or not there is a cure.
- List the methods for the transmission of the HIV virus.
- Explain what makes some sexual behaviors high risk.
- "Discuss the influence the media have on attitudes and beliefs about relationships and sexuality." [1]

"The purpose of this chapter is to familiarize students with the female and male anatomy."[1] Methods of contraception, their effectiveness, and advantages and disadvantages for each will be discussed. "Additional material will be presented detailing various sexually transmitted infections (STIs), the health risks associated with contraction of STIs, and various preventative measures and techniques in sexually transmitted infections and pregnancy."[1]

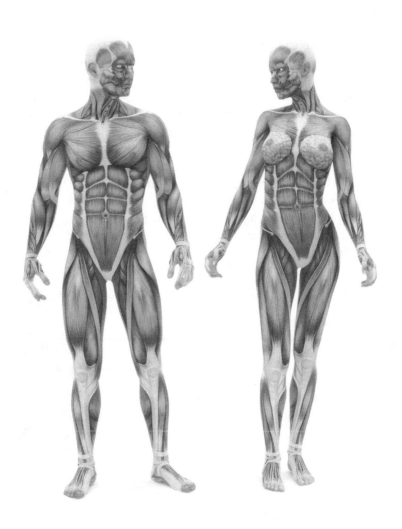

© Digital Storm/Shutterstock.com

ANATOMY

Female Sexual Anatomy

"The female anatomy consists of multiple integral parts both externally and internally (see Figure 7.1 a & b). The **vulva** includes visible external genitalia. The **mons pubis** is the soft fatty tissue covering the pubic symphysis (joint of the pubic bones). This area is covered with pubic hair that begins growing during puberty. The **labia majora** include two longitudinal folds of skin that extend on both sides of the vulva and serve as protection for the inner parts of the vulva. The **labia minora** are the delicate inner folds of skin that enclose the urethral opening and the vagina. These skin flaps, which contain sweat and oil glands, extensive blood vessels, and nerve endings, are hairless and sensitive to touch. When sexually stimulated, the labia minora swell and darken. The **clitoris** is usually the most sensitive part of the female genitalia and consists of erectile tissue, which becomes engorged with blood, resulting in swelling during sexual arousal that enables it to double in size. The **clitoral hood** consists of inner lips, which join to form a soft fold of skin, or hood, covering and connecting to the clitoris. The **urethra** is approximately 2.5 centimeters below the clitoris and functions as the opening for urine to be excreted from the bladder. Because the urethra is located close to the vaginal opening, some irritation may result from vigorous or prolonged sexual activity. The most common problem associated with this is the development of urinary tract infections. The **vagina** is located between the urethral opening and the anus. The **hymen** is the small membrane around the vaginal opening that is believed to tear during initial intercourse, tampon use, while riding a horse, or other various types of athletic activities. The only function of the hymen is to protect the vaginal tissues early in life. The **perineum** is the smooth skin located between the labia minora and the anus. During childbirth this area may tear or be cut (episiotomy) as the newborn passes out of the vagina. The anal canal is located just behind the perineum and allows for elimination of solid waste. The **anal canal** is approximately an inch long with two sphincter muscles, which open and close like valves."[1]

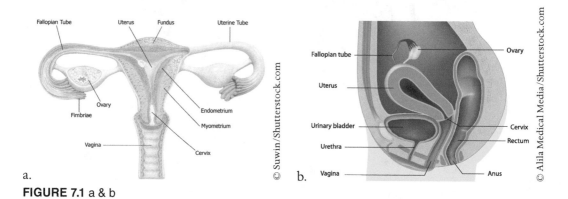

a.   b.

© Suwin/Shutterstock.com   © Alila Medical Media/Shutterstock.com

FIGURE 7.1 a & b

"Internally, just past the vagina, is the cervix, which connects the vagina and the uterus. The uterus is the hollow, pear-shaped muscular organ about the size of a fist when a female is not pregnant. This is the organ in which the fetus develops during pregnancy. The upper expanded portion is referred to as the fundus and the lower constricted part is the cervix. On each side of the uterus are **fallopian tubes**, which are quite narrow and approximately four inches in length. Because of the narrow passageway within these tubes, infection and scarring may cause fertility problems. Most women have a right and a left fallopian tube. These tubes extend from the ovaries to the uterus and transport mature ovum. Fertilization usually takes place within the fallopian tubes. The opening between the fallopian tube and the uterus is only about as wide as a needle. On each end of the fallopian tubes are the **ovaries**, where eggs are produced and released usually once a month. Each ovary is about the size of a large olive. At birth, a female's ovaries contain 40,000 to 400,000 immature ova, of which approximately 450 will mature and be released during the reproductive years. The ovaries also produce the hormones estrogen and progesterone, both of which help regulate the menstrual cycle (Crooks and Baur, 2009)."[1]

"**The female *sexual response* consists of four phases:**

1. Excitement:
   Vaginal lubrication begins and the vagina, clitoris, labia majora and minora fill with blood. The nipples swell, and there is increased tension in many voluntary muscles.

2. Plateau:
   The vaginal opening usually decreases in diameter due to swelling, the uterus usually increases in size, and the labia majora and minora become more swollen and engorged.

3. Orgasm:
   The muscles of the vaginal wall undergo rhythmic contractions. The number of contractions may range from three to as many as twelve. Involuntary contraction of other muscles may take place as well.

4. Resolution:
   Blood rapidly returns to the rest of the body from the vagina, clitoris, labia majora, and minora, resulting in reduced swelling. At this time the breasts also return to their original size."[1]

Menstrual Cycle

"The menstrual cycle typically lasts twenty-eight days, with a range of twenty-five to forty days. Day one of the cycle is the first day of menstruation. The cycle ends with the next menstruation (See Figure 7.2) The follicular phase begins with menstruation and terminates when ovulation occurs. The follicular phase can be very unpredictable (typically fourteen days, but can be as little as ten or as long as twenty-five). Stress, illness, and many other factors can change when a female ovulates. This can cause problems when individuals are trying to control whether they become pregnant or not. The length of the luteal phase is much more predictable (typically thirteen to fifteen days), beginning with ovulation and ending when the next menstrual cycle begins. Premenstrual syndrome (PMS) can oc-

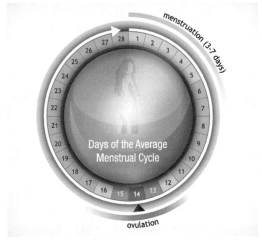

© Janos Levente/Shutterstock.com

Figure 7.2

cur from one to ten days before a woman's period. This syndrome can consist of feeling bloated, diarrhea, nausea, backache, and/or cramping. Behaviors that can help ease PMS symptoms include:

- decrease salt and sugar intake,
- do not consume caffeine, and
- exercise regularly."[1]

Ovarian Cycle

"During the ovarian cycle immature eggs (follicles) are maturing and moving toward the surface of the ovary. The follicle and the ovarian surface open and allow the egg to float out. At the time of ovulation some women may feel a twinge or pain in the lower abdomen or back. After ovulation, the egg is swept into a fallopian tube (where fertilization typically occurs) by fimbriae and the cilia (tiny hairs) and travels to the uterus. If the egg is not fertilized, it simply disintegrates or flows out with vaginal secretions, usually before menstruation. If the egg is fertilized, it will attach itself to the endometrium (internal lining of the uterus) in order to develop."[1]

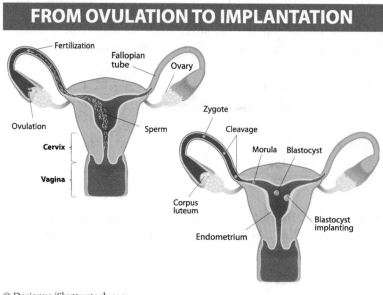

© Designua/Shutterstock.com

Endometrial Cycle

"The endometrial cycle consists of three phases:

1. Menstrual

2. Proliferative

3. Progestational (secretory).

"The menstrual phase lasts approximately four to seven days, when the lining of the uterus is sloughed off and flows out of the uterus through the vagina, along with blood and other vaginal secretions. The proliferative phase lasts from the completion of the menstrual phase until a day or two after ovulation. During this time the endometrium is regenerating the layer that was sloughed off with new epithelial cells. During the progestational phase the endometrium becomes twice as thick as it did during the proliferative phase. It develops a cushion-like surface, thereby possessing the ability to nourish an implanted fertilized ovum. During the end of the progestational phase, if fertilization has not occurred, the endometrium begins to deteriorate. These phases repeat throughout the reproductive years until fertilization or menopause occurs."[1]

Male Sexual Anatomy

"The external male sexual structures include the penis and scrotum. The **penis** is an organ through which semen and urine pass, and is structured into three main sections: the root, the shaft, and the glans penis (see Figure 7.3 a & b). The root attaches the penis within the pelvic cavity at the base, while the shaft, or the tube-shaped body of the penis, hangs freely. The **glans penis** is covered by a loose portion of tissue called the **foreskin**, which may be removed during a surgery known as circumcision. A penis without foreskin is circumcised, while one with the foreskin intact is uncircumcised. Uncircumcised men should gently pull the foreskin back when they bathe to wash the foreskin and tip of the penis. At the base of the glans is a rim known as the corona. On the underside is a triangular area of highly sensitive skin called the frenulum, which attaches the glans to the foreskin. The glans penis is the soft, fleshy, enlarged tissue at the end of the shaft, with the urethral opening at the tip. The **scrotum** is the pouch of skin, which hangs from the root of the penis and holds the two testicles. Covered sparsely with hair, the scrotum is divided in the middle by a ridge of skin, showing the separation of the testes. The surface changes of the scrotum help maintain a moderately constant temperature within the testes (93 degrees Fahrenheit), which is important for maintaining good sperm production (Crooks and Baur, 2009).[1]

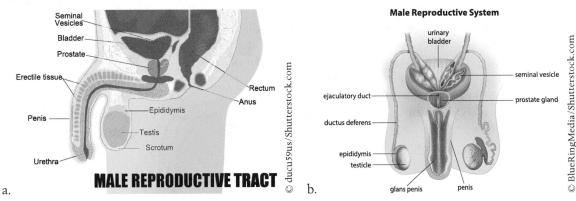

Figure 7.3 a & b

"The male internal sexual structures include the testes, epididymis, vas deferens, seminal vesicles, and prostate and Cowper's glands. The **testes** are the reproductive ball-shaped glands inside the scrotum, which are also referred to as testicles. Sperm and hormone production are the two main functions of the testes (Crooks and Baur, 2007). Sperm are formed constantly, beginning during puberty, inside the highly coiled thin tubes called seminiferous tubules within each testis. Between the seminiferous tubules are cells that produce sex hormones. One such important sex hormone is testosterone, which stimulates the production of sperm. On top of each testis is another tightly coiled tube, the **epididymis**, where nearly mature sperm complete the maturation process (Crooks and Baur, 2009). Mature sperm are stored in the epididymis until they are released during ejaculation. The **vas deferens** is a long tube through which sperm travel during ejaculation. The epididymis is connected to the seminal vesicle via the vas deferens, which is responsible for contracting and pushing the sperm to the seminal vesicle. Located beneath the bladder are the two small seminal vesicles, which secrete a fluid that provides nourishment as well as an environment conducive to sperm mobility. After the sperm have combined with the seminal fluid, they reach the prostate where another substance is added. A thin, milky fluid is produced by the prostate and secreted into the urethra during the time of emission of semen, which enhances the swimming environment for the sperm (Crooks and Baur, 2009). Below the prostate and attached to the urethra are the two pea-sized **Cowper's glands**, responsible for depositing a lubricating fluid for sperm and a coating for the urethra. If there are sperm in the urethra from a previous ejaculation, they will mix with the Cowper's fluid and become a pre-ejaculate lubricant fluid. Ejaculation occurs at peak sexual excitement when the prostate muscle opens and sends the seminal fluid to the urethra where it is then forced out through the urethral opening, forming semen."[1]

"The shaft of the penis can change dramatically during sexual arousal."[1] "The average penis is approximately 3 to 4 inches when flaccid (soft). One study noted that , when erect, the average length among subjects was found to be 6.02 inches, with a variation from 3.4 to 9.44 inches. Average penis girth (circumference) at erection was found to be 4.96 inches with a variation from 2.24 to 7.4 inches (Harding

& Golombok, 2002). Most of the variation in penis size occurs during erection. Erection has been called "the great equalizer" because smaller penises seem to grow more during erection than larger ones, so the extremes tend to equalize when erect."[5]

> ### Did you know . . .
>
>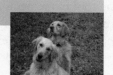
>
> Courtesy of Shelley Hamill
>
> According to Dr. Laura Burman:
>
> - Sperm can live in a woman's body for up to five days after intercourse!
> - There are many ingredients in semen, and its makeup is similar for every man. Some of the components are vitamin C, calcium, chlorine, cholesterol, citric acid, creatine, fructose, lactic acid, magnesium, nitrogen, phosphorus, potassium, sodium, vitamin B12, and zinc.
> - An average human ejaculate contains about 180 million sperm (66 million/ml), but some ejaculates contain as many as 400 million sperm
> - A man can actually improve the taste of his sperm by avoiding dairy, coffee, and potent herbs like onions and garlic. He can make his sperm taste sweeter by enjoying fruits and by drinking plenty of water.

"During sexual excitement, tiny muscles inside the shaft tissue called corpus spongiosum and corpus cavernosa relax and open, allowing inflow of blood. As these tissues fill with blood, the penis becomes longer, thicker, and less flexible, resulting in an erection. Although sexual sensitivity is unique among individuals, the glans penis is particularly important in sexual arousal due to its high concentration of nerve endings. When a man is either sexually aroused or cold, the testes are pulled close to the body (Crooks and Baur, 2009)."[1]

SEXUAL ORIENTATION

According to the American Psychological Association (APA), sexual orientation refers to an enduring pattern of emotional, romantic and/or sexual attractions to men, women or both sexes. Sexual orientation also refers to a person's sense of identity based on those attractions, related behaviors and membership in a community of others who share those attractions. Research over several decades has demonstrated that sexual orientation ranges along a continuum, from exclusive attraction to the other sex to exclusive attraction to the same sex. However, sexual orientation is usually discussed in terms of three categories: heterosexual (having emotional, romantic or sexual attractions to members of the other sex), gay/lesbian (having emotional, romantic or sexual attractions to members of one's own sex) and bisexual (having emotional, romantic or sexual attractions to both men and women). This range of behaviors and attractions has been described in various cultures and nations throughout the world. Many cultures use identity labels to describe people who express these attractions. In the United States the most frequent labels are lesbians (women attracted to women), gay men (men attracted to men), and bisexual people (men or women attracted to both sexes). However, some people may use different labels or none at all.

"Sexual orientation is distinct from other components of sex and gender, including biological sex (the anatomical, physiological and genetic characteristics associated with being male or female), gender identity (the psychological sense of being male or female)* and social gender role (the cultural norms that define feminine and masculine behavior).

"Alfred Kinsey, a sex researcher in the mid-1900s, developed a 7-point continuum representing sexual orientation (See Figure 7.4). He used this scale to study the sexual behaviors and preferences of the American population. The scale ranges from 0 to 6, with 0 representing exclusive heterosexual behavior, 3 representing bisexual behavior, and 6 representing exclusive homosexual behavior. This scale recognizes that many individuals do not fit solely into one of the three previously described sexual orientations."[1]

0	1	2	3	4	5	6
Exclusive heterosexual experience	Heterosexual with incidental homosexual experience	Heterosexual with substantial homosexual experience	Equal heterosexual and homosexual experience	Homosexual with incidental heterosexual experience	Homosexual with substantial heterosexual experience	Exclusively homosexual experience

Figure 7.4 Kinsey Scale of Sexual Behavior Kinsey believed that come people did not fit into strict same gender opposite-gender sexual behavior. His scale of sexual behavior reflects this belief.

There is no consensus among scientists about the exact reasons that an individual develops a heterosexual, bisexual, gay or lesbian orientation. Although much research has examined the possible genetic, hormonal, developmental, social and cultural influences on sexual orientation, no findings have emerged that permit scientists to conclude that sexual orientation is determined by any particular factor or factors. Many think that nature and nurture both play complex roles; most people experience little or no sense of choice about their sexual orientation (APA).

Lesbian, gay and bisexual people in the United States encounter extensive prejudice, discrimination and violence because of their sexual orientation. Intense prejudice against lesbians, gay men, and bisexual people was widespread throughout much of the 20th century. Public opinion studies over the 1970s, 1980s and 1990s routinely showed that, among large segments of the public, lesbian, gay and bisexual people were the target of strongly held negative attitudes. More recently, public opinion has increasingly opposed sexual orientation discrimination, but expressions of hostility toward lesbians and gay men remain common in contemporary American society. Prejudice against bisexuals appears to exist at comparable levels. In fact, bisexual individuals may face discrimination from some lesbian and gay people as well as from heterosexual people.

Sexual orientation discrimination takes many forms. Severe antigay prejudice is reflected in the high rate of harassment and violence directed toward lesbian, gay and bisexual individuals in American society. Numerous surveys indicate that verbal harassment and abuse are nearly universal experiences among lesbian, gay and bisexual people. Also, discrimination against lesbian, gay, and bisexual people in employment and housing appears to remain widespread (APA).

READINESS FOR SEXUAL ACTIVITY

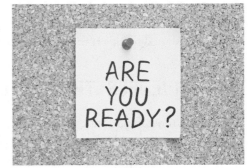

© Ivelin Radkov/Shutterstock.com

"Deciding whether you are ready for sexual activity is a very important and personal decision. It is a decision that has numerous physical, spiritual, and emotional implications and should not be taken lightly. Typically individuals have very different timelines at which they feel comfortable participating in different types of sexual activity. Different sexual activities include: vaginal/penal, anal/penal, oral/vaginal, or oral/penal intercourse. Some individuals consider themselves 'virgins' if they have not had vaginal/penal intercourse, but have participated in other sexual activities. It is important to realize there are very real risks associated with all forms of sexual activity, which include and are not limited to sexually transmitted infections (STIs). It is also important that you decide what you would like out of a relationship and when you feel comfortable with beginning a specific sexual activity. Some individuals view sexual activity as a very casual event and others wait until they are married to participate in any sexual activity.

Sexually transmitted infections do not discriminate based on your sexual orientation. If they are present, they can be spread from mucus membrane to mucus membrane based on the sexual activity partners decide to participate in. Gay, straight, bisexual or lesbian, anyone is at risk if you do not know the status of your partner and you do not use a barrier method to prevent transmission.

"One of the most important tools to use with your partner is communication. An individual must be able to talk openly and honestly to their prospective sexual partner about their wishes and beliefs on this subject. Talking can bring you closer because it develops a sense of trust. It can also help you learn more about your partner and remind both of you about the risks of sexual activity.

"If you decide the time is right to become sexually active, you should stay informed about and decide which contraception method and STI protection makes sense for you and your partner. Think about how an unplanned pregnancy, STI, or a break-up would affect you and your long-term plans. Learn the difference between "YES" and "NO." If you hear "no," "maybe," or if you hear nothing, STOP and talk to your partner. Always respect and adhere to what a person is saying. Make sure any "yes" is absolute and certain. Do not use mind-altering substances such as drugs and alcohol (including beer). These substances decrease your decision-making ability."[1]

Contraception

"Many people use the terms birth control, contraception, and family planning interchangeably. Although the terms are similar because they refer to strategies for preventing unintended pregnancy, they are vastly different in terms of their nature and scope.

"**Family planning** implies the desire to have children at some point in time. Planning a family involves postponing childbearing until it is desired, spacing subsequent births and avoiding pregnancy at other times. Family planning may also include all the reproductive technologies available to facilitate a pregnancy as well as adoption. Family planning does not refer to specific methods or techniques to avoid unintended pregnancy.

"**Contraception** refers to all methods designed to prevent conception or fertilization. Contraceptive methods work by preventing the sperm and egg from uniting to cause fertilization. These methods include noninsertive sexual activity, barrier methods, hormonal contraception, withdrawal, fertility awareness, and sterilization. How effective these methods are ranges from 'not very' to 'almost complete' at the other end of the spectrum.

"**Birth control** is a broad term encompassing all methods designed to prevent pregnancy and birth. It includes all contraceptive methods, what may be considered post conceptive methods, and abortion, which is designed to interrupt an established pregnancy."[5]

EFFECTIVENESS: THEORETICAL AND ACTUAL USE

"One of the most important questions regarding any method of fertility control is 'How effective is it?' Effectiveness is measured in two ways: theoretical use and actual use.

"The **theoretical effectiveness** (also called perfect use) of any fertility control method estimates how it should work if it is used consistently and correctly. It is the ideal effectiveness of the method, determined through laboratory research and experimental studies. Theoretical effectiveness research designs attempt to control for as many variables as possible that may interfere with correct and consistent use. Failure of the method accounts for most of the ineffectiveness. Theoretical effectiveness is the lowest expected percentage of women who will get pregnant while using the method.

"The actual-use effectiveness (also called typical use) of any fertility control method is how it actually works when real people use it under normal circumstances. This is observed effectiveness of the method, determined by following a group of actual users for 1 year to see how many get pregnant (Blonna & Carter, 2013)."[5]

Of course, not everyone engaging in sexual behavior is concerned about pregnancy. Protection from sexually transmitted infections has to also be a part of the consideration when choosing a contraceptive method.

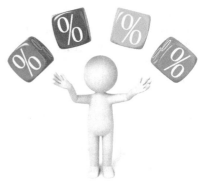

© Jane0606/Shutterstock.com

Pregnancy

"Pregnancy is usually divided into three trimesters, each of which lasts approximately three months or thirteen weeks. Typically, fertilization occurs twelve to eighteen days after the beginning of the menstrual cycle. There are many variables that can impact the timing of fertilization, including irregular periods, extreme exercise, illness, stress, a missed contraceptive pill, as well as many other factors. As soon as fertilization occurs, the cells begin to divide and multiply. The fertilized egg implants in the uterus after

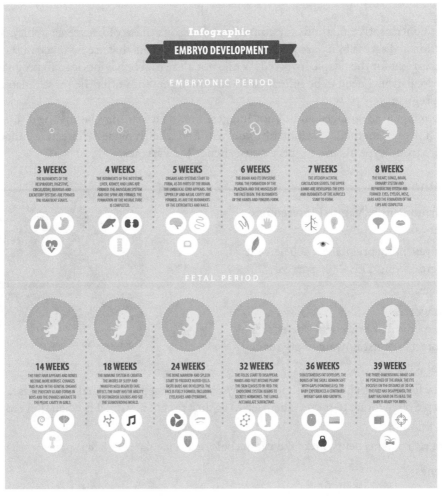

© twins_nika/Shutterstock.com

Figure 7.5

approximately one week after fertilization. For most women the first sign(s) of pregnancy include a missed period, nausea, or excessive fatigue. Home pregnancy kits are 97 to 99 percent accurate if used correctly. These tests can detect human chorionic gonadotropin (HCG) within two to three weeks of fertilization. HCG is the hormone secreted by the placenta to help sustain the pregnancy for the first trimester. During the second and third trimesters the HCG levels decrease and the levels of estrogen and progesterone are sufficient to sustain the pregnancy to term. This is believed to be the reason morning sickness ends for most women after the first trimester. The embryo develops very rapidly during the first trimester. During these three months, all of the major organs are formed. Therefore, it is imperative to see a physician as soon as an individual thinks she may be pregnant to begin and change any habits that could be harmful to the developing embryo. It is also important to remember that no amount of alcohol during pregnancy is safe (CDC). The pregnancy is dated utilizing the first day of the last menstrual period (LMP). The heartbeat can be seen during a sonogram as early as the sixth or seventh week when the embryo is approximately 5 millimeters long. During the second and third trimesters the fetus is growing larger and stronger in preparation for delivery. Typically the mother will begin to feel the movements of the fetus between the sixteenth and twentieth weeks. This is referred to as 'quickening.' After an additional month or so, these movements can be felt externally by friends or family members. Thirty-six weeks is considered a full-term pregnancy, but a typical delivery does not occur until around the fortieth week."[1]

Pregnancy Prevention

Partners select contraceptive methods for a number of reasons. Ease of use, reversibility, knowledge of, disease protection and accessibility are just some of the many factors that are involved in the decision as to which method is right for the people involved. While not all sexual behaviors lead to pregnancy concerns, for those that do, partners need to be informed about which methods offer the most reliability to prevent an unwanted pregnancy.

When looking at advantages and disadvantages, many factors may be involved. Listed below are some of those for each method. Additionally, you will find a fairly wide % effective range. Remember, these ranges are from "typical" use to "perfect use, hence the variance.

"Natural Methods

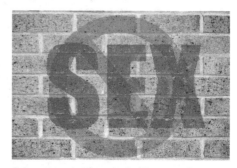

© SergeBertasiusPhotography/Shutterstock.com

"Abstinence from Penile/Vaginal Intercourse

Effectiveness:

- in preventing pregnancy: 100 percent
- in preventing STIs—100 percent

Advantages:

- No worries
- No medical or hormonal side effects
- Protects against unwanted pregnancy

Disadvantages:

- Very few people choose lifetime celibacy or abstinence from sexual intercourse.
- People often forget to protect themselves against pregnancy or STIs when they stop abstaining."[1]

"Withdrawal Method

The man will pull his penis out of the vagina before he ejaculates to keep sperm from joining an egg.

Effectiveness:

- in preventing pregnancy: 73–96 percent
- in preventing STIs—NONE

Advantage:

- Can be used when no other method is available

Disadvantages:

- Requires great self-control, experience, and trust
- Not for men who ejaculate prematurely
- Not for men who do not know when to pull out
- Not recommended for teenagers"[1]

"Fertility Awareness-based Methods (FAMs)

- A woman must chart her menstrual cycle and must be able to detect certain physical signs in order to predict 'unsafe' days.
- She must abstain from intercourse or use barrier contraceptives during nine or more 'unsafe' days each menstrual cycle.
- Check temperature daily. Before ovulation waking temperatures remain low, after ovulation temperatures rise until the next menstrual cycle begins.
- Check cervical mucus daily. Before ovulation the mucus is wet and similar to a raw egg white, after ovulation the cervical fluid dries up quickly.
- Record menstrual cycles on calendar to determine if she has regular or irregular cycles. This method is more effective for those with regular menstrual cycles.
- Remember that the sperm can live up to 120 hours after ejaculation. If a female ovulates within 120 hours after unprotected sexual intercourse the possibility of pregnancy exists.

Effectiveness:

- in preventing pregnancy: 75–99 percent
- in preventing STIs—NONE

Advantages:

- No medical or hormonal side effects
- Calendars, thermometers, and charts are easy to obtain

Disadvantages:

- Requires expert training before effective use
- Taking risks during 'unsafe' days
- Poor record keeping
- Illness and lack of sleep affect body temperatures
- Vaginal infections and douches change mucus
- Cannot use with irregular periods or temperature patterns"[1]

"Barrier Methods

"Male Condom

The male condom is a latex sheath, placed over the penis prior to intercourse (see Figure 7.6).

Effectiveness:

- in preventing pregnancy: 83–98 percent
- in preventing STIs—85–98 percent

To increase pregnancy prevention effectiveness also use spermicide or have female utilize another form of contraception. Do not use oil-based lubricants such as Vaseline or lotion, which will cause the condom to break. Use only water-based lubricants such as KY jelly once the condom is on the penis.

Advantages:

- Most effective way to prevent STIs besides abstinence
- Easy to buy (inexpensive)
- Easy to carry
- Only way for male to protect himself from unplanned pregnancy
- Can help relieve premature ejaculation

Disadvantages*:

- Possible allergies to latex
- Less sensation
- Condom breakage
- Sometimes interrupts 'the mood'
- Human error: withdrawal without holding the condom in place; using after the expiration date; opening the package with teeth, fingernails, or sharp objects can damage the condom; storage of condoms in a warm place such as a wallet in a back pocket can decrease effectiveness."[1]

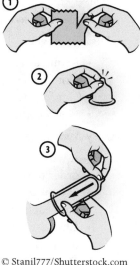

© Stanil777/Shutterstock.com

Figure 7.6

"Diaphragm and Femcap

Latex cup (diaphragm) or silicone cup (Femcap) requires fitting by a clinician. The diaphragm or cap is coated with spermicide before placement in the vagina. The diaphragm or cervical cap combined with spermicide act by destroying the sperm and preventing the sperm from reaching the egg. After intercourse, the Femcap should be left in place for eight hours.

Effectiveness:

in preventing pregnancy:

- Diaphragm with spermicide—86–94 percent
- Femcap with spermicide—84–91 percent for women who have never given birth; 68–74 percent for women who have given birth
- in preventing STIs—NONE

Advantages:

- Femcap can be inserted many hours before sexual intercourse
- Diaphragm can be inserted two hours before sexual intercourse
- Does not alter the menstrual cycle; easy to carry with you, comfortable
- No major health concerns
- Can last several years

Disadvantages:

- Can be messy
- Possibility of allergies to latex, silicone, or spermicide
- Cannot use with vaginal bleeding or an infection
- Diaphragm—can only be left in place for up to twenty-four hours
- Diaphragm—increased risk of bladder infection
- Femcap—difficult for some women to use
- Femcap—can only be left in place for up to forty-eight hours"[1]

Diaphragm
Barrier method of birth control

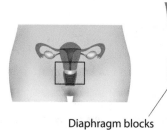
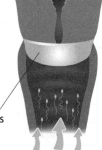

Diaphragm blocks sperm

Sperm

© Tefi/Shutterstock.com

"Over-the-Counter Contraceptives for Women

- Female condom—insert vaginal pouch deep into vagina prior to intercourse
- Spermicide, foam, jelly, or cream—insert deep into vagina prior to intercourse

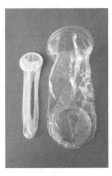

© Image Point Fr /Shutterstock.com

Effectiveness:

in preventing pregnancy:

- Female condom—79–95 percent
- Spermicide, foam, jelly, or cream—71–82 percent in preventing STIs:
- Female condom—similar to the male condom, but not quite as effective, due to possible folding
- Spermicides, foam, jelly, and cream in preventing STIs—NONE

Advantages:

- Easy to purchase in drugstores, supermarkets, etc.
- Increased sensation compared to the male condom
- Erection not necessary to keep female condom in place

Disadvantages:

- Outer ring of female condom may slip into vagina during intercourse
- Possible difficulty inserting the pouch
- More difficult preparation
- Possible allergies to spermicide"[1]

"Hormonal Methods

"The Pill

The pill (oral contraceptive pills) is a prescription medication containing the hormones estrogen and/or progesterone, which usually prevents the release of the egg, thickens the cervical mucus, and reduces the buildup of the endometrial lining within the uterus. The sperm is thus unable to penetrate the egg, and/or the fertilized egg is prevented from implanting in the uterus.

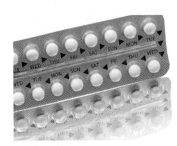

© areeya_ann/Shutterstock.com

Effectiveness:

- in preventing pregnancy: 92–99.7 percent
- in preventing STIs—NONE

Advantages:

- Nothing to put into place before intercourse
- Regular and shorter periods
- Decreases chances of developing ovarian and endometrial cancers, non-cancerous breast tumors, ovarian cysts, pelvic inflammatory disease, and osteoporosis
- Decreased incidence of tubal pregnancies
- Ability to become pregnant returns quickly when use is stopped

Disadvantages:

- Less effective when taken with some drugs
- Must be taken daily (within the same two hour period)
- Rare but serious health risks, including: blood clots, heart attack, and stroke, which are more common for women over 35 and/or who smoke cigarettes (ARHP, 2008). This increased risk is found in most of the hormonal contraceptive methods. This is due to an increased correlation of cardiovascular disease most likely from the formation of atherosclerosis in women who smoke and use hormonal contraceptive methods. This risk also increases as women age, smoke, and use hormonal contraceptive methods.
- Side effects can include temporary irregular bleeding, weight gain, breast tenderness, and nausea.

Women who experience any of the following symptoms while taking the pill should call their physician immediately:

- Abdominal pains (severe)
- Chest pain or shortness of breath
- Headaches (severe)
- Eye problems, such as blurred vision
- Severe leg or arm pain or numbness"[1]

"Mini-pills

Mini-pills (oral contraceptive pills) are a prescription medication containing progesterone only, which usually prevents the release of the egg, thickens the cervical mucus, and reduces the buildup of the endometrial lining within the uterus. The sperm is thus unable to penetrate the egg, and/or the fertilized egg is prevented from implanting in the uterus.

Effectiveness:

- in preventing pregnancy: 87–99.7 percent (slightly less than regular birth control pills)
- in preventing STIs—NONE

Advantages:

- Nothing to put into place before intercourse
- Avoids typical side effects of regular birth control pills
- Has no estrogen
- Ability to become pregnant returns quickly when use is stopped

Disadvantages:

- Less effective when taken with some drugs
- MUST be taken at the same time every day
- Increased risk of ectopic pregnancy
- Increased risk of functional ovarian cysts"[1]

"Vaginal Ring

The female will insert a small, flexible ring deep into the vagina for three weeks and take it out for the fourth week. It releases combined hormones that protect against pregnancy for one month. The ring uses hormones similar to the estrogen and progesterone made by a woman's ovaries to prevent the ovaries from releasing an egg, thickens the cervical mucus, and reduces the buildup of the endometrial lining within the uterus. The sperm is thus unable to penetrate the egg, and/ or the fertilized egg is prevented from implanting in the uterus.

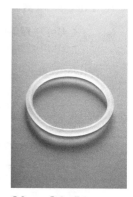

© Image Point Fr
/Shutterstock.com

Effectiveness:

- in preventing pregnancy: 92–99.7 percent
- in preventing STIs—NONE

Advantages:

- Protects against pregnancy for one month
- No pill to take daily
- Does not require a "fitting" by a clinician
- Does not require the use of spermicide
- Ability to become pregnant returns quickly when use is stopped
- Nothing to put into place before intercourse
- More regular and shorter periods
- Reduces the risk of ovarian and endometrial cancers, pelvic inflammatory disease, non-cancerous growths of the breasts, ovarian cysts, and osteoporosis
- Fewer occurrences of ectopic pregnancy

Disadvantages:

- Increased vaginal discharge
- Vaginal irritation or infection
- Cannot use a diaphragm or cap for a backup method of birth control
- Rare but serious health risks, including blood clots, heart attack, and stroke—women who are 35 and older and/or smoke are at a greater risk. This increased risk is found in most of the hormonal contraceptive methods. This is due to an increased correlation of cardiovascular disease most likely from the formation of atherosclerosis in women who smoke and use hormonal contraceptive methods. This risk also increases as women age, smoke, and use hormonal contraceptive methods.
- Temporary irregular bleeding, weight gain, breast tenderness, and nausea

Women who experience any of the following symptoms while using the ring should call their physician immediately:

- Abdominal pains (severe)
- Chest pain or shortness of breath
- Headaches (severe)
- Eye problems, such as blurred vision
- Severe leg or arm pain or numbness"[1]

"Contraceptive Patch

The female will place a thin plastic patch on the skin of the buttocks, stomach, upper outer arm, or upper torso once a week for three weeks in a row. Use a new patch each week. Do not use a patch for the fourth week. The patch releases combined hormones that protect against pregnancy for one month. The patch uses hormones similar to the estrogen and progesterone made by a woman's ovaries to prevent the ovaries from releasing an egg, thickens the cervical mucus, and reduces the buildup of the endometrial lining within the uterus. The sperm is thus unable to penetrate the egg, and/or the fertilized egg is prevented from implanting in the uterus.

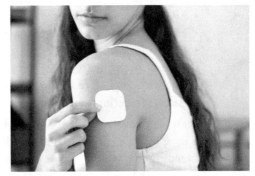

© Image Point Fr/Shutterstock.com

Effectiveness:

- in preventing pregnancy: 99 percent (for women who weigh 197 pounds or less) 92 percent (for women who weigh 198 pounds or more)
- in preventing STIs—NONE

Advantages:

- Protects against pregnancy for one month
- No pill to take daily
- Nothing to put into place before intercourse
- Ability to become pregnant returns quickly when use is stopped
- More regular and shorter periods
- Reduce the risk of ovarian and endometrial cancers, pelvic inflammatory disease, non-cancerous growths of the breasts, ovarian cysts, and osteoporosis
- Fewer occurrences of ectopic pregnancy

Disadvantages:

- Skin reaction at the site of application
- Menstrual cramps
- May not be effective for women who weigh more than 198 pounds
- Rare but serious health risks, including blood clots, heart attack, and stroke— women who are 35 and older and/or smoke are at a greater risk. This increased risk is found in most of the hormonal contraceptive methods. This is due to an increased correlation of cardiovascular disease most likely from the formation of atherosclerosis in women who smoke and use hormonal contraceptive methods. This risk also increases as women age, smoke, and use hormonal contraceptive methods.
- Temporary irregular bleeding, weight gain, breast tenderness, and nausea

Some women may not be able to use contraceptive patches because of the risk of serious health problems. Women over 35 who smoke or have any of the following conditions should not use the patch:

- History of heart attack or stroke
- Chest pain
- Blood clots
- Unexplained vaginal bleeding
- Severe high blood pressure
- Diabetes with kidney, eye, nerve, or blood vessel complications
- Known or suspected cancer
- Known or suspected pregnancy
- Liver tumors or liver disease
- Headaches with neurological symptoms
- Hepatitis or jaundice
- Disease of the heart valves with complications
- Require long bed rest following surgery
- Allergic reaction to the patch

Women who have a family history of breast cancer, diabetes, high blood pressure, high cholesterol, headaches or epilepsy, depression, gallbladder disease, kidney disease, heart disease, irregular periods, or are breast-feeding may not be able to use the patch. Women who experience any of the following symptoms while using the contraceptive patch should call their physician immediately:

- Abdominal pains (severe)
- Chest pain or shortness of breath

- Headaches (severe)
- Eye problems, such as blurred vision
- Severe leg or arm pain or numbness"[1]

"Depo-Provera

Depo-Provera is a hormone shot injected into the arm or buttocks every twelve weeks, which will prevent the release of the egg, less often thickens the cervical mucus and reduces the buildup of the endometrial lining within the uterus thereby preventing conception, and/or the fertilized egg from implanting in the uterus.

Effectiveness:

- in preventing pregnancy: 97–99.7 percent
- in preventing STIs—NONE

Advantages:

- Protects against pregnancy for twelve weeks
- No daily pill
- Nothing to put into place before intercourse
- Can be used by some women who cannot take the pill (oral contraceptive)
- Decreases incidence of endometrial and ovarian cancer, as well as iron deficiency anemia (ARHP, 2008)
- Can be used while breast-feeding

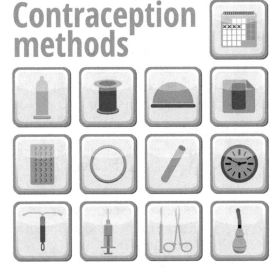

© vadim-design/Shutterstock.com

Figure 7.7

Disadvantages:

- Studies released in 2004 show that Depo-Provera is associated with a loss of bone density resulting in an increased risk of osteoporosis. The bone loss appears not to be reversed when the woman stops the Depo-Provera injections (U.S. Department of Health and Human Services).
- Side effects include irregular bleeding, headaches, depression, nausea, loss of monthly period, weight gain, nervousness, and dizziness
- Side effects cannot be reversed until medication wears off (up to twelve weeks)
- May cause delay in getting pregnant after shots are stopped (up to twelve to eighteen months)
- Should not be used continuously for more than two years."[1]

"IUD

The intrauterine device (IUD) requires a health care professional to insert a small plastic device through the cervix and into the uterus. The IUD contains copper or hormones that impede conception or rarely prevent implantation of a fertilized egg. IUDs can last one to ten years.

Effectiveness:

- in preventing pregnancy: 99.2–99.9 percent
- in preventing STIs—NONE

Advantages:

- Nothing to put into place before intercourse
- Para Gard (copper IUD) may be left in place for up to ten years; Mirena (hormone IUD) may be left in place for up to five years
- No daily pills
- Ability to become pregnant returns quickly when use is stopped

Disadvantages:

- May cause cramping (copper IUD)
- Spotting between periods
- Heavier and longer periods
- Increased risk of tubal infection, which may lead to infertility if inserted when a women has an STI
- Rarely, the wall of the uterus is punctured"[1]

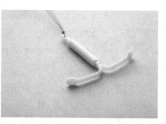

© Image Point Fr/Shutterstock.com

"Contraceptive Implant

Contraceptive implants are soft capsules, about 1.5 inches long, placed under the skin in a woman's upper inner arm. The capsules release progestin, which usually prevents the release of the egg, thickens the cervical mucus, and reduces the buildup of the endometrial lining within the uterus. The sperm is thus unable to penetrate the egg, and/or the fertilized egg is prevented from implanting in the uterus. Implanon is currently being used in the United States and is a single rod that releases a hormone called etonogestrel which lasts three years. Contraceptive implants can be removed at any time.

Effectiveness:

- in preventing pregnancy: 99 percent
- in preventing STIs—NONE

Advantages:

- Can be worn for three years
- Affects fertility one month at a time
- Has no estrogen

Disadvantages:

- Increased risk of heart attack
- Increased risk of stroke"[1]

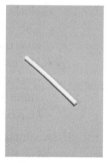

© Michael Kraus /Shutterstock.com

"Sterilization

Sterilization is an operation performed on the female (tubal ligation) or male (vasectomy). The tubal ligation is intended to permanently block a woman's fallopian tubes, where sperm typically unite with the eggs. A vasectomy is performed to permanently block a man's vas deferens tubes, which transport sperm.

Effectiveness:

- in preventing pregnancy: 99.5–99.9 percent
- in preventing STIs—NONE

Advantages:

- Permanent protection against pregnancy
- No lasting side effects
- No effects on sexual pleasure
- Protects woman whose health would be seriously threatened by a pregnancy

Disadvantages:

- Mild bleeding or infection after the surgery
- Some people eventually regret being unable to have children later in life
- Reaction to anesthetic
- Not usually reversible if you change your mind

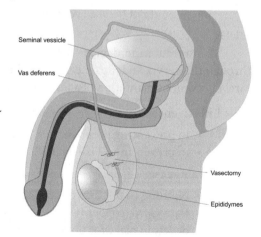

© ellepigrafica/Shutterstock.com

- Rarely, tubes reopen, allowing pregnancy to occur
- Rare complications with tubal ligation include bleeding and injury to the bowel
- Vasectomy—infection or blood clot can occur in or near the testicles; often there is temporary bruising, swelling, or tenderness of the scrotum

Go to www.arhp.org/Method Match and use this interactive program to help you choose the birth control method that is right for you."[1]

EMERGENCY CONTRACEPTION "THE MORNING AFTER PILL"

"There is considerable public confusion about the difference between emergency contraception (EC) pills and medication abortion (RU-486). Pregnancy begins when a pre-embryo completes implantation into the lining of the uterus (ACOG, 1998). EC helps prevent pregnancy, whereas medication abortion terminates pregnancy. Hormonal methods of contraception, including EC, prevent pregnancy by inhibiting ovulation and fertilization (ACOG, 2011). More specifically, EC works by delaying or inhibiting ovulation, and/or altering tubal transport of sperm and/or ova (thereby inhibiting fertilization), and/or altering the endometrium (thereby inhibiting implantation) (Trussell and Jordan, 2006). After un-

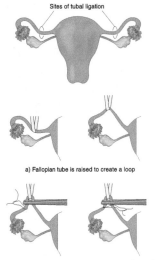

a) Fallopian tube is raised to create a loop

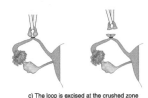

b) The loop is crushed with forceps, then ligated in a figure-of-eight

c) The loop is excised at the crushed zone

© Blamb/Shutterstock.com

protected intercourse, emergency contraception may be utilized. This treatment has been in place for several years in other countries, but only recently became available in the United States. The medication should be taken within 120 hours of unprotected sexual intercourse. The sooner the medication is begun, the higher the effectiveness for pregnancy prevention. There are two types of ECs. The first one contains both estrogen and progestin. When taken within seventy-two hours of unprotected intercourse, ECs that contain both estrogen and progestin reduce the risk of pregnancy by 75 percent. The combination pills are taken in two doses, twelve hours apart. The other type of ECs only contains progestin. When taken within twenty-four hours of unprotected intercourse, progestin-only ECs were found to reduce the risk of pregnancy by 95 percent (Ellertson et al., 2003). The progestin-only ECs are taken in two doses, twelve hours apart or at the same time. The emergency contraceptive method is typically used in cases of unanticipated sexual intercourse, contraceptive failure, or sexual assault. Some common side effects include substantial nausea and vomiting. These side effects generally subside within forty-eight hours. This is not to be used as a regular method of birth control. As with many of the other pregnancy prevention methods, this one offers no protection against the contraction of STIs."[1]

Did you know . . .

According to Huffpost:

Courtesy of Shelley Hamill

- Every year, fewer than 1 in 100 women will become pregnant if they take the pill every day, but 9 in 100 will if they don't manage to take the pill daily.
- Early versions of birth control pills had higher doses of hormones and caused many women to gain weight, but most modern iterations do not.
- Researchers say that both hormonal and non-hormonal birth control options are on the way!

PREGNANCY PREVENTION CHART

		Effectiveness	Advantages	Disadvantages
Natural Methods:	Abstinence from Penile/ Vaginal Intercourse	• In preventing pregnancy: 100% • In preventing STIs: 100%	• No worries • No medical or hormonal side effects • Protects against unwanted pregnancy	• People often forget to protect themselves against pregnancy or STIs when they stop abstaining
	Withdrawal Methods	• In preventing pregnancy: 73-96% • In preventing STIs: NONE	• Can be used when no other method is available	• Requires great self-control, experience, and trust • Not for men who ejaculate prematurely • Not recommended for teenagers
	Fertility Awareness-based Methods (FAMs)	• In preventing pregnancy: 75-99% • In preventing STIs: NONE	• No medical or hormonal side effects • Calendars, thermometers, and charts are easy to obtain	• Taking risks during 'unsafe' days • Illness and lack of sleep affect body temperatures • Cannot use with irregular periods or temperature patterns
Barrier Methods:	Male Condom	• In preventing pregnancy: 83-98% • In preventing STIs: 85-98%	• Most effective way to prevent STIs besides abstinence • Easy to buy (inexpensive); easy to carry • Can help relieve premature ejaculation	• Possible allergies to latex • Condom breakage • Sometimes interrupts 'the mood' • Human error
	Diaphragm	• In preventing pregnancy: 86-94% • In preventing STIs: NONE	• Diaphragm: Can be inserted 2 hours before sexual intercourse • Femcap: Can be inserted many hours before sexual intercourse • No major health concerns • Does not alter the menstrual cycle • Can last several years	• Can only be left in place for up to 24 hrs. • Increased risk of bladder infection
	Femcap	• In preventing pregnancy: 84-91% • In preventing STIs: NONE		• Difficult for some women to use • Can only be left in place for up to 48 hrs.
Over-the-Counter Contraceptives for Women:	• Female Condom • Spermicide, foam, jelly or cream	• In preventing pregnancy: • Female Condom 79-95% • Spermicide 71-82% • In preventing STIs: NONE	• Easy to purchase • Increased sensation compared to male condom • Erection not necessary to keep female condom in place	• Outer ring of female condom may slip into vagina during intercourse • Possible difficulty inserting the pouch • Possible allergies to spermicide

		Effectiveness	**Advantages**	**Disadvantages**
Hormonal Methods:	The Pill	• In preventing pregnancy: 92-99.7% • In preventing STIs: NONE	• Regular and shorter periods • Nothing to put in place before intercourse	• Less effective when taken with some drugs • Must be taken daily
	Mini-pills	• In preventing pregnancy: 87-99.7% • In preventing STIs: NONE	• Nothing to put into place before intercourse • Has no estrogen • Avoids typical side effects of regular birth control pills	• Less effective when taken with some drugs • MUST be taken at the same time every day • Increased risk of ectopic pregnancy
	Vaginal Ring	• In preventing pregnancy: 92-99.7% • In preventing STIs: NONE	• Protects against pregnancy for one month • No daily pill	• Increased vaginal discharge • Vaginal irritation or infection
	Contraceptive Patch	• In preventing pregnancy: 99% (197 lbs or less) • 92% (198 lbs or more) • In preventing STIs: NONE	• Protects against pregnancy for one month • No daily pill • Nothing to put in place before intercourse	• Skin reaction at the site of application • Menstrual cramps • Temporary irregular bleeding, weight gain, breast tenderness, and nausea
	Depo-Provera	• In preventing pregnancy: 97-99.7% • In preventing STIs: NONE	• Protects pregnancy for 12 weeks • No daily pill • Can be used while breast-feeding	• Increased risk for osteoporosis • Side effects cannot be reversed until medication wears off
	IUD	• In preventing pregnancy: 99.2-99.9% • In preventing STIs: NONE	• Para Gard may be left in up to 10 years, Mirena may be left in up to 5 years	• Increased risk of tubal infection, which can lead to infertility • Rarely, the wall of the uterus is punctured
	Contraceptive Implant	• In preventing pregnancy: 99% • In preventing STIs: NONE	• Can be worn for 3 years • Affects fertility one month at a time • Has no estrogen	• Increased risk of heart attack • Increased risk of stroke
	Sterilization	• In preventing pregnancy: 99.5-99.9% • In preventing STIs: NONE	• Permanent protection against pregnancy • No effects on sexual pleasure	• Some people eventually regret being unable to have children later in life • Mild bleeding or infection after surgery

Courtesy of Caylee King

Unplanned Pregnancy

"This can be a very exciting and/or frightening time in an individual's life. The thought of pregnancy conjures up many emotions, such as the realization of life changes, increased responsibility, happiness, and worry all at the same time. Pregnancy and the responsibilities of parenthood are tremendous. It is important to realize these potential consequences of unprotected intercourse or failed pregnancy prevention. It is a good idea to discuss how you might handle this situation with your potential sexual partner. In the event of an unplanned pregnancy, there are several options, none of which are easy and all can be life altering. These will be discussed in the following sections."[1]

Parenthood

"Parenthood has been described in many words. Many agree it is one of the best things that can happen, while for others parenthood is quite difficult and challenging. For most, this phase of life (given its rewards and demands) is a blend of these two perspectives. These differences of opinion are often influenced by the stage of life during which the individual becomes a parent, combined with factors such as other life circumstances (whether the parent will be a single

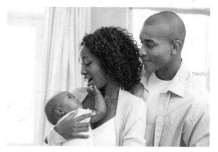

© wavebreakmedia/Shutterstock.com

parent or not), as well as the personality and financial situation of the new parent. Parenthood usually will dramatically alter the lifestyle to which an individual has become accustomed. Initially, it is an end to restful nights, spur-of-the-moment trips, and many social activities. New parents now have an individual who is solely dependent upon them twenty-four hours a day for attention, love, food, clothing, safety, and shelter. This can be overwhelming physically, mentally, and financially even for the most prepared parents. It is also a time of tremendous joy, as well as many special moments, such as your baby's first smile, giggle, word, or step. As the child grows they are less dependent upon you for the basic necessities, but those needs change into dance lessons, soccer practice, and slumber parties, to name a few. The commitment to becoming a parent is large and one that never ends and can be very difficult to face alone."[1]

Adoption

For some, life circumstances may not support becoming a parent at that time. Adoption may be an option for the parent or parents and may be part of the discussion during the pregnancy. There are many factors involved in the decision. While it may be a very difficult one to make, it can be one that is beneficial to both the parent(s) and the child.

"Many adoption agencies exist to help make this option as painless as possible. There are many different types of adoptions. Some allow the biological parents to remain a part of the child's life; others do not, but provide a mechanism whereby the child can eventually obtain information regarding the biological parents. Often this information can be made available only after the adopted child enters adolescence or adulthood."[1]

Abortion

"Some individuals cannot (due to medical reasons) or do not want to carry the embryo to term, and therefore choose abortion. This decision is reached for various reasons. Sometimes this is felt to be the best decision because of the circumstances of conception (such as a rape resulting in pregnancy). Some believe they cannot disclose a pregnancy to their parents or partner and see no other alternative. Others are not ready to become parents and do not want to complete the pregnancy.

"Abortion was made legal throughout the United States in 1973. Today, abortion is about ten times safer than giving birth. There are some potential complications associated with abortion. The complications can include an incomplete abortion, which means the procedure would need to be repeated; an infection, which can usually be treated with antibiotics; or perforation of the uterine wall. There are several types of abortion procedures available, depending on the stage of the pregnancy. Medical abortion (Mifepristone, RU-486, or nonsurgical abortion) is an option up to eight weeks since the last menstrual period (LMP). Surgical vacuum aspiration abortion is the procedure used to empty the uterus and can be performed between six and twelve weeks since the LMP. Last, the dilation and evacuation procedure can be performed between thirteen and twenty-four weeks since the LMP. After and during an abortion there is typically mild to very strong cramping for one to three hours, as well as bleeding and/or spotting for three to six weeks. A normal menstrual period should begin within four to eight weeks. Usually clinics will offer counseling before and after an abortion. Due to the emotional nature of any decision associated with pregnancy, counseling is highly recommended. As mentioned earlier, pregnancy is accompanied by many emotions and lasting effects for both partners. There is no easy route once pregnancy has occurred. It is a good idea to discuss your values and ideas of what you would do in the event of an unplanned pregnancy with your prospective sexual partner. It is best to fully consider all of the options before making a decision."[1]

SEXUALLY TRANSMITTED INFECTIONS (STIs)

According to the Center for Disease Control, (CDC), the number of sexually transmitted infections, sometimes called sexually transmitted diseases, is on the rise.

STIs are a substantial health challenge facing the United States. CDC estimates that nearly 20 million new sexually transmitted infections occur every year in this country, half among young people aged 15–24, and account for almost $16 billion in health care costs. Incidence and prevalence estimates suggest that young people aged 15–24 years acquire half of all new STDs and that 1 in 4 sexually active adolescent females have an STD, such as chlamydia or human papillomavirus (HPV). Each of these infections is a potential threat to an individual's immediate and long-term health and well-being. In addition to increasing a person's risk for acquiring and transmitting HIV infection, STIs can lead to se-

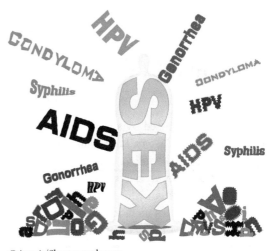

© jcwait/Shutterstock.com

vere reproductive health complications, such as infertility and ectopic pregnancy. In 2014, there was an increase in number of reported cases of chlamydia, gonorrhea and syphilis. STDs continue to affect young people—particularly women—most severely, but increasing rates among men contributed to the overall increases in 2014 across all three diseases.

"STIs are transmitted during vaginal, oral, anal sexual activity, or in some cases by simply touching an infected area. STIs can be transferred not only to the genitalia area, but also to the mouth, eyes, nose, and other orifices of the body. You can become infected if someone's blood, semen, vaginal secretions, or precum goes into your body during vaginal, anal, or oral sex. Many individuals who become infected with STIs are asymptomatic (without symptoms) and thus become silent carriers. This is one of the reasons STIs have reached epidemic proportions. There are many health problems that can result if an asymptomatic STI carrier is not treated. Some of these health problems include infertility, ectopic pregnancies, and genital cancers, particularly cervical cancer in women. Therefore, it is very important to know your sexual history and be tested for STIs regularly."[1]

Levels of Risk

"Sexual behaviors have different levels of risk for different STIs. Using condoms lowers the risk of transmitting STIs in association with anal, oral, or vaginal intercourse. The following list depicts risk, assuming no protection is used for the following behaviors.

High Risk

- Anal intercourse
- Vaginal intercourse
- Oral sex on a man with ejaculation
- Oral sex on a man without ejaculation
- Oral sex on a woman
- Oral-anal contact

© Vertes Edmond Mihai/Shutterstock.com

Low Risk

- Intimate kissing
- Casual kissing
- Touching, massage

© Lack-O'Keen/Shutterstock.com

No Risk

- Masturbation
- Talking, fantasy"[1]

BACTERIAL STIs

Chlamydia

"Chlamydia is caused by a bacteria-like intracellular parasite called *Chlamydia trachomati*. Chlamydia is typically spread during vaginal, oral, or anal sex and can infect other body parts such as the eyes, nose, or throat where chlamydia can also be contracted. Symptoms in males include a thin, clear-whitish urethral discharge, itching or burning during urination, pain, or swelling in the testes and a low-grade fever. In females, symptoms include moderate vaginal discharge, itching or burning during urination, abdominal pain, bleeding between periods, nausea, head-

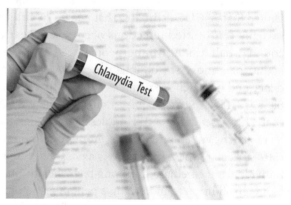

© Jarun Ontakrai/Shutterstock.com

aches, and a low-grade fever. If symptoms occur, they will typically begin one to three weeks after infection. 75 percent of infected females and 51 percent of infected males are asymptomatic (without symptoms). The long-term effects of untreated chlamydia can include infertility in both males and females from scarring in the testicles and fallopian tubes. Chlamydia infections are the leading cause of preventable infertility and ectopic pregnancies. In up to 40 percent of women with untreated chlamydia, infection can spread into the uterus and fallopian tubes, causing pelvic inflammatory disease (PID). Most infections respond to tetracycline, doxycycline, or erythromycin, but not penicillin. It is very important that all partners be treated to decrease the spread of infection, as well as prevent reinfection. Chlamydia is estimated to be the most common bacterial STI in the United States, with approximately three million new cases occurring each year (ASHA, 2009). Adolescents and young adults have the highest infection rates College students account for over 10 percent of the infected cases which are on the rise (Donatelle, 2010)."[1]

Gonorrhea

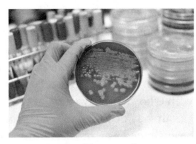

"Gonorrhea is caused by the bacterium called *Neisseria gonorrhea*. Infection is found primarily in the linings of the urethra, vagina, mouth, and rectum (Crowley, 2009). Symptoms in males include a foul-smelling thick, creamy white, yellow, or yellow-green discharge from the penis, painful urination, blood or pus in the urine, and enlarged lymph nodes in the groin area. In females, the symptoms include similar discharge from the vagina, pain during urination, pelvic pain, or irregular and painful menstruation. If symptoms are present, they usually appear

© Jarun Ontakrai/Shutterstock.com

about one week after exposure. Many individuals are asymptomatic (5 to 20 percent of infected males and 60 to 80 percent of females). The long-term effects of untreated gonorrhea can cause infertility in both males and females, as a result of infection and scarring in both testicles and in the fallopian tubes. Gonorrhea remains one of the major causes of PID. Most infections respond to penicillin, tetracycline, spectinomycin, cefixime, or ceftriaxone. It is very important that all partners be treated to decrease the spread of the infection, as well as to prevent reinfection."[1]

Pelvic Inflammatory Disease (PID)

"PID is a general term that refers to an infection of the uterus, fallopian tubes, or other reproductive organ. Untreated sexually transmitted infections can cause PID. Chlamydia and gonorrhea are the most common STIs (if left untreated) that lead to PID. Damage to the fallopian tubes and tissues in and near the uterus and ovaries can result from PID. This damage occurs from the inflammation and results in scarring of these tissues. This scarring can lead to serious consequences including infertility, ectopic pregnancy, abscess formation, and chronic pelvic pain."[1]

Pelvic Inflammatory Disease

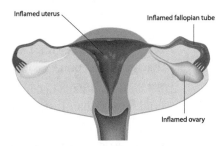

© Alila Medical Media/Shutterstock.com

Unprotected vaginal or anal intercourse:

Bacterial Vaginosis
Chlamydia
Cytomegalovirus (CMV)
Gonorrhea
Hepatitis B
Herpes Simplex
Human Immunodeficiency Virus (HIV)
Human Papilloma Virus (HPV, Warts)
Pelvic Inflammatory Disease (PID)
Pubic Lice
Scabies
Syphilis
Trichomoniasis
*Safer Sex Tip: Always use condoms.

Unprotected oral sex:
("blow job," "giving head," "going down," "rimming")

Cytomegalovirus (CMV)
Gonorrhea
Hepatitis B

Herpes (including cold sores)
Human Immunodeficiency Virus (HIV)
Human Papilloma Virus (HPV, Warts)
Syphilis
*Safer Sex Tip: Use dental dams, non-lubricated or flavored condom, or female condoms.

Unprotected manual sex:
("hand job" or "fingering")

Bacterial Vaginosis
Cytomegalovirus (CMV)
Herpes Simplex
Human Papilloma Virus (HPV, Warts)
Pubic Lice
Scabies
*Safer Sex Tip: Use gloves or condoms.

Source: Adapted from www.scarleteen.com.

©Kendall Hunt Publishing Company

Figure 7.8 STI Risk Sheet

"The more sexual partners a woman has had, the higher her risk of developing PID. This is because of the potential for more exposure to STIs. Most of the time there are no symptoms associated with PID. Meanwhile, the infection is causing serious long-term damage to the woman's reproductive organs. If symptoms exist, they can include lower abdominal pain, fever, unusual vaginal discharge, painful intercourse or urination, irregular menstrual bleeding, or pain in the right upper abdomen. PID can be cured with Ofloxacin, Levo- floxacin, or Metronidazole. "Antibiotic treatment does not reverse any damage that has already occurred to the reproductive organs. It is critical for any woman who has symptoms of PID to be evaluated by a physician immediately. The longer treatment is delayed for PID the more likely she is to become infertile due to the damage to the reproductive organs."[1]

Syphilis

"Syphilis is a serious bacterial infection caused by the *spirochete Treponema pallidum*. Syphilis can be contracted and spread through vaginal, oral, or anal sex, as well as through blood and blood products. This disease can be debilitating and even fatal if left untreated. A person may be unknowingly infected with syphilis and transmit it to others. It is estimated that for every case of syphilis that is reported, three are not (Crooks and Baur, 2009). This disease has three stages.

1. "During the first stage, a painless sore (chancre) about the size of a dime may appear at the point where the bacteria first entered the body, usually three weeks after contact. This sore may appear around or in the vagina, on the penis, or inside the mouth or anus. Sores inside the vagina or anus are often unnoticed and may disappear on their own if not treated; however, the bacterial infection remains.

2. "The second stage occurs two to eight weeks after the exposure and includes flu-like symptoms and possible hair loss, a rash on the palms of hands and soles of feet, as well as over the entire body

3. "The tertiary (third stage) syphilis can appear five to twenty-five years after the initial exposure. Symptoms of this stage may include skin lesions, mental deterioration, loss of balance and vision, loss of sensation, shooting pains in the legs, and heart disease (Crooks and Baur, 2009)."[1]

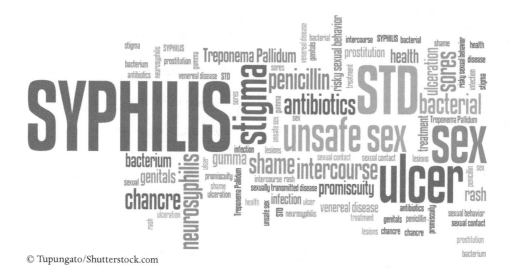

© Tupungato/Shutterstock.com

"See a physician immediately if there is any chance you have been exposed to syphilis. A simple blood test can usually determine whether or not you have the disease. However, if you become infected two to three weeks prior to testing, the blood test may not be sensitive enough to detect the antibodies. Syphilis can be treated with the proper antibiotics, most commonly penicillin injections. There have been several resistant strains that have developed when individuals did not take the full prescription dose. Always take all of the antibiotics that are prescribed to you; don't save them for later or stop them just because you feel better and NEVER take someone else's medication. Go to www.thebody.com/surveys/sex-survey.html to take this absolutely anonymous test and discover your risk for HIV or other STIs."[1]

VIRAL STIs

Genital Herpes

"Genital herpes is a chronic, life-long infection caused by the herpes simplex virus (HSV). There are two types of HSV (Type 1 and Type 2), both of which can infect any area of the body, producing lesions (sores) in and around the vaginal area, on the penis, around the anal opening, on the buttocks or thighs, in or around the mouth, and in the eyes possibly causing blindness (Donatelle, 2010). Herpes can be

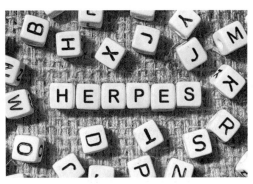

© schatzie/Shutterstock.com

contracted and spread through vaginal, oral, or anal sex, as well as skin-to-skin contact. A newborn may be infected with genital herpes while passing through the birth canal (Crooks and Baur, 2009). Infection in the newborn can cause mental retardation, blindness, or even death (Crooks and Baur, 2009). Therefore, it is important that an infected pregnant female inform her physician of the infection so that the physician can watch for an outbreak and perform a cesarean section (C-section) if necessary."[1]

In the United States, about one out of every six people aged 14 to 49 years have genital herpes. Each year there are approximately 750,000 new herpes infections. "There are many more individuals who have genital herpes and are asymptomatic. The symptoms vary, and many people have no noticeable symptoms. Symptoms will most commonly occur within two to twenty days after infection. Early symptoms may include a tingling or burning sensation in the genitals, lower back pain, pain when urinating, and flu-like symptoms. A few days later, small red bump(s) may appear in the genital area. Later, these bumps can develop into painful blisters, which then crust over, form a scab, and heal. Sometimes the diagnosis can be made by physical examination alone. For testing, the physician collects a small amount of fluid from the sores to see if the herpes virus is present. It may take up to two weeks to receive the results. If no sores are present, testing may be difficult. However, a blood test does exist to determine if an individual does have the herpes virus. It is expensive and does not indicate the location of the infection. Although herpes is a chronic, lifelong viral infection, the symptoms can be treated. Treatment of genital herpes outbreaks, especially when begun early, shortens the duration of the outbreak and reduces the symptoms (Marr, 2007)."[1]

HIV/AIDS

"Human Immunodeficiency Virus (HIV)/Acquired Immune Deficiency Syndrome (AIDS) was first identified in the United States in June 1981 by the Centers for Disease Control and Prevention (CDC). HIV is the virus that causes AIDS and is transmitted in one of four ways: 1. vaginal, oral, or anal sex; 2. sharing a needle for piercing, tattoos, or drugs including steroids; 3. blood products infected with HIV; 4. from mother to child during pregnancy, delivery or breast milk. The highest concentrations of HIV are found in bodily fluids such as blood, semen, vaginal secretions, and breast milk (Floyd et al., 2007). Infection can occur when any of these fluids from an infected person comes into direct contact with the bloodstream or mucous membranes of another person. Trace amounts are found in tears, saliva, and other body fluids but have not been found to transmit infection. HIV is not spread by casual contact. It is not known if all individuals infected with this virus will develop AIDS. Women are more likely to become infected with HIV during heterosexual sex than males, because the concentration of virus is higher in semen than it is in vaginal secretions (Floyd et al., 2007). An individual may be asymptomatic or may have some of the symptoms, which include:

- fatigue,
- dry cough,
- fever,
- night sweats,
- diarrhea,
- skin rashes,
- swollen lymph nodes,
- recurrent vaginal yeast infections,
- unexplained weight loss.

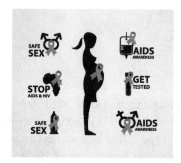

© jennylipets/Shutterstock.com

"Typically six weeks to six months is required after the initial infection to detect the HIV antibodies in a blood test (Floyd et al., 2007). There are numerous drugs/cocktails (mixture of different types of drugs) that exist to boost the immune system and interfere with the replication of the virus, therefore delaying the onset of AIDS. The best way to avoid contracting HIV is to abstain from vaginal, oral, or anal sex or have a mutually monogamous relationship with an uninfected partner. Other ways to protect yourself include HIV testing before becoming sexually active, consistent and correct use of latex condoms with all sexual acts (vaginal, oral, and anal), avoid sharing needles for anything, and do not have sex with anyone known or suspected of using injectable drugs including steroids."[1]

CDC estimates that 1,218,400 persons aged 13 years and older are living with HIV infection, including 156,300 (12.8%) who are unaware of their infection. Over the past decade, the number of people living with HIV has increased, while the annual number of new HIV infections has remained relatively stable. The estimated incidence of HIV has remained stable overall in recent years, at about 50,000 new HIV infections per year.

HPV

HPV is the most common sexually transmitted infection (STI). HPV is a different virus than HIV and HSV (herpes). HPV is so common that nearly all sexually active men and women get it at some point in their lives. There are many different types of HPV. Some types can cause health problems including genital warts and cancers. But there are vaccines that can stop these health problems from happening.

You can get HPV by having vaginal, anal, or oral sex with someone who has the virus. It is most commonly spread during vaginal or anal sex. HPV can be passed even when an infected person has no signs or symptoms. Anyone who is sexually active can get HPV, even if you have had sex with only one person. You also can develop symptoms years after you have sex with someone who is infected making it hard to know when you first became infected.

About 79 million Americans are currently infected with HPV. About 14 million people become newly infected each year. HPV is so common that most sexually-active men and women will get at least one type of HPV at some point in their lives. There is no test to find out a person's "HPV status." Also, there is no approved HPV test to find HPV in the mouth or throat.

There are HPV tests that can be used to screen for cervical cancer. These tests are recommended for screening only in women aged 30 years and older. They are not recommended to screen men, adolescents, or women under the age of 30 years.

Most people with HPV do not know they are infected and never develop symptoms or health problems from it. Some people find out they have HPV when they get genital warts. Women may find out they have HPV when they get an abnormal Pap test result (during cervical cancer screening). Others may only find out once they've developed more serious problems from HPV, such as cancers.

HPV Vaccine

"In 2006, the FDA approved Gardasil, the first vaccine developed to prevent certain types (16 and 18) of HPV, which cause 70 percent of cervical cancers and against types 6 and 11, which cause approximately 90 percent of genital warts. Gardasil has also been shown to protect against anal, vaginal, and vulvar cancers (CDC, 2011). The vaccine is designed for females and males age 9–26. Ideally, the vaccine would be given before an individual becomes sexually active and is exposed to the viruses. In order for the vaccine to be effective, it must be given in three different doses over a six month period."[1]

Hepatitis B

Hepatitis B is a contagious liver disease that results from infection with the Hepatitis B virus. When first infected, a person can develop an "acute" infection, which can range in severity from a very mild illness with few or no symptoms to a serious condition requiring hospitalization. **Acute** Hepatitis B refers to the first 6 months after someone is exposed to the Hepatitis B virus. Some people are able to fight the infection and clear the virus. For others, the infection remains and leads to a "chronic," or lifelong, illness. **Chronic** Hepatitis B refers to the illness that occurs when the Hepatitis B virus remains in a person's body. Over time, the infection can cause serious health problems.

In the United States, approximately 1.2 million people have chronic Hepatitis B. Unfortunately, many people do not know they are infected. The number of new cases of Hepatitis B has decreased more than 80% over the last 20 years. An estimated 40,000 people now become infected each year. Many experts believe this decline is a result of widespread vaccination of children.

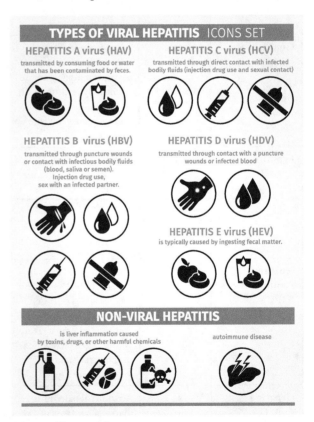

© Leyasw/Shutterstock.com

Hepatitis B is usually spread when blood, semen, or other body fluids from a person infected with the Hepatitis B virus enter the body of someone who is not infected. This can happen through sexual contact with an infected person or sharing needles, syringes, or other injection drug equipment. Hepatitis B can also be passed from an infected mother to her baby at birth.

Hepatitis B is *not* spread through breastfeeding, sharing eating utensils, hugging, kissing, holding hands, coughing, or sneezing. Unlike some forms of hepatitis, Hepatitis B is also not spread by contaminated food or water.

In the United States, Hepatitis B is most commonly spread through sexual contact. The Hepatitis B virus is 50–100 times more infectious than HIV and can be passed through the exchange of body fluids, such as semen, vaginal fluids, and blood.

TABLE 7.1 What Are the Common Sexually Transmitted Infections (STIs)?

STI/D	Pathogen	Symptoms	How Transmitted	Cure?
Herpes	Virus	Fever, headache, blisters at the site of exposure.	Contact with viral shedding at mucus membrane sites.	No, but there are medications to help suppress outbreaks and lesson severity.
Chlamydia	Bacteria	Initially, women in particular may be asymptomatic; painful urination, low back pain; men may experience a discharge.	Vaginal intercourse, oral sex, anal sex and vulva to vulva contact.	Yes, with appropriate antibiotics.
Gonorrhea	Bacteria	Initially for women this is another that may be asymptomatic before eventually leading to PID; men may have discharge, and frequency/urgency of urination.	Vaginal intercourse, oral sex, anal sex and vulva to vulva contact.	Yes, with appropriate antibiotics.
Syphilis	Bacteria	There are 3 stages for syphilis (see chapter for details). Primary, secondary, and tertiary.	Vaginal intercourse, oral sex, anal sex and vulva to vulva contact.	In the first or second stages, yes, with appropriate antibiotics. However, once the third stage has occurred there may be no repairing the damage already done.
Human Papillomavirus (HPV)	Virus	There are more than 40 types of HPV. Depending on the type of infection will determine the symptoms. Some of the strains create wart like growths which may be undetectable if located internally.	Vaginal intercourse, oral sex, anal sex and vulva to vulva contact.	There are various treatments available (see text). There is also a vaccine to help prevent infection.
Hepatitis A, B, C	Virus	Abdominal pain, fatigue, diarrhea, and loss of appetite; jaundice can also appear along with headaches, enlarged liver, and vomiting.	Hep A is typically spread by fecal contaminated food, though it can be spread through anal/oral. Hep B is typically through sexual contact. Hep C can be spread through sexual contact but is more commonly spread through blood transfusions.	There are vaccines for both A and B; treatment is available for all three to reduce viral load and assist the body with an immune response.

STI/D	Pathogen	Symptoms	How Transmitted	Cure?
Pubic Lice "crabs"	Parasite	Itching unless the person infected is not allergic to the insect's saliva.	Contact with person, bedding or clothing infected with lice; they do crawl.	Yes but there are multiple things that must be done to remove the lice and their eggs. There are also creams to help with itching.
Scabies "mites"	Parasite	Rash and intense itching.	Usually spread via skin to skin contact.	Yes but there are multiple things that must be done to remove the lice and their eggs. There are also creams to help with itching.
HIV	Virus	Initial flu like symptoms may appear. However, this virus gradually deteriorates the immune system so additional symptoms will vary (see chapter).	Can be spread through blood, semen, vaginal secretions, breast milk, and perinatal.	There is currently no cure for HIV but there are medications to suppress the viral load.

Courtesy of Shelley Hamill

This chart is designed as a "quick glance" for information on the most common sexually transmitted infections. Further details about each one, along with ways to diagnose, can be found in this chapter.

PARASITIC STIs

Pubic Lice and Scabies

"Pubic lice (often called 'crabs') and scabies (itch mites) are parasitic insects that live on the skin. They are sometimes spread sexually, but are also transmitted by contact with infected bed linens, clothes, or towels. Pubic lice infect hairy parts of the body, especially around the groin area and can be transmitted by fingers to the armpits or scalp (Crooks and Baur, 2009). With scabies, an itchy rash is the result of a female mite burrowing into a person's skin to lay her eggs. The eggs can be seen on the hair close to the skin, where they hatch in five to ten days.

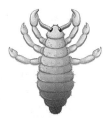

© Matthew Cole /Shutterstock.com

"Some individuals infected with pubic lice have no symptoms, while others may experience considerable itching in the area infected. Yellowish-gray insects the size of a pinhead moving on the skin or oval eggs attached to body hair may be visible. The primary symptom of scabies is itching, especially at night. A rash may appear in the folds of skin between the fingers or on the wrists, elbows, abdomen, or genitals.

"If you think you may have pubic lice or scabies, see your physician. They can determine whether treatment is necessary or not. The most effective treatments include shampoos and creams that contain lindane or a related compound. Pubic lice can be treated at home with special creams, lotions, and shampoos that are available in drugstores without a prescription. Be certain to follow the instructions carefully and do not exceed the recommended applications. The infestation may be stubborn, requiring an additional treatment.

"Avoid close contact with others if you have pubic lice or scabies until it is treated. Wash clothes, bed linens, and any other materials that may have been infected in hot water and dry on the hottest setting. If you have pubic lice or scabies, be sure to tell your sexual partner(s) or anyone with whom you have had close contact or who has shared your bed linens, clothes, or towels. These individuals should be seen by a physician even if they do not have an itch or rash. The best way to protect yourself is to know your partner's sexual history, don't share towels, swimsuits, or underwear and thoroughly wash any materials that you think may carry pubic lice or scabies in hot water."[1]

Trichomoniasis

"Trichomoniasis is caused by a protozoan parasite, Trichomonas vaginalis. The most common sites of infection are the vagina (in women) and the urethra (in men). The parasite is sexually transmitted through the penis to the vagina during intercourse or vulva to vulva contact with an infected partner. Most men infected with trichomoniasis are asymptomatic, but have the parasites and can infect their sexual partners. Some women will have signs or symptoms from the infection which include a yellowish-green vaginal discharge, a slight burning after urination, or itching in the genital area. These signs or symptoms typically appear five to twenty-eight days after exposure. A health care provider must perform a physical exam and laboratory tests to diagnose trichomoniasis. The treatment for trichomoniasis is a prescription drug (either Metronidazole or Tinidazole) taken by mouth in a single dose. It is important for both partners to be treated at the same time to eliminate the parasite. The best way to avoid contracting trichomoniasis is to abstain from vaginal, oral, or anal intercourse or have a mutually monogamous relationship with an uninfected partner. Utilizing male condoms consistently and correctly can reduce the risk of transmission of trichomoniasis."[1]

STI Prevention

There are several ways to avoid or reduce your risk of sexually transmitted infections.

- **Abstain.** The most effective way to avoid STIs is to abstain from sex.
- **Stay with 1 uninfected partner.** Another reliable way of avoiding STIs is to stay in a long-term mutually monogamous relationship with a partner who isn't infected.
- **Wait and verify.** Avoid vaginal and anal intercourse with new partners until you have both been tested for STIs. Oral sex is less risky, but use a latex condom or dental dam—a thin, square piece of rubber made with latex or silicone—to prevent direct contact between the oral and genital mucous membranes. Keep in mind that no good screening test exists for genital herpes for either sex, and human papillomavirus (HPV) screening isn't available for men. Different STI's require different screenings (see Table 7.2).
- **Get vaccinated.** Getting vaccinated early, before sexual exposure, is also effective in preventing certain types of STIs. Vaccines are available to prevent human papillomavirus (HPV), hepatitis A and hepatitis B. The Centers for Disease Control and Prevention (CDC) recommends the HPV vaccine for girls and boys ages 11 and 12. If not fully vaccinated at ages 11 and 12, the CDC recommends that girls and women through age 26 and boys and men through age 26 receive the vaccine. The hepatitis B vaccine is usually given to newborns, and the hepatitis A vaccine is recommended for 1-year-olds. Both vaccines are recommended for people who aren't already immune to these diseases and for those who are at increased risk of infection, such as men who have sex with men and IV drug users.

- **Use condoms and dental dams consistently and correctly.** Use a new latex condom or dental dam for each sex act, whether oral, vaginal or anal. Never use an oil-based lubricant, such as petroleum jelly, with a latex condom or dental dam. Condoms made from natural membranes are not recommended because they're not as effective at preventing STIs. Keep in mind that while condoms reduce your risk of exposure to most STIs, they provide a lesser degree of protection for STIs involving exposed genital sores, such as human papillomavirus (HPV) or herpes. Also, nonbarrier forms of contraception, such as oral contraceptives or intrauterine devices, don't protect against STIs.

- **Don't drink alcohol excessively or use drugs.** If you're under the influence, you're more likely to take sexual risks.

- **Communicate.** Before any serious sexual contact, communicate with your partner about practicing safer sex. Reach an explicit agreement about what activities will and won't be OK.

TABLE 7.2 STI Screenings

STI	Type of Test
Chlamydia	Urine test and/or culture
Genital Herpes	Visual inspection, culture and/or blood test
Gonorrhea	Urine test and/or culture
Hepatitis B	Blood test
HIV	Blood test
HPV	Visual inspection
Pubic Lice/Scabies	Visual inspection
Syphilis	Blood test

Are you a wise consumer?

If you are or plan on becoming sexually active, are you aware of the different types of contraceptive methods that can prevent pregnancy and or sexually transmitted infections (STI's)? How do you know what works best for you? Are you aware of some of the signs and symptoms of STI's? If you have been sexually active, have you ever been tested to see if you might have been infected, as some may be asymptomatic? We are responsible for our own health, as health literate individuals and wise consumers.

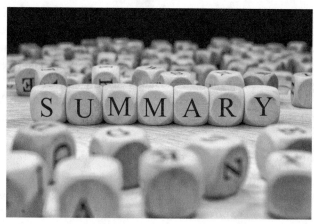

© Fabrik Bilder/Shutterstock.com

Deciding whether you are ready for sexual activity is a very important and personal decision. No one should be pressured in to an action or behavior they are unwilling to engage in nor should they be forced. If you decide the time is right to be sexually active, knowing what forms of protection are available is important. If a pathogen should present itself, knowing where to go and what to do for treatment is equally important.

Personal Reflections . . . so, what have you learned?

1. In your own words, what is the difference in family planning, contraception and birth control?

2. What is the difference between "theoretical effectiveness" and "actual effectiveness"? Do you think most people actually know the difference? Why or why not?

3. Do you agree with the statement "If you are not mature enough to talk about sex, you are not mature enough to have it?" Why or why not?

NOTES

RESOURCES ON CAMPUS FOR YOU!

Health Services

Health Services is designed to provide confidential, professional, quality, cost-effective, acute, and routine medical care for all enrolled students. The staff of Health Services is committed in obtaining optimum personal health for each student through services and programs provided.

Counseling Services

Counseling Services will provide quality mental health service to enhance the overall mental health of students along cognitive, emotional, personal, and interpersonal dimensions.

Office of Victims Assistance

The Office of Victims Assistance is committed to providing quality services and advocacy to victims and survivors of sexual assault, stalking, and domestic and dating violence through a concentrated community response. Support and provide programming and education directed at eradicating sexual violence both on campus and in the community.

Office of Disability Services

The Office of Disability Services helps to create an accessible campus community where students with disabilities have equal opportunity to fully participate in their educational experience.

Wellness Services

Wellness Services provides a collaborative, evidence-based approach to individual and community wellness through health promotion, educational programming, and service to the community. Wellness Services promotes the physical, emotional, social, intellectual, occupational, and spiritual well-being of students by enabling them to make informed choices conducive to healthy lifestyles.

REFERENCES

American Cancer Society. (2005.)

American College Health Association (ACHA). (2005). *Sexually Transmitted Infections: What Everyone Should Know.*

American College Health Association (ACHA). (2004).

American College of Obstetricians and Gynecology (ACOG). (2011).

American Phycology Association (APA) Retrieved January, 5, 2016 from http://www.apa.org/topics/lgbt /orientation.aspx.

American Psychology Association. *Sexual orientation and homosexuality.* Retrieved January 5, 2016 from http://www.apa.org/topics/lgbt/orientation.aspx.

American Social Health Association (ASHA). (2009).

Association of Reproductive Health Professionals (ARHP). (2008). Retrieved from www.arhp.org

Berman, L. (2012) Everyday Health. *Facts about male ejaculation.* Retrieved 2016 from http://www .everydayhealth.com/sexual-health-pictures/dr-laura-berman-male-ejaculation-facts.aspx#19

Blonna, R., & Carter, L.C. (2013). *Healthy sexuality.* Dubuque, IA: Kendall Hunt Publishing Company.

Cedar River Clinics Women's Health Specialist. (2016). *Birth control comparison chart.* Retrieved from http://www.birth-control-comparison.info/

Centers for Disease Control and Prevention (CDC). (2015.) www.cdc.gov/ std/syphilis/STDFact-syphilis .htm www.cdc.gov/std/herpes/STDFact-herpes.htm www.cdc.gov/std/PID/STDFact-PID.htm

Center for Disease Control and Prevention. (2015). *HIV in the United States at a glance.* Retrieved 2016 from http://www.cdc.gov/hiv/statistics/overview/ataglance.html.

Center for Disease Control and Prevention. (2015). *Genital herpes - CDC fact sheet.* Retrieved 2016 from http://www.cdc.gov/std/herpes/stdfact-herpes.htm

Center for Disease Control and Prevention. *Genital HPV infection-fact sheet.* Retrieved 2016 from http://www.cdc.gov/STD/HPV/STDFact-HPV.htm

Centers for Disease Control and Prevention (CDC). (2006). *Guidelines for treatment of sexually transmitted infections.* Retrieved from http://www.cdc.gov/std/treatment/.

Centers for Disease Control and Prevention (CDC). (2016). *Guidelines for treatment of sexually transmitted infections.* Retrieved from http://www.cdc.gov/std/treatment/.

Centers for Disease Control and Prevention. *Hepatitis B.* Retrieved 2016 from http://www.cdc.gov /hepatitis/HBV/PDFs/HepBGeneralFactSheet.pdf

Center for Disease Control and Prevention. (2015). *HIV basics.* Retrieved 2016 from http://www.cdc.gov /hiv/basics

Centers for Disease Control and Prevention (CDC). (2006). *HIV/AIDS surveillance report: Cases of HIV infection and AIDS in the United States and dependent areas.* http://www.cdc.gov/hepatitis/HBV/PDFs/HepBGeneralFactSheet.pdf

Center for Disease Control and Prevention. (2014). *STDs in adolescence and young adults.* Retrieved 2016 from http://www.cdc.gov/std/stats14/adol.htm#foot1.

Centers for Disease Control and Prevention (CDC). (2007). *Youth risk behavior survey.* Retrieved from www.cdc.gov/nchhstp/Newsroom/WADPressrelease-112408.htm

Crooks, R. and Baur, K. (2009). *Our Sexuality* (11th ed). Pacific Grove, CA: Brooks/Cole.

Crowley, L. (2009). *An Introduction to human disease: Pathology and pathophysiology correlations* (8th ed). Boston: Jones and Bartlett Publishers, Inc.

Donatelle, R. (2010). *Access to health* (12th ed). San Francisco: Benjamin Cummings.

Ellertson, C. et al. (2003). Extending the fine limit for starting the Yuzpe regimen of emergency contraception to 120 hours. *Obstetrics and Gynecology,* 101, 1168–1171.

ETR Associates. (2007). *Men's health: What's normal, what's not.*

ETR Associates. (2007). *Not ready for sex: Talking with your partner.*

ETR Associates. (2007). *Women's health: What's normal, what's not.*

ETR Associates. (2008). *Nine sexually responsible behaviors.*

Floyd, P. et al. (2007). *Personal health: perspectives & lifestyles* (4th ed). Englewood, CO: Morton Publishing Co.

Herek, G. et al. (1999). Psychological sequelae of hate-crime victimization among lesbian, gay, and bisexual adults. *Journal of Consulting and Clinical Psychology, 67,* 6.

Huffpost Women. (2013). *Birth control facts: 10 things you should absolutely know.* Retrieved 2016 from http://www.huffingtonpost.com/2013/06/27/birth-control-facts_n_3416638.html

Mayo Clinic. (2014). *Sexually transmitted diseases (STDs).* Retrieved 2016 from http://www.mayoclinic.org/diseases-conditions/sexually-transmitted-diseases-stds/basics/prevention/CON-20034128

Marr, L. (2007). *Sexually transmitted siseases: A physician tells you what you need to know.* (2nd ed). Baltimore: Johns Hopkins University Press.

Sexuality Information and Education Council of the United States (SIECUS). (2008.) Retrieved from www. siecus.org/index.cfm?fuseaction=Page.viewPage+pageId=598+ ParentID=477

Trussell, J. and Jordan, B. (2006). Mechanism of action of emergency contraceptive pills. Contraception, 74, 87–89.

U.S. Department of Health and Human Services. (2004). *Bone health and osteoporosis: A report of the surgeon general.* Retrieved from www.cdc.gov/STD/HPV/STDFact-HPV.htm

www.cdc.gov/vaccines/recs/acip/downloads/mtg-slides-feb08/15-4-hpv.pdf

6 modes of HBV transmission in early childhood. Retrieved from www.fwhc.org/birth-control

CREDITS

Chapter 8   Drugs ╋━━━━━━━━

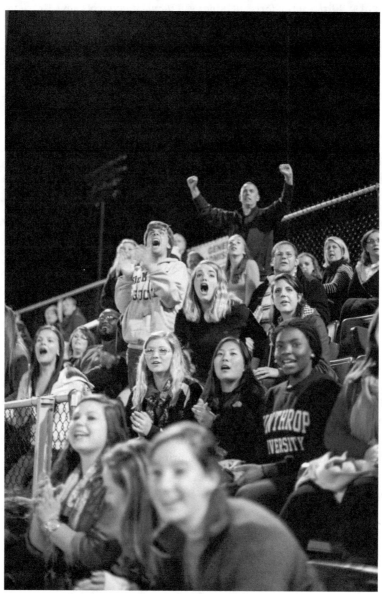

© Winthrop University

Pre-assessment

THINGS TO THINK ABOUT. . .

Tobacco

1. Have you ever tried smoking cigarettes, even one or two puffs?
   A. Yes
   B. No

2. How old were you when you smoked a whole cigarette for the first time?
   A. I have never smoked a whole cigarette
   B. 8 years old or younger
   C. 9 or 10 years old
   D. 11 or 12 years old
   E. 13 or 14 years old
   F. 15 or 16 years old
   G. 17 years old or older

3. During the past 30 days, on how many days did you smoke cigarettes?
   A. 0 days
   B. 1 or 2 days
   C. 3 to 5 days
   D. 6 to 9 days
   E. 10 to 19 days
   F. 20 to 29 days
   G. All 30 days

4. During the past 30 days, on the days you smoked, how many cigarettes did you smoke per day?
   A. I did not smoke cigarettes during the past 30 days
   B. Less than 1 cigarette per day
   C. 1 cigarette per day
   D. 2 to 5 cigarettes per day
   E. 6 to 10 cigarettes per day
   F. 11 to 20 cigarettes per day
   G. More than 20 cigarettes per day

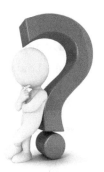

©3dmask
/Shutterstock.com

5. During the past 30 days, how did you usually get your cigarettes? (Select only one response.)

   A. I did not smoke cigarettes during the past 30 days

   B. I bought them in a store such as a convenience store, supermarket, discount store, or gas station

   C. I got them on the Internet

   D. I gave someone else money to buy them for me

   E. I borrowed (or bummed) them from someone else

   F. A person 18 years old or older gave them to me

   G. I took them from a store or family member

   H. I got them some other way

6. During the past 12 months, did you ever try to quit smoking cigarettes?

   A. I did not smoke during the past 12 months

   B. Yes

   C. No

7. During the past 30 days, on how many days did you use chewing tobacco, snuff, or dip, such as Redman, Levi Garrett, Beechnut, Skoal Bandits, or Copenhagen?

   A. 0 days

   B. 1 or 2 days

   C. 3 to 5 days

   D. 6 to 9 days

   E. 10 to 19 days

   F. 20 to 29 days

   G. All 30 days

8. During the past 30 days, on how many days did you smoke cigars, cigarillos, or little cigars?

   A. 0 days

   B. 1 or 2 days

   C. 3 to 5 days

   D. 6 to 9 days

   E. 10 to 19 days

   F. 20 to 29 days

   G. All 30 days

The next 2 questions ask about electronic vapor products, such as blu, NJOY, or Starbuzz. Electronic vapor products include e-cigarettes, e-cigars, e-pipes, vape pipes, vaping pens, ehookahs, and hookah pens.

9. Have you ever used an electronic vapor product?

   A. Yes

   B. No

10. During the past 30 days, on how many days did you use an electronic vapor product?

    A. 0 days

    B. 1 or 2 days

    C. 3 to 5 days

    D. 6 to 9 days

    E. 10 to 19 days

    F. 20 to 29 days

    G. All 30 days

The next 6 questions ask about drinking alcohol. This includes drinking beer, wine, wine coolers, and liquor such as rum, gin, vodka, or whiskey. For these questions, drinking alcohol does not include drinking a few sips of wine for religious purposes.

11. During your life, on how many days have you had at least one drink of alcohol?

    A. 0 days

    B. 1 or 2 days

    C. 3 to 9 days

    D. 10 to 19 days

    E. 20 to 39 days

    F. 40 to 99 days

    G. 100 or more days

12. How old were you when you had your first drink of alcohol other than a few sips?

    A. I have never had a drink of alcohol other than a few sips

    B. 8 years old or younger

    C. 9 or 10 years old

    D. 11 or 12 years old

    E. 13 or 14 years old

    F. 15 or 16 years old

    G. 17 years old or older

13. During the past 30 days, on how many days did you have at least one drink of alcohol?

    A. 0 days

    B. 1 or 2 days

    C. 3 to 5 days

    D. 6 to 9 days

    E. 10 to 19 days

    F. 20 to 29 days

    G. All 30 days

14. During the past 30 days, on how many days did you have 5 or more drinks of alcohol in a row, that is within a couple of hours?

    A. 0 days

    B. 1 day

    C. 2 days

    D. 3 to 5 days

    E. 6 to 9 days

    F. 10 to 19 days

    G. 20 or more days

15. During the past 30 days, what is the largest number of alcoholic drinks you had in a row, that is, within a couple of hours?

    A. I did not drink alcohol during the past 30 days

    B. 1 or 2 drinks

    C. 3 drinks

    D. 4 drinks

    E. 5 drinks

    F. 6 or 7 drinks

    G. 8 or 9 drinks

    H. 10 or more drinks

16. During the past 30 days, how did you usually get the alcohol you drank?

    A. I did not drink alcohol during the past 30 days

    B. I bought it in a store such as a liquor store, convenience store, supermarket, discount store, or gas station

    C. I bought it at a restaurant, bar, or club

    D. I bought it at a public event such as a concert or sporting event

    E. I gave someone else money to buy it for me

    F. Someone gave it to me

    G. I took it from a store or family member

    H. I got it some other way

The next 3 questions ask about marijuana use. Marijuana also is called grass, weed, or pot.

17. During your life, how many times have you used marijuana?

    A. 0 times

    B. 1 or 2 times

    C. 3 to 9 times

    D. 10 to 19 times

    E. 20 to 39 times

    F. 40 to 99 times

    G. 100 or more times

18. How old were you when you tried marijuana for the first time?

    A. I have never tried marijuana

    B. 8 years old or younger

    C. 9 or 10 years old

    D. 11 or 12 years old

    E. 13 or 14 years old

    F. 15 or 16 years old

    G. 17 years old or older

19. During the past 30 days, how many times did you use marijuana?

    A. 0 times

    B. 1 or 2 times

    C. 3 to 9 times

    D. 10 to 19 times

    E. 20 to 39 times

    F. 40 or more times

The next 10 questions ask about other drugs.

20. During your life, how many times have you used any form of cocaine, including powder, crack, or freebase?

    A. 0 times

    B. 1 or 2 times

    C. 3 to 9 times

    D. 10 to 19 times

    E. 20 to 39 times

    F. 40 or more times

21. During your life, how many times have you sniffed glue, breathed the contents of aerosol spray cans, or inhaled any paints or sprays to get high?

    A. 0 times

    B. 1 or 2 times

    C. 3 to 9 times

    D. 10 to 19 times

    E. 20 to 39 times

    F. 40 or more times

22. During your life, how many times have you used heroin (also called smack, junk, or China White)?

    A. 0 times

    B. 1 or 2 times

    C. 3 to 9 times

    D. 10 to 19 times

    E. 20 to 39 times

    F. 40 or more times

23. During your life, how many times have you used methamphetamines (also called speed, crystal, crank, or ice)?

    A. 0 times

    B. 1 or 2 times

    C. 3 to 9 times

    D. 10 to 19 times

    E. 20 to 39 times

    F. 40 or more times

24. During your life, how many times have you used ecstasy (also called MDMA)?

    A. 0 times

    B. 1 or 2 times

    C. 3 to 9 times

    D. 10 to 19 times

    E. 20 to 39 times

    F. 40 or more times

25. During your life, how many times have you used synthetic marijuana (also called K2, Spice, fake weed, King Kong, Yucatan Fire, Skunk, or Moon Rocks)?

    A. 0 times

    B. 1 or 2 times

    C. 3 to 9 times

    D. 10 to 19 times

    E. 20 to 39 times

    F. 40 or more times

26. During your life, how many times have you taken steroid pills or shots without a doctor's prescription?

    A. 0 times

    B. 1 or 2 times

    C. 3 to 9 times

    D. 10 to 19 times

    E. 20 to 39 times

    F. 40 or more times

27. During your life, how many times have you taken a prescription drug (such as OxyContin, Percocet, Vicodin, codeine, Adderall, Ritalin, or Xanax) without a doctor's prescription?

    A. 0 times

    B. 1 or 2 times

    C. 3 to 9 times

    D. 10 to 19 times

    E. 20 to 39 times

    F. 40 or more times

28. During your life, how many times have you used a needle to inject any illegal drug into your body?

    A. 0 times

    B. 1 time

    C. 2 or more times

29. During the past 12 months, has anyone offered, sold, or given you an illegal drug on school property?

    A. Yes

    B. No

These questions were adapted from the National Youth Risk Behavior Survey (CDC, 2015).

Chapter 8 +

Tobacco, Alcohol and Other Drugs

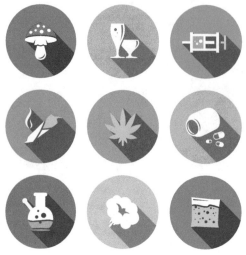

© Steinar/Shutterstock.com

OBJECTIVES:

Students will be able to:

- Identify types of tobacco products and the adverse effects associated with each.
- Discuss the concerns with E cigarettes.
- "Identify types of alcoholic beverages and the alcohol content for each.
- "Identify the physiological and societal effects of alcohol.
- "Identify risks of drinking and driving.
- "Identify factors relating to binge drinking and alcohol poisoning.
- "Identify common sources of caffeine.
- "Identify types of drugs and their physiological effects.
- "Identify the adverse effects of club drugs
- "Identify commonly abused prescription drugs.

'First we form habits, and then they form us. Conquer your bad habits, or they'll eventually conquer you.' –Rob Gilbert"[1]

INTRODUCTION

"America has always had some opposition to the non-medicinal use of drugs. Alcohol and tobacco created outcries throughout the country during colonial times and through the Civil War, which provoked prohibition legislation. Warnings of alcohol and tobacco use did not seem to deter the prevalence in American society.

"Early prohibitionists were the precursors to the twentieth century 'war on drugs' but it was hard to categorize the variety of substances until Congress passed The Controlled Substance Act in 1970. Richard Evans, a Professor from the University of Houston, created a model that included teaching students to resist social influences and peer pressure. The slogan 'Just Say No' was adopted and the National Institutes of Health supported this model. This program that emerged from the substance abuse model created by Evans became a campaign throughout college campuses. First Lady Nancy Reagan became involved in the program in 1980 during her husband's presidency. This campaign had a positive outcome with a significant decline in drug use during the late 70's and 80's. However, illicit drug use continues to rise in our country. The World Health Organization's survey of legal and illegal drug use in 17 countries, including the Netherlands and other countries with less stringent drug laws shows Americans report the highest level of cocaine and marijuana use. Despite tough anti-drug laws, this survey shows the U.S. has the highest level of illegal drug use in the world.

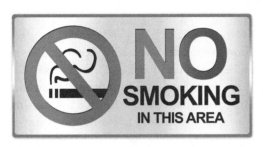

© DeiMosz/Shutterstock.com

'Understanding what drugs can do to your children, understanding peer pressure and understanding why they turn to drugs is . . . the first step in solving the problem.' Nancy Reagan"[1]

TOBACCO

"The U.S. Surgeon General reported in 1970 that cigarette smoking is dangerous to your health. Over the years we have come to realize just how dangerous."[1] According to the Center for Disease Control (CDC), tobacco use remains the single largest preventable cause of death and disease in the United States. Cigarette smoking kills more than 480,000 Americans each year, with more than 41,000 of these deaths from exposure to secondhand smoke.1 In addition, smoking-related illness in the United States costs more than $300 billion a year, including nearly $170 billion in direct medical care for adults and $156 billion in lost productivity (CDC, 2015).

Tobacco use is started and established primarily during adolescence. Nearly 9 out of 10 cigarette smokers first tried smoking by age 18, and 99% first tried smoking by age 26. If smoking continues at the current rate among youth in this country, 5.6 million of today's Americans younger than 18 will die early from a smoking-related illness. That's about one of every 13 Americans aged 17 years or younger alive today (CDC).

Tobacco Components

"The toxic components of tobacco include tar, nicotine, and carbon monoxide. **Tar** is a by-product of burning tobacco. Its composition is a dark, sticky substance that can be condensed from cigarette smoke. Tar contains many potent carcinogens and chemicals that irritate tissue in the lungs and promote chronic bronchitis and emphysema. These substances paralyze and destroy the cilia that line the bronchi, causing 'smoker's cough.' Long-term exposure of extremely toxic tar to lung tissue can lead to the development of cancer."[1]

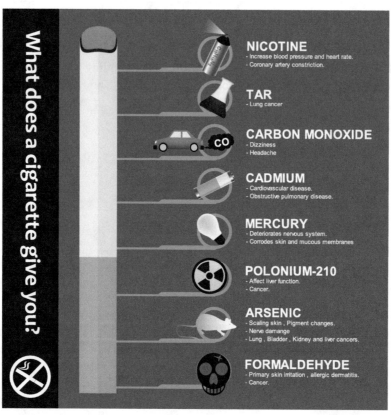

© Wikrom Kitsamritchai/Shutterstock.com

"**Nicotine** is a colorless, oily compound that is extremely poisonous in concentrated amounts. This highly addictive drug is a major contributor to heart and respiratory diseases causing short-term increases in blood pressure, heart rate, and blood flow from the heart, resulting in narrowing of the arteries. A strong dependence on nicotine can occur after as little as three packs of cigarettes, and it is more addictive than cocaine or heroin. Because of its addictive effects, the Food and Drug Administration (FDA) has determined nicotine should be regulated.

"At first, nicotine acts as a stimulant and then it tends to tranquilize the nervous system. The effects depend largely on how one chooses to smoke. Shallow puffs seem to increase alertness because low doses of nicotine facilitate the release of acetylcholine, which creates feelings of alertness. Long, deep drags tend to relax the smoker because high doses of nicotine block the flow of acetylcholine. Ninety percent of the nicotine inhaled while smoking is absorbed into the body, while 20 to 30 percent of nicotine is absorbed if the smoke is drawn only into the mouth, not the lungs.

"Other side effects include inhibiting formation of urine, discoloration of the fingers, dulling the taste buds, and irritating the membranes in the mouth and throat. Because nicotine constricts blood vessels, it causes the skin to be clammy and have a pallid appearance, as well as reducing body temperature. The highly addictive nature of nicotine can cause withdrawal symptoms to occur quite suddenly. These symptoms include irritability, anxiousness, hostility, food cravings, headaches, and the inability to concentrate. Carbon monoxide is an odorless, tasteless gas that is highly toxic. It reduces the amount of oxygen the blood can carry, causing shortness of breath.

"**Cigarette smoking** greatly impairs the respiratory system and is a major cause of chronic obstructive pulmonary diseases (COPD), including emphysema and chronic bronchitis. Problems associated with cigarette smoking include mouth, throat, and other types of cancer, cirrhosis of the liver, stomach, duodenal ulcers, gum and dental disease, decreased HDL cholesterol and decreased platelet survival and clotting time, as well as increased blood thickness. Cigarette smoking increases problems such as heart disease, atherosclerosis, and blood clots. It increases the amount of fatty acids, glucose, and various hormones in the blood, cardiac arrhythmia, allergies, diabetes, hypertension, peptic ulcers, and sexual impotence. Smoking doubles the risk of heart disease, and those who smoke have only a 50 percent chance of recovery. Smokers also have a 70 percent higher death rate from heart disease than non-smokers (CDC, 2006). Smoking also causes cardiomyopathy, a condition that weakens the heart's ability to pump blood.

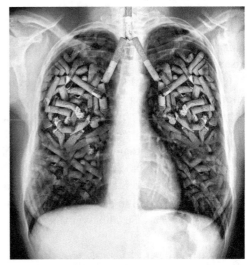

© Protasov AN/Shutterstock.com

"Life expectancy of smokers parallels smoking habits in that the younger one starts smoking and the longer one smokes, the higher the mortality rate. Also, the deeper smoke is inhaled and the higher the tar and nicotine content, the higher the mortality rate. On average, smokers die 13–14 years earlier than non-smokers (CDC, 2012). The risk and mortality rates for lip, mouth, and larynx cancers for **pipe and cigar smoking** are higher than for cigarette smoking. Pipe smoke, which is 2 percent carbon monoxide, is more irritating to the respiratory system than cigarette smoking, but for those who do not inhale, the risk for developing cancer is just as likely. Cigars have recently gained popularity in the United States among younger men and women with approximately 4.5 billion cigars consumed yearly."[1]

Electronic cigarettes, or e-cigarettes, are battery-powered devices that provide doses of nicotine and other additives to the user in an aerosol. Depending on the brand, e-cigarette cartridges typically contain nicotine, a component to produce the aerosol (e.g., propylene glycol or glycerol), and flavorings (e.g., fruit, mint, or chocolate) (1). Potentially harmful constituents also have been documented in some e-cigarette cartridges, including irritants, genotoxins, and animal carcinogens. E-cigarettes that are not marketed for therapeutic purposes are currently unregulated by the Food and Drug Administration, and in most states there are no restrictions on the sale of e-cigarettes to minors. Use of e-cigarettes has increased among U.S. adult current and former smokers in recent years however, the extent of use among youths is uncertain.

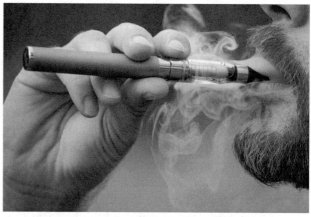

© Marc Bruxelle/Shutterstock.com

Kretekes, sometimes referred to as clove cigarettes are "erroneously believed to be safer because they do not contain as much tobacco. In actuality, clove cigarettes are most harmful because they contain **eugenol**, which is an active ingredient of clove. Eugenol deadens sensations in the throat, which allows smokers to inhale more deeply and hold smoke in the lungs longer. Kretekes also contain twice as much tar, nicotine, and carbon monoxide as most moderate brands of American cigarettes."[1]

Bidis are small, thin, hand-rolled cigarettes imported to the United States, primarily from India and other Southeast Asian countries. They comprise tobacco wrapped in a tendu or temburni leaf (plants native to Asia) and may be secured with a colorful string at one or both ends. Bidis can be flavored (e.g., chocolate, cherry, mango) or unflavored (CDC). Though their use is relatively low in the United States, those who do partake are inhaling three to five times the amount of nicotine as regular cigarette users and increasing both the risks of addiction and chronic diseases associated with tobacco use (CDC).

Hookahs are water pipes that are used to smoke specially made tobacco that is usually flavored. They are also called a number of different names, including waterpipe, narghile, argileh, shisha, hubble-bubble, and goza. Hookah smoking is typically practiced in groups, with the same mouthpiece passed from person to person.

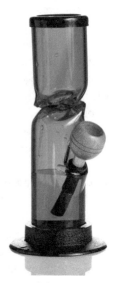

Similar to cigarettes, hookah smoking delivers the addictive drug nicotine and it is at least as toxic as cigarette smoking. While many hookah smokers may consider this practice less harmful than smoking cigarettes, hookah smoking carries many of the same health risks as cigarettes.

In recent years, there has been an increase in hookah use around the world, most notably among youth and college students. The Monitoring the Future survey found that in 2014, about 23% of 12th grade students in the United States had used hookahs in the past year, up from 17% in 2010. In 2014, this rate was slightly higher among boys (25%) than girls (21%). CDC's National Youth Tobacco Survey found that from 2013 to 2014, hookah smoking roughly doubled for middle and high school students in the United States. Current hookah use among high school students rose from 5.2% (770,000) to 9.4% (1.3 million) and for middle school students from 1.1% (120,000) to 2.5% (280,000) over this period.

© Yurchyks
/Shutterstock.com

Environmental Tobacco Smoke

"Environmental tobacco smoke (ETS), or secondhand smoke, contains more than 7,000 chemicals, including hundreds that are toxic and 70 carcinogens. Secondhand smoke exposure to non-smoking adults can cause heart disease, a 20–30 percent increased risk of lung cancer, and a 25–30 percent increased risk of heart attacks. Approximately 126 million non-smokers are exposed to secondhand smoke in homes,

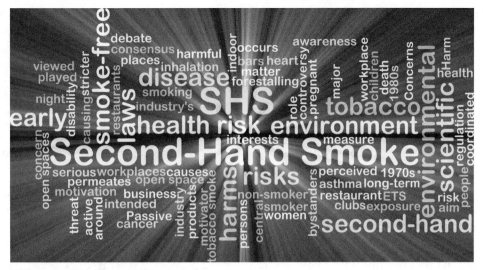

© Kheng Guan Toh/Shutterstock.com

workplaces, and public places, resulting in an estimated 38,000 deaths and healthcare costs exceeding $10 billion annually. To those individuals with existing health issues, second-hand smoke exposure is an extremely high risk. There is no 'risk-free' exposure to secondhand smoke; even brief exposure can be dangerous (CDC, 2006). Secondhand smoke is especially dangerous to infants and children. In the United States, almost 22 million children are exposed to secondhand smoke. Globally almost half of the world's children breathe air polluted by tobacco smoke. This exposure can cause sudden infant death syndrome, acute respiratory infections, ear problems, slow lung growth, and severe asthma attacks. Each year in the United States, secondhand smoke is responsible for an estimated 150,000–300,000 new cases of bronchitis and pneumonia in children less than 18 months, resulting in nearly 15,000 hospitalizations annually (CDC, 2012)."[1]

Smoking Cessation

"Each year an estimated 1.3 million smokers quit successfully. More than four out of five smokers say they want to quit (AHA, 2006). Although there are various pharmacological agents used to aid smokers in quitting, nicotine replacement therapy has been shown to be the most effective. The transdermal nicotine patch is safe, as well as nicotine gum, although the patch appears to be preferred by most. In addition to the patch and gum, a nicotine nasal spray and nicotine inhalers are also available.

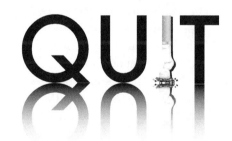

© Jane Rix/Shutterstock.com

"Of the 46 million Americans who currently smoke cigarettes, most are either actively trying to quit or want to quit (CDC, 2012). Quitting can bring a major reduction in the occurrence of coronary heart disease and other forms of cardio-vascular diseases. Quitting reduces the risk for repeat heart attacks and death from heart disease by 50 percent or more (CDC, 2012). Quitting can also aid in the management of contributors to heart attacks such as atherosclerosis, thrombosis, and cardiac arrhythmia.

"The American Heart Association (AHA) reports that after one year off cigarettes, risk for heart attacks is reduced by 50 percent. After fifteen years of abstinence from smoking, your risks are similar to that of a person who never smoked. In five to fifteen years of being smoke-free, the risk of stroke is the same as for non-smokers. The National Center for Chronic Disease Prevention and Control (part of the CDC) has shown that these five steps will help you quit and quit for good. You have the best chance if you use these together:"[1]

1. "Get ready—set a quit date, get rid of all your cigarettes, do not let people smoke in your home; once you quit, do not smoke!

2. "Get support and encouragement—tell family, friends, and co-workers. Ask them not to smoke around you.

3. "Learn new skills and behaviors—change your routine, get busy with new tasks, reduce stress."[1]

4. "Get medication and use it correctly—ask your healthcare provider for advice; FDA approved medications."[1] Gum, nicotine patches, inhalers, spray, and prescription drugs are current options to assist those wishing to quit smoking.

5. "Be prepared for relapse or difficult situations—most relapses occur within the first three months after quitting. Don't be discouraged, most people try several times before they finally quit. Keep trying! For more information, visit smokefree.gov."[1]

"There is some irreversible damage to virtually every organ system in the body. There are dangers from smoking that remain even after quitting. Although it is never too late to quit smoking, the damage that has been done may never entirely disappear. It is best to choose to never light up! For more information on smoking and the health problems associated with tobacco products, contact these agencies:"[1]

Smokeless tobacco is not a safe alternative to cigarette smoking. It comes in multiple forms: chewing tobacco (loose leaf, plug or twists and may be flavored); snuff (moist, dry, or in packets); and dissolvables (lozenges, strips, stick, or orbs). Users place the tobacco product in their mouth and typically suck on the tobacco juices, spitting out the saliva. The sucking allows the nicotine to be absorbed in the bloodstream. This can be equally as dangerous and harmful. Just as cigarette smoking is addictive, so is smokeless tobacco. "According to the Centers for Disease Control and Prevention (CDC) estimates, 5.5% percent of high school students are current smokeless tobacco users (CDC, 2014)."[1]

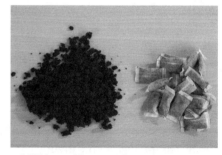

© bildfokus.se/Shutterstock.com

"The National Cancer Institute reports there are three thousand chemical compounds in smokeless tobacco. Nicotine is the addictive drug in all forms of tobacco. Holding one pinch of smokeless tobacco in your mouth for thirty minutes delivers as much nicotine as three to four cigarettes (National Cancer Institute, 2011)."[1]

"**There have been at least twenty-eight cancer-causing agents found in smokeless tobacco:**

- Nitrosamines—20 to 43,000 more nitrosamines are found in smokeless tobacco. Other consumer products like beer or bacon only contain five parts per billion

- Polonium 210—radioactive particles that turn into radon

- Formaldehyde—embalming fluid

- Cadmium—metallic element; its salts are poisonous

- Arsenic—poisonous element"[1]

"Immediate effects from chewing tobacco are bad breath and stains on your teeth. Mouth sores also accompany smokeless tobacco users. The complications of long-term use can be very serious. These

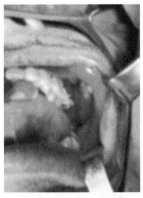

© ScofieldZa/Shutterstock.com

complications include increased gum and teeth problems, increased heart rate, irregular heartbeat, heart attacks, and cancer. Oral cancer can occur in the mouth, lips, tongue, cheeks, or gums. Other cancer possibilities resulting from smokeless tobacco can be stomach cancer, bladder cancer, and cancer of the esophagus.

"Another major problem caused by smokeless tobacco is **leukoplakia**, a precancerous condition that produces thick, rough white patches on the gums, tongue, and inner cheeks. A variety of cancers such as lip, pharynx, larynx, esophagus, and tongue can be attributed to smokeless tobacco. Dental and gum problems are major side effects as well. Smokeless tobacco used during pregnancy increases the risk for preeclampsia, a condition that includes high blood pressure, fluid retention, and swelling. It also puts the mother and newborn at higher risk for premature birth and low birth weight. In men, smokeless tobacco reduces sperm count and increases the likelihood of abnormal sperm cell (CDC, 2010)."[1]

ALCOHOL

Approximately 52.7% of Americans age twelve and over (139.7 million people) reported being current drinkers in the 2014 National Survey on Drug Use and Health (SAMHSA, 2015). "**Ethyl alcohol**, or ethanol, has been prevalent in our society for centuries. Except for the Prohibition Era in the United States from 1917 to 1932 when alcohol was considered an illegal substance, it has become the legal and accepted drug of choice. There are three major types of alcoholic beverages: distilled spirits (hard liquor), wine or wine coolers, and beer."[1]

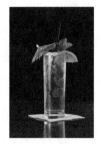

© Wollertz/ Shutterstock.com

"Distilled spirits include scotch, gin, rum, vodka, tequila, and whiskey. The alcohol content varies according to the proof of the beverage, which is twice the percent of alcohol. For example, if whiskey is 80 proof, then that particular beverage is 40 percent alcohol by volume. The average mixed drink contains a one-ounce shot of hard liquor."[1] Of course, some mixed drinks have multiple shots of hard liquor. A "Long Island Ice Tea" for example may have 4–5 shots of different liquors making one drink the equivalent of 4–5 drinks!

"Wine usually averages 12 percent alcohol by volume, and wine coolers average approximately 5 percent alcohol by volume. The average glass of wine is four ounces, and wine coolers are usually served in twelve-ounce bottles."[1]

"Beer is usually served in twelve-ounce cans or bottles, although some pubs sell pints, which are 16 ounces. The average alcohol content of beer is 4.5 percent by volume. To be considered a beer, the alcohol content must not exceed 5 percent by weight and volume. If the amount of alcohol is greater, it is considered ale."[1] **Craft beer** has become a booming industry. According to Fortune.com (2015), 1 out of every 10 beers sold is a craft beer. The average alcohol content of craft beer is 5.9 percent. However, that number is increasing. According consumer research group Mintel, the amount of beers released with more than 6.5 percent alcohol by volume increased by 319 percent in North America from 2011 to 2014, with 46 percent of new beer releases falling into this category (CNN.com, 2015).

Physiological Effects

"Alcohol is a drug that has two major effects on the body. Being a depressant, it slows down the nervous system (respiratory and cardiovascular systems). Alcohol and its by-products also irritate the nerve endings and eventually sedate or deaden them. Vision is another sense that alcohol affects quickly. This is an important ability for driving because 90 percent of the information we receive is obtained through vision. Alcohol has a direct effect on our vision by causing the loss of fine muscle control in the eyes accounting for eye focus, visual acuity, peripheral vision, color distinction, night vision, distance judgment, and double vision (Dennis and the Texas Commission on Alcohol and Drug Abuse, 2005). Other physiological effects are impaired mental and physical reflexes, increased risk of diseases such as cancer of the brain, tongue, mouth, esophagus, larynx, liver, and the bladder. Heart and blood pressure problems are also associated with alcohol consumption."[1]

Blood Alcohol Concentration (BAC)

"BAC is a measure of the concentration of alcohol in blood, expressed in grams per 100 milliliter. An example would be 100 milligrams of alcohol in 10 milliliter of blood would be reported as .10 percent. The higher the alcohol content of the drink, the higher BAC it will produce.

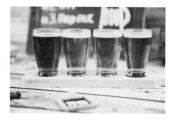

© MaxyM/Shutterstock.com

"Factors influencing a person's BAC are body weight, alcohol content of the drink, size of the drink, time spent drinking, and food. Gender is also a factor in determining one's BAC. Women do not process alcohol as well as men because of the enzyme alcohol dehydrogenase, which breaks down alcohol. Men produce more alcohol dehydrogenase than women; therefore, men can eliminate alcohol at a slightly faster rate (Dennis and the Texas Commission on Alcohol and Drug Abuse, 2005). Women also have less water content, so a woman at the same weight as a man will have a higher BAC. The higher alcohol content of a drink, the higher BAC it will produce. For example, a one-ounce shot of a 100 proof beverage has more alcohol than a one-ounce shot of an 80 proof beverage. The larger an alcoholic drink, the more alcohol it will contain and produce a higher BAC. For example, a twenty-four ounce beer will have twice the amount of alcohol of a twelve-ounce beer. The liver begins to process alcohol shortly after it is absorbed into the bloodstream. The longer time factor will result in a lower BAC. For example, if a person drinks a six-pack in three hours, they will have a lower BAC than if they had consumed a six-pack in one hour. Having food in the stomach may coat the lining of the stomach, therefore slowing down the absorption of alcohol. However, food will not absorb or soak up the alcohol, so the alcohol will eventually reach the bloodstream.

"There are three ways that alcohol is removed or eliminated from the body. Ninety percent of alcohol is eliminated through the oxidation process of the liver at .015 percent per hour. The alcohol dehydrogenase then converts alcohol to acetaldehyde. Alcohol is then metabolized at approximately .25 to .30 ounces per hour, regardless of the blood alcohol concentration. The rate of metabolism is

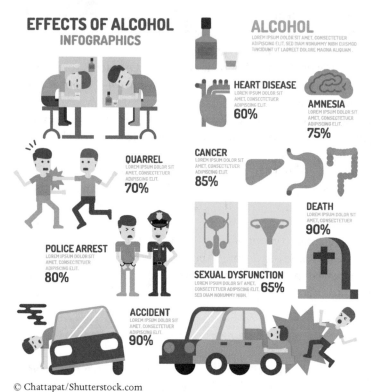

EFFECTS OF ALCOHOL
INFOGRAPHICS

ALCOHOL
LOREM IPSUM DOLOR SIT AMET, CONSECTETUER
ADIPISCING ELIT. SED DIAM NONUMMY NIBH EUISMOD
TINCIDUNT UT LAOREET DOLORE MAGNA ALIQUAM.

HEART DISEASE
LOREM IPSUM DOLOR SIT
AMET, CONSECTETUER
ADIPISCING ELIT.
60%

AMNESIA
LOREM IPSUM DOLOR SIT
AMET, CONSECTETUER
ADIPISCING ELIT.
75%

QUARREL
LOREM IPSUM DOLOR SIT
AMET, CONSECTETUER
ADIPISCING ELIT.
70%

CANCER
LOREM IPSUM DOLOR SIT
AMET, CONSECTETUER
ADIPISCING ELIT.
85%

DEATH
LOREM IPSUM DOLOR SIT
AMET, CONSECTETUER
90%

POLICE ARREST
LOREM IPSUM DOLOR SIT
AMET, CONSECTETUER
ADIPISCING ELIT.
80%

SEXUAL DYSFUNCTION
LOREM IPSUM DOLOR SIT AMET,
CONSECTETUER ADIPISCING ELIT.
SED DIAM NONUMMY NIBH. **65%**

ACCIDENT
LOREM IPSUM DOLOR SIT
AMET, CONSECTETUER
ADIPISCING ELIT.
90%

© Chattapat/Shutterstock.com

based on the activity of alcohol dehydrogenase, working at its own pace (Ray and Kisr, 1999). Eight percent of alcohol is eliminated through breath, which is why a breath test is used to determine BAC. A small amount of alcohol, approximately 2 percent, is eliminated through sweat. For the average individual, elimination will reduce a given blood alcohol concentration by .015 per hour. Contrary to popular belief, cold showers, black coffee, aspirin, or exercise will not speed up this elimination process."[1]

Tolerance is when an individual adapts to the amount consumed so that larger quantities are needed to achieve the same effect. (This can apply to alcohol as well as other drugs). "This can take place over several months or years of consuming alcohol, depending on the amount consumed and at what age the individual begins to drink. At some point, after a person's tolerance has increased over a period of time, it begins to drop, allowing the effects of alcohol to be felt after only a few drinks. This reverse tolerance is caused by the natural aging process or liver disease after years of abusive drinking (Dennis and the Texas Commission Alcohol and Drug Abuse, 2005). **Intoxication** is defined as a transient state of physical and mental disruption due to the presence of a toxic substance, such as alcohol (Maisto, 2005). As BAC increases, the central nervous system alters behavior and physical function. Change can occur as low as .02 BAC in some people, while everyone is impaired to some degree at .05 BAC."[1]

Societal Problems

"The dangers of alcohol consumption are a major problem in our society. Drinking too much alcohol can cause a range of very serious problems, in addition to the obvious health issues. Alcohol is a contributing factor in motor vehicle accidents, violence, and school/work problems, as well as family problems."[1]

Drinking and Driving

The National Highway Traffic Safety Administration (NHTSA) reported in 2013 that 10,076 people were killed in alcohol impaired driving crashes. This is 31 percent of the nation's total traffic fatalities for the year and represents one alcohol-impaired driving fatality every 52 minutes. In 2013, the 21–24 age group had the highest percentage of drivers in fatal crashes. The rate of alcohol impairment among drivers involved in fatal crashes in 2013 was nearly four times higher at night than during the day (NHTSA).

"Drunk driving is no accident; it is a crime. The greatest tragedy is that these crashes are preventable, predictable, and 100 percent avoidable. Although most drivers involved in fatal crashes have no prior convictions for DUI, about one-third of all drivers arrested for driving under the influence are repeat offenders, which

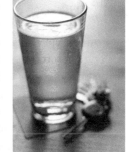

© Arjuna Kodisinghe /Shutterstock.com

greatly increases their risk of causing a drunk driving accident. As a nation, we have seen a downward trend in alcohol-related fatalities. Today, all states have lowered their legal level of intoxication to .08 BAC. All states have some form of the zero tolerance law, as well as an open container law. These laws, in addition to stricter enforcement of existing laws, have helped in changing behavior. High school and university education programs, such as non-alcoholic activities for prom nights and designated driver organizations, have also contributed in raising awareness to combat such a serious problem."[1]

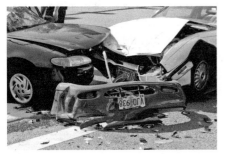

© TFoxFoto/Shutterstock.com

"The NHTSA and the Advertising Council's Innocent Victims public service campaign stresses the need to get the keys from someone who is about to drive.

Here are some tips:

- If it is a close friend, try to use a soft, calm approach. Suggest to them that they have had too much to drink and it would be better if someone else drove, or call a cab.
- Be calm. Joke about it. Make light of it.
- Try to make it sound like you are doing them a favor.
- If it is somebody you do not know well, speak to their friends; usually they will listen.
- If it is a good friend, tell them if they insist on driving, you are not going with them.
- Locate their keys while they are preoccupied and take them away. Mostly they will think they lost them and will be forced to find another mode of transportation.
- Avoid embarrassing the person or being confrontational."[1]

Alcohol Use in College

"The legal drinking age in all states is 21 years old, but that does not mean individuals under 21 do not consume alcohol. Studies suggest that substance use, including alcohol, tobacco, and other drug use, is common among college-aged youth. Students who use any of these substances are at significantly greater risk than non-substance using peers to: drive after drinking and with a driver who has been drinking, and are less likely to use a seatbelt. These consistently poor and risky choices increase their risk of being in a motor vehicle crash and having crash-related injuries (Everett, 1999). College students and ad-

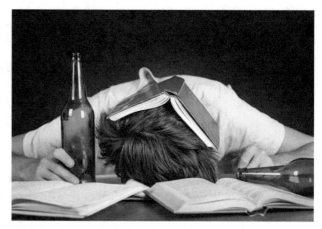

© Sabphoto/Shutterstock.com

ministrators struggle with the problems associated with alcohol abuse, binge drinking, and drunk driving. These actions put students at risk for many serious problems, such as date rape violence and possibly death.

"The National Institute on Alcohol Abuse and Alcoholism (NIAAA) reports that 1,825 college students die annually from alcohol-related unintentional injuries, including motor vehicle crashes, with 3.36 million students driving under the influence of alcohol. Another 599,000 between the ages of 18 and 24 are injured, and approximately 690,000 students per year are assaulted by a drinking student. Also, approximately 400,000 students between 18 and 24 years old reported having unprotected sex as a result of drinking. More than 97,000 students are victims of alcohol-related sexual assault or date rape (NIAAA, 2015)."[1]

About 23% of college students report academic consequences of their drinking including missing class, falling behind, doing poorly on exams or papers, and receiving lower grades overall. "More than 150,000 college students develop an alcohol-related health problem, with 1.5 percent attempting suicide because of alcohol (NIAAA, 2015)."[1]

Binge Drinking

"College presidents agree that **binge drinking** is the most serious problem on campus. The National Institute on Alcohol Abuse and Alcoholism defines **binge drinking** as a pattern of drinking that brings a person's blood alcohol concentration to .08 or above. This typically happens when men consume five or more drinks and women consume four or more drinks in about two hours (NIAAA, 2010)."[1] According to a national survey, almost 60% of college students ages 18–22 drank alcohol in the past month and almost 2 out of 3 of them engaged in binge drinking during that same time frame (SAMSA 2014).

"Binge drinkers usually experience more alcohol-related problems than their non-drinking counterparts. These problems affect their health, education, safety, and interpersonal relationships. According to the Harvard School of Public Health College Alcohol Study, these problems include driving after drinking, damaging property, getting injured, missing classes, and getting behind in school work. According to the same Harvard study, one in five students surveyed experienced five or more different alcohol-related problems and more than one-third of the students reported driving after drinking.

"The study also found that the vast majority of non-binge drinking students are negatively affected by the behavior of binge drinkers. It was reported that four out of five students who were non-binge drinkers and who lived on campus experienced secondary effects of binge drinking such as being the victim of a sexual assault or an unwanted sexual advance, having property vandalized, and having sleep or study interrupted."[1]

Did you know . . .

Binge Drinking

According to the National Institute on Alcohol Abuse and Alcoholism:

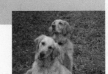
Courtesy of Shelley Hamill

- **Death:** 1,825 college students between the ages of 18 and 24 die each year from alcohol-related unintentional injuries.
- **Assault:** More than 690,000 students between the ages of 18 and 24 are assaulted by another student who has been drinking.
- **Sexual Abuse:** More than 97,000 students between the ages of 18 and 24 are victims of alcohol-related sexual assault or date rape.
- **Injury:** 599,000 students between the ages of 18 and 24 receive unintentional injuries while under the influence of alcohol.
- **Academic Problems:** About 25 percent of college students report academic consequences of their drinking including missing class, falling behind, doing poorly on exams or papers, and receiving lower grades overall.
- **Health Problems/Suicide Attempts:** More than 150,000 students develop an alcohol-related health problem and between 1.2 and 1.5 percent of students indicate that they tried to commit suicide within the past year due to drinking or drug use.

Alcohol Poisoning

"The most serious consequence of binge drinking is alcohol poisoning. This results when an overdose of alcohol is consumed. When excessive amounts of alcohol are consumed, the brain is deprived of oxygen, which causes it to shut down the breathing and heart rate functions. Many think that the only deadly mix is alcohol and driving, but an alcohol overdose can be lethal. It can happen to anyone."[1]

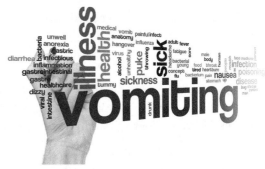
© ibreakstock/Shutterstock.com

"Some symptoms of alcohol poisoning are:

- Person does not respond to talking, shouting, or being shaken.
- Person cannot stand up.
- Person has slow, labored, or abnormal breathing—less than eight breaths/minute or ten or more seconds between each breath.
- Person's skin feels clammy.
- Person has a rapid pulse rate and irregular heart rhythm.
- Person has lowered blood pressure.
- Vomiting"[1]

"If you think a friend is experiencing alcohol poisoning, seek medical attention immediately"[1] by calling 911. (**The Good Samaritan** law protects individuals who offer assistance to someone in danger from prosecution. Winthrop University supports that law and urges individuals to seek help should an overdose occur).You should stay "with the person until help arrives. Turn the victim onto one side in case of vomiting. Choking to death on one's own vomit after an alcohol overdose is quite common. Death by asphyxiation occurs when alcohol depresses and inhibits the gag reflex to the point that the person cannot vomit properly. **Do not leave the victim alone.** Be honest in telling medical staff exactly how much alcohol the victim consumed. This is an extreme medical emergency and one that is a matter of life and death."[1]

"Colleges are attempting to make progress in preventing some of these problems. Many sororities and fraternities as well as other student organizations have taken action by banning alcohol at many functions. By implementing alcohol awareness programs, stronger hazing policies, and tougher enforcements on drinking violations and alcohol restrictions on campus and with the student body, some of these tragedies may be prevented."[1]

Drinking Problems

In 2013, 86.8 percent of people ages 18 or older reported they drank alcohol at some point in their lifetime; 70.7 percent of those reported that they drank in the past year; 56.4 reported that they drank in the past month (NIAA, 2015). "The National Institute on Alcohol Abuse and Alcoholism (NIAAA) found that the earlier young people begin to drink alcohol, the more likely they are to become an alcohol abuser or alcoholic. According to the report:

- Young people who start drinking before age 15 are four times more likely to become an alcoholic than if they start after age 21.
- Forty percent who drink before age 15 become alcohol dependent; 10 percent if they wait until 21.
- Fourteen percent decreased risk of alcoholism for each year drinking is delayed until age 21."[1]

Alcoholism

"**Alcoholism**, also known as alcohol dependence, is a chronic, progressive disease with symptoms that include a strong need to drink and continued drinking despite repeated negative alcohol-related consequences. There are four symptoms generally associated with alcoholism:

1. a craving or a strong need to drink,
2. impaired control or the inability to limit one's drinking,

3. a physical dependence accompanied by withdrawal symptoms such as nausea, sweating, shakiness, and anxiety when alcohol use is stopped, and

4. an increased tolerance.

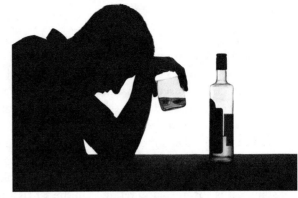

© thaumatr0pe/Shutterstock.com

"Can alcoholism be hereditary? Alcoholism has a biological base. The tendency to become an alcoholic is inherited. Men and women are four times more likely to become alcoholics if their parents were (NIAAA, 2008). Currently, researchers are finding the genes that influence vulnerability to alcohol. A person's environment may also play a role in drinking and the development of alcoholism. This is not destiny. A child of an alcoholic parent will not automatically develop alcoholism, and a person with no family history of alcohol can become alcohol dependent."[1]

Alcohol and Pregnancy

There is no known safe amount of alcohol use during pregnancy or while trying to get pregnant (CDC). There is also no safe time during pregnancy to drink. All types of alcohol are equally harmful, including all wines and beer. When a pregnant woman drinks alcohol, so does her baby.

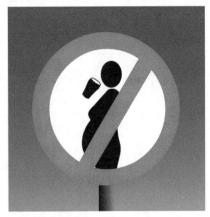

© Stephen Finn/Shutterstock.com

Women also should not drink alcohol if they are sexually active and do not use effective contraception (birth control). This is because a woman might get pregnant and expose her baby to alcohol before she knows she is pregnant. Nearly half of all pregnancies in the United States are unplanned. Most women will not know they are pregnant for up to 4 to 6 weeks.

Chronic Effects

"Drinking too much alcohol can cause a wide range of chronic health problems including liver disease, cancer, heart disease, nervous system problems, as well as alcoholism. Although moderate amounts of alcohol may not be harmful, there are some major health issues associated with chronic alcohol use and abuse."[1]

Laws Relating to Alcohol

"In every state in the United States, it is illegal for a person under the age of 21 to attempt to purchase, possess, or consume alcohol.

"By operating a motor vehicle in a public place, the driver has given consent to take a breath/blood test to determine alcohol in their system. Refusing or failing the test is considered a violation, and penalties will result in loss of license, regardless of the outcome of the violation. In many states, the legal definition of **driving while intoxicated** (DWI) is not having normal use of your mental or physical faculties because of alcohol or other drugs; or a blood alcohol concentration of .08 or more. It is, however, illegal in all states to drink and drive. In addition, in most states, it is also illegal for anyone in the vehicle to possess an **open container** of alcohol regardless of age."[1]

Cannabinoids

"**Marijuana** is a naturally occurring plant called Canna-bis sativa, whose leaves and stems can be dried, crushed, and rolled in cigarettes (joints) to be smoked. The fibers of this plant are also used to manufacture hemp rope and paper. The resins scraped from the flowering tops of the plant yield **hashish**, a form of marijuana that can be smoked in a pipe. The amount of the active ingredient, tetrahydrocannabinol (THC), determines the potency of the hallucinogenic effect. Because THC is a fat-soluble substance, it is absorbed and retained in the fat tissues of the body for up to a month. Drug tests can detect trace

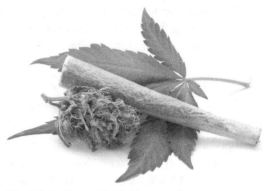

© Luis Carlos Jimenez del rio/Shutterstock.com

amounts of THC for up to three weeks after consumption. Medicinal uses include relief of the nausea caused by chemotherapy, improvement of appetite in AIDS patients, and the relief of pressure in the eyes of glaucoma patients. The effects of marijuana use vary from user to user, but usually result in some simi-lar experiences. Acute effects include euphoria, relaxation, slowed reaction time, distorted sensory percep-tion, impaired balance and coordination, increased heart rate and appetite impaired learning and memory, anxiety, panic attacks and psychosis (NIDA, 2011)."[1]

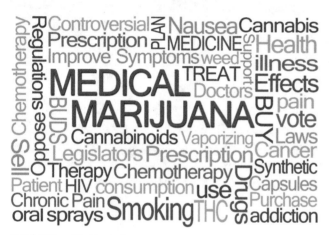

© Rob Wilson/Shutterstock.com

Prior to 2015, marijuana was the most commonly used illicit drug in the United States (SAMHSA, 2014). There are currently 23 states, as well as the District of Columbia, who have laws legalizing marijuana in some form. (It is still illegal in South Carolina). Its use is wide-spread among young people. According to a yearly survey of middle and high school stu-dents, rates of marijuana use have steadied in the past few years after several years of in-crease. However, the number of young people who believe marijuana use is risky is decreas-ing (Johnston, 2014).

"The long-term effects are still being studied; however, chronic abuse may lead to a motivational syndrome in some. Marijuana smoke is irritating to the lung tissues and may be more dam-aging than cigarette smoke. There are four hundred chemicals in marijuana linked to lung cancer devel-opment. In addition, the immune system and reproductive systems are damaged. There is an increase in birth defects among children whose mothers smoke marijuana during pregnancy. The biggest concern related to marijuana use is the perception that there is no risk or harm associated with occasional use. Other health risks include possible mental health decline and addiction."[1]

Synthetic Cannabinoids

Synthetic cannabinoids refer to a growing number of man-made mind-altering chemicals that are either sprayed on dried, shredded plant material so they can be smoked (herbal incense) or sold as liquids to be vaporized and inhaled in e-cigarettes and other devices (liquid incense) (NIDA, 2015).

These chemicals are called *cannabinoids* because they are related to chemicals found in the marijuana plant. Because of this similarity, synthetic cannabinoids are sometimes misleadingly called "synthetic marijuana" (or "fake weed"), and are often marketed as "safe," legal alternatives to that drug. In fact, they may affect the brain much more powerfully than marijuana; their actual effects can be unpredictable and, in some cases, severe or even life-threatening.

Manufacturers sell these herbal incense products in colorful foil packages and sell similar liquid incense products, like other e-cigarette fluids, in plastic bottles. They market these products under a wide variety of specific brand names; in past years, K2 and Spice were common. Hundreds of other brand names now exist, such as Joker, Black Mamba, Kush, and Kronic.

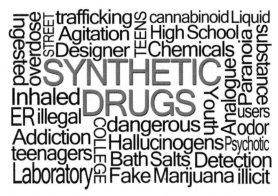

© Rob Wilson/Shutterstock.com

Did you know . . .

According to the National Institute on Drug Abuse:

- Marijuana, including synthetic cannabinoids, can be addictive.
- After alcohol, marijuana is the drug most often linked to car accidents, including those involving deaths.
- Marijuana is linked to school failure.
- High doses of marijuana can cause psychosis or panic when you're high.
- The effects of synthetic cannabinoids can be unpredictable and life-threatening.

Courtesy of Shelley Hamill

Opioids

"Derived from poppy seeds, **opium** is the base compound used for all narcotics. Opiates, which are narcotics, include opium and other drugs derived from opium, such as morphine, codeine, and heroin. Methadone is a synthetic chemical that has a morphine-like action, and also falls into this category of drugs."[1]

Heroin

"**Heroin** is derived from a naturally occurring substance in the Oriental poppy plant called opium. It is a highly effective, fast-acting analgesic (painkiller) if injected when used medicinally; however, its benefits are outweighed by its risk of toxicity and high dependence rate. Heroin can be injected, snorted, or smoked. When heroin enters the brain it produces a dream-like euphoria (NIDA, 2010). Abuse is common because this drug creates a strong physical and psychological dependence and tolerance. Recently heroin has become more popular among young people. The risks of heroin use are increased due to the use of needles for injection. There is an increased likelihood of transmission of communicable diseases like HIV and hepatitis due to the practice of sharing needles. Although abrupt withdrawal from heroin is rarely fatal, the discomfort associated with going 'cold turkey' is extremely intense.

"Heroin users are at high risk for addiction. It is estimated that approximately 23% of heroin users become dependent. Anyone can become dependent, and life expectancy of the heroin

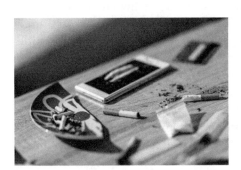

© Photographee.eu/Shutterstock.com

addict who injects the drug intravenously is significantly lower than that of one who does not. Overdosing on heroin can result in death within minutes."[1]

Heroin use has increased across the US among men and women, most age groups, and all income levels. Some of the greatest increases occurred in demographic groups with historically low rates of heroin use: women, the privately insured, and people with higher incomes. Not only are people using heroin, they are also abusing multiple other substances, especially cocaine and prescription opioid painkillers. As heroin use has increased, so have heroin-related overdose deaths. Between 2002 and 2013, the rate of heroin-related overdose deaths nearly quadrupled, and more than 8,200 people died in 2013 (CDC, 2015).

STIMULANTS

Caffeine

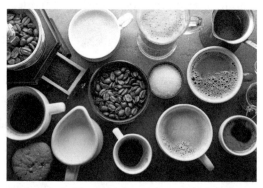

© Africa Studio/Shutterstock.com

"**Caffeine** is a stimulant as well as a psychotropic (mind affecting) drug. Caffeine is generally associated with coffee, tea, and cola, but can also be found in chocolate, cocoa, and other carbonated beverages, as well as some medications, both prescription and non-prescription, i.e., Excedrin®. Approximately 65–180 milligrams of caffeine is found in one cup of coffee, compared to tea, which contains 40–100 mg per cup, and cola, which contains 30–60 mg per twelve ounce serving. Caffeine is readily absorbed into the body and causes stimulation of the cerebral cortex and medullary centers in the brain, resulting in mental alertness. Moderation is the key when using caffeine. Researchers agree that 300 milligrams of caffeine is considered moderate intake, which is equivalent to approximately three cups of coffee. Some individuals are more sensitive to caffeine than others and may feel the effects at smaller doses. According to research, caffeine in beverage form is not dehydrating, but if ingesting caffeine from food or tablets, be sure to rehydrate from the drug's diuretic action.

"Excessive consumption of caffeine increases plasma levels of epinephrine, norepinephrine, and renin. It can also cause serious side effects, such as tremors, nervousness, irritability, headaches, hyperactivity, arrhythmia, dizziness, and insomnia. It can elevate the blood pressure and body temperature, increase the breathing rate, irritate the stomach and bowels, and dehydrate the body."[1]

Energy drink use has grown steadily over that past several years with some brands selling billions of dollars' worth of product. While some may use them as an energy boost, the amount of caffeine in some drinks can create some of the side effects listed above. Energy drinks are beverages like Red Bull, Rock Star, and Monster contain large doses of caffeine and other legal stimulants like guarana and ginseng. The amount of caffeine in an energy drink can range from 75 milligrams to over 200 milligrams per serving. This compares to 34 milligrams in Coke and 55 milligrams in Mountain Dew (Brown.edu).

"Excessive amounts of caffeine may increase the incidence of premenstrual syndrome (PMS) in some women and may increase fibrocystic breast disease (noncancerous breast lumps) as well. The U.S. Surgeon General recommends that women avoid or restrict caffeine

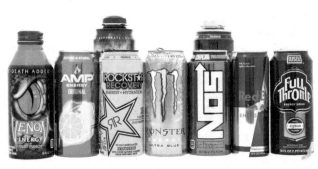

© Keith Homan/Shutterstock.com

intake during pregnancy. Withdrawal symptoms from caffeine may include headaches, depression, drowsiness, nervousness, and a feeling of lethargy.

"College students have been known to use caffeinated products like these for extra energy when studying, driving long distances, or needing more energy in general. A common practice of mixing energy drinks and alcohol is of special concern. Drinking large amounts of caffeine (a stimulant) combined with large amounts of alcohol (a depressant) can cause people to misjudge their level of intoxication. The combination of drugs may mask symptoms such as headache, weakness, and muscle coordination, but in reality visual reaction time and motor coordination are still negatively affected by alcohol. Driving or making any other important decisions under these circumstances can be extremely dangerous."[1]

Cocaine

Cocaine is a powerfully addictive stimulant drug made from the leaves of the coca plant native to South America. It produces short-term euphoria, energy, and talkativeness in addition to potentially dangerous physical effects like raising heart rate and blood pressure.

The powdered form of cocaine is either inhaled through the nose (snorted), where it is absorbed through the nasal tissue, or dissolved in water and injected into the bloodstream.

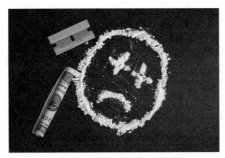

© Christopher Slesarchik/Shutterstock.com

Crack is a form of cocaine that has been processed to make a rock crystal (also called "freebase cocaine") that can be smoked. The crystal is heated to produce vapors that are absorbed into the blood-stream through the lungs. (The term "crack" refers to the crackling sound produced by the rock as it is heated.)

The intensity and duration of cocaine's pleasurable effects depend on the way it is administered. Injecting or smoking cocaine delivers the drug rapidly into the bloodstream and brain, producing a quicker and stronger but shorter-lasting high than snorting. The high from snorting cocaine may last 15 to 30 minutes; the high from smoking may last 5 to 10 minutes.

Cocaine affects the body in a variety of ways. It constricts blood vessels, dilates pupils, and increases body temperature, heart rate, and blood pressure. It can also cause headaches and gastrointestinal complications such as abdominal pain and nausea. Because cocaine tends to decrease appetite, chronic users can become malnourished as well.

Most seriously, people who use cocaine can suffer heart attacks or strokes, which may cause sudden death. Cocaine-related deaths are often a result of the heart stopping (cardiac arrest) followed by an arrest of breathing.

Cocaine is more dangerous when combined with other drugs or alcohol (poly-drug use). For example, the combination of cocaine and heroin (known as a "speedball") carries a particularly high risk of fatal overdose (http://www.drugabuse.gov/publications/drugfacts/cocaine). Cited*

Amphetamines

"Amphetamines are drugs that speed up the nervous system. They do not occur naturally and must be manufactured in a laboratory. When used in moderation, amphetamines stimulate receptor sites for two naturally occurring neurotransmitters, having the effect of elevated mood, increased alertness, and feelings of well-being. In addition, the activity of the stomach and intestines may be slowed and appetite suppressed. When amphetamines are eliminated from the body, the user becomes fatigued. With abuse, the user

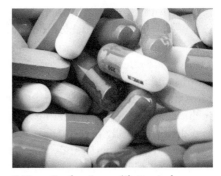

© Nenov Brothers Images/Shutterstock.com

will experience rapid tolerance and a strong psychological dependence, along with the possibility of impotence and episodes of psychosis. When use stops, the abuser may experience periods of depression."[1]

Methamphetamines

"An extremely addictive and powerful drug that stimulates the central nervous system is commonly known as 'meth.' In its smoked form, it is called 'crystal,' 'crank,' or 'ice.' It is chemically similar to amphetamines, but much stronger. The effects from methamphetamine can last up to eight hours or in some cases even longer. It comes in many forms and can be injected, inhaled, orally ingested, or snorted. Methamphetamine is considered to be the fastest growing drug in the United States. According to the director of the Substance Abuse and Mental Health Services Administration (SAMHSA), the growth and popularity of this drug is because of its wide availability, easy production, low cost, and highly addictive nature. Methamphetamine is a psychostimulant but different than others like cocaine or amphetamine. Methamphetamine, like cocaine, results in an accumulation of dopamine. Dopamine is a neurotransmitter in regions of the brain that deal with emotion, movement, motivation, and pleasure. The large release of dopamine is presumed to help the drug's toxic effects on the brain. However, unlike cocaine, which is removed and metabolized quickly from the body, methamphetamine has a longer duration of action, which stays in the body and brain longer, leading to prolonged stimulant effects. Chronic methamphetamine abuse significantly changes the way the brain functions (NIDA, 2010).

"Methamphetamine abusers may display symptoms that include violent behavior, confusion, hallucinations, and possible paranoid or delusional feelings, also causing severe personality shifts. These feelings of paranoia can lead to homicidal or suicidal thoughts or tendencies. Methamphetamines are highly addictive and can be fatal with a single use. Deadly ingredients include antifreeze, drain cleaner, fertilizer, battery acid, or lantern fuel. The results when overused can cause heart failure and death. Long-term physical effects can lead to strokes, liver, kidney, and lung damage. Abuse can also lead to permanent and severe brain and psychological damage."[1]

Club Drugs /Street Drugs

The evolution of chemical substances to create an altered effect on the body or mind is ongoing. New combinations appear regularly with some causing catastrophic effects. Even substances designed for other uses, (remember bath salts?) can be used inappropriately leading to death. Some are given "friendly" street names masking their potentially harmful effects.

For example, "Smiles" is a hallucinogen whose effects are not immediately felt, increasing the risk of overdose. It can be taken as small tables, on blotter paper, or in powder form, often mixed with something else—chocolate, for instance. Side effects include loss of control, panic, heart palpitations and memory loss. "Wet" can refer to a marijuana cigarette dipped in liquid PCP, or to the PCP itself. Side effects include hostile behavior, feelings of detachment from reality, and distorted body perception. "Weed candy" is just what it sounds like—ordinary candy that's laced with marijuana, and oftentimes other dangerous ingredients (NIDA, 2015).

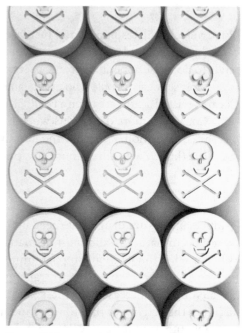

© ancroft/Shutterstock.com

MDMA

"**MDMA**, also known as **ecstasy**, has a chemical structure similar to methamphetamines and mescaline, causing hallucinogenic effects. As a result, it can produce both stimulant and psychedelic effects. In addition to its euphoric effects, MDMA can lead to disruptions in body temperature and cardiovascular regulation causing panic, anxiety, and rapid heart rate. It also damages nerves in the brain's serotonin system and possibly produces long-term damage to brain areas that are critical for thought and memory (NIDA, 2010). Physical effects can include muscle tension, teeth clenching, nausea, blurred vision, and faintness. The psychological effects can include confusion, depression, sleep disorders, anxiety, and paranoia that can last long after taking the drug. It is most often available in tablet form and usually taken orally. Occasionally it is found in powder form and can be snorted or smoked, but it is rarely injected. An overdose can be lethal, especially when taken with alcohol or other drugs, such as heroin ("H-bomb")."[1]

2C-B

"This is a psychedelic drug synthesized by a chemist in 1974 and is considered both a psychedelic and a drug similar to MDMA. 2C-B is a white powder found in tablets or gel caps and is taken orally. The visual effects can be more intense than those created by LSD and can cause nausea, trembling, chills, and nervousness."[1]

Rohypnol

"Flunitrazepam is an illegal drug in the United States, but an approved medicine in other parts of the world where it is generally prescribed for sleep disorders. A 2-mg tablet is equal to the potency of a six-pack of beer. Rohypnol is a tranquilizer, similar to Valium, but ten times more potent, producing sedative effects including muscle relaxation, dizziness, memory loss, and blackouts. The effects occur twenty to thirty minutes after use and lasts for up to eight hours. Rohypnol, more commonly known as "roofies," is a small, white, tasteless, pill that dissolves in food or drinks. It is most commonly used with other drugs, such as

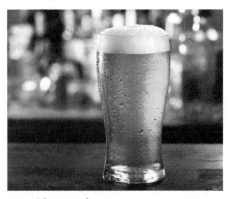

© Nitr/Shutterstock.com

alcohol, ecstasy, heroin, and marijuana to enhance the feeling of the other drug. Although Rohypnol alone can be very dangerous, as well as physically addicting, when mixed with other drugs it can be fatal. It is also referred to as the "date rape" drug because there have been many reported cases of individuals giving Rohypnol to someone without their knowledge. The effects incapacitate the victim, and therefore they are unable to resist a sexual assault. It produces an 'anterograde amnesia,' meaning they may not remember events experienced while under effects of the drug (NIDA, 2010)."[1]

Gamma Hydroxybutyrate (GHB)

"GHB is a fast-acting, powerful drug that depresses the nervous system. It occurs naturally in the body in small amounts. Commonly taken with alcohol, it depresses the central nervous system and induces an intoxicated state. GHB is commonly consumed orally, usually as a clear liquid or a white powder. It is odorless, colorless, and slightly salty to taste. Effects from GHB can occur within fifteen to thirty minutes. Small doses (less than 1 g) of GHB act as a relaxant with larger doses causing strong feelings of relaxation, slowing heart rate, and respiration. There is a very fine line to cross to find a lethal dose, which can lead to seizures, respiratory distress, low blood pressure, and comas.

"According to the Drug Abuse Warning Network, The Drug Induced Rape Prevention and Punishment Act of 1996 was enacted into federal law in response to the abuse of Rohypnol. This law makes it a crime to give someone a controlled substance without his/her knowledge and with the intent to commit a crime. The law also stiffens the penalties for possession and distribution of Rohypnol and GHB. Used in Europe as a general anesthetic and treatment for insomnia, GHB is growing in popularity and is widely available underground. Manufactured by non-professional "kitchen" chemists, concerns about quality and purity should be considered."[1]

DISSOCIATIVE DRUGS

Ketamine Hydrochloride

"'Special K' or 'K' was originally created for use in a medical setting on humans and animals. Ninety percent is legally sold for veterinary use. Ketamine usually comes in liquid form and is cooked into a white powder for snorting. Higher doses produce a hallucinogenic effect and may cause the user to feel far away from his or her body. This is called a "K-hole" and has been com-

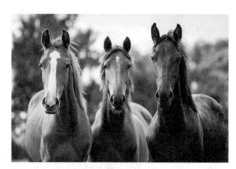

© Rita Kochmarjova/Shutterstock.com

pared to near-death experiences. Low doses can increase heart rate and numbness in the extremities with higher doses depressing consciousness and breathing. This makes it extremely dangerous if combined with other depressants such as alcohol or GHB."[1]

Phencyclidine Hydrochloride

"Also known as PCP or angel dust, phencyclidine hydrochloride is sometimes considered a hallucinogen, although it does not easily fit into any category. First synthesized in 1959, it is used intravenously and as an anesthetic that blocks pain without producing numbness. Taken in small doses, it causes feelings of euphoria. The harmful side effects include depression, anxiety, confusion, and delirium. High doses of PCP cause mental confusion, hallucinations, and can cause serious mental illness and extreme aggressive and violent behavior, including murder."[1]

Hallucinogens

"**Hallucinogens**, also called psychedelics, are drugs that affect perception, sensation, awareness, and emotion. Changes in time, space, and hallucinations may be mild or extreme depending on the dose, and may vary on every occasion. There are many synthetic as well as natural hallucinogens in use. Synthetic groups include LSD, which is the most potent; mescaline, which is derived from the peyote cactus, and psilocybin, derived from mushrooms, have similar effects."[1]

"Magic" Mushrooms

Psilocybin, also more widely known as magic mushrooms, is a psychedelic compound that is produced by a wide range of mushroom species. The more than 200 species of mushrooms that are responsible for the production of psilocybin are collectively known on the streets to

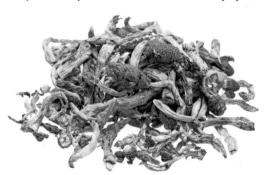

© robtek/Shutterstock.com

recreational drug users as magic mushrooms. These psychedelic hallucinogens produce mind-altering effects when they are consumed.

Like other types of hallucinogenic drugs, psilocybin can produce a wide range of euphoric and psychedelic effects. Psilocybin can produce euphoria, hallucinations, and a distorted sense of time for the user. It is very common for those under the influence of magic mushrooms to act erratically and irrationally. Behavior may include odd reactions to normal events, distinct outbursts and panic attacks.

Lysergic Acid Diethylamide (LSD)

According to the National Survey on Drug Use and Health conducted in 2014, 16.60 percent of the people aged 18–25 had used a hallucinogenic substance with 7% of those using LSD (drugabuse.gov). "LSD is a colorless, odorless, and tasteless liquid that is made from lysergic acid, which comes from the ergot fungus. It was first converted to lysergic acid diethylamide (LSD) in 1938. In 1943, its psychoactive properties accidentally became known (NIDA, 2009). Hallucinations and illusions often occur, and effects vary according to the dosage, personality of the user, and conditions under which the drug is used. A flashback is a recurrence of some hallucinations from a previous LSD experience days or months after the dose. Flashbacks can occur without reason, occurring to heavy users more frequently. After taking LSD, a person loses control over normal thought process. Street LSD is often mixed with other substances and its effects are quite uncertain (NIDA, 2009)."[1]

OTHER DRUGS

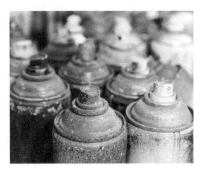

© dimbar76/Shutterstock.com

"**Inhalants** are poisonous chemical gases, fumes, or vapors that produce psychoactive effects when sniffed."[1] They are easy to access and inexpensive to purchase. Inhalants are often among the first drugs that young adolescents use. In fact, they are one of the few classes of drugs that are used more by younger adolescents than older ones. Inhalant use can become chronic and continue into adulthood (teens. drugabuse.gov). "When inhaled, the fumes take away the body's ability to absorb oxygen. Inhalants are considered deleriants, which can cause permanent damage to the heart, brain, lungs, and liver. Common inhalants include model glue, acetone, gasoline, kerosene, nail polish, aerosol sprays, Pam™ cooking spray, Scotchgard™ fabric protectant, lighter fluids, butane, and cleaning fluids, as well as nitrous oxide (laughing gas). These products were not created to be inhaled or ingested. They were designed to dissolve things or break things down, which is exactly what they do to the body."[1]

"Inhalants reach the lungs, bloodstream, and other parts of the body very quickly. Intoxication can occur in as little as five minutes and can last as long as nine hours. Inhaled lighter fluid/butane displaces the oxygen in the lungs, causing suffocation. Even a single episode can cause asphyxiation or cardiac arrhythmia and possibly lead to death. The initial effects of inhalants are similar to those of alcohol, but they are very unpredictable. Some effects include dizziness and blurred vision, involuntary eye movement, poor coordination, involuntary extremity movement, slurred speech, euphoric feeling, nosebleeds, and possible coma.

"Health risks involved with the use of inhalants may include hepatitis, liver and/or kidney failure, as well as the destruction of bone marrow and skeletal muscles. Respiratory impairment and blood abnormalities, along with irregular heartbeat and/or heart failure, are also serious side effects of inhalants. Regular use can lead to tolerance, the need for more powerful drugs, and addiction (NIDA, 2011)."[1]

Prescription Drugs

According to SAMHSA, in 2010 over 52 million people over the age of 12 have used prescription drugs non-medicinally. Over 6 Million people have used them non-medically in the past month and 5 percent of the United States is the world's population and consumes 75 percent of the world's prescription drugs. "It is not that these drugs should not be used for the purpose intended, as 'they have an important place in the treatment of debilitating conditions,' says Richard Brown, M.D., associate professor at the University of Wisconsin (FDA, 2005)."[1] The following are more frequently used/abused prescription drugs.

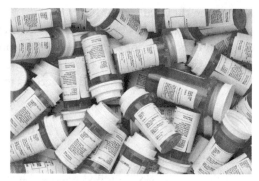

© David Smart/Shutterstock.com

OPIUM/OPIOID PAIN RELIEVERS

The opioid crisis in the United States has reached epidemic proportions. According to the Department of Health and Human Services (HHS) in 2015:

- 12.5 million people misused prescription opioids
- 2.1 million misused opioids for the first time
- 33,091 died from opioid overdose
- 828,000 used heroin
- 135,000 used heroin for the first time
- 12,989 died from a heroin overdose

The impact has affected the economy by over $78 billion dollars (www.hhs.gov).

With so many prescription drugs available, it is imperative that those we use them as prescribe, store them safely and securely, and dispose of them properly. Do not share your prescription drugs as you do not know how they may affect someone they have not be prescribe for. The following are examples of a few of the most overused opioids.

"This is the main alkaloid found in opium. It is ten times stronger than opium and brings quick relief from pain. It is most effectively used as an anesthetic during heart surgery, to relieve pain in post-operative patients, and sometimes used to relieve pain for cancer patients.

"**Hydrocodone** is a narcotic used to relieve pain and suppress cough. This drug, which can lead to both physiological and psychological dependence, saw a dramatic increase in legal sales between 1991 and 2010 with prescriptions topping 100 million (NIDA, 2011).

"**Codeine** is a natural derivative of opium. Codeine is medically used as a mild painkiller or a cough suppressant. Although widely used, there is potential for physical dependence.

"**Oxycodone**, a drug used for moderate to severe pain relief, has a high potential for abuse. Tablets should be taken orally, but when crushed and injected intravenously or snorted, a potentially lethal dose is released (FDA, 2004)."[1]

Stimulants

"According to recent reports from the FDA, a highly abused stimulant among middle and high school students is methylphenidate, commonly known as **Ritalin**. This drug is more powerful than caffeine but not as potent as amphetamines and is prescribed for individuals with attention-deficit/hyperactivity disorders, ADHD, and sometimes to treat narcolepsy. Researchers speculate that Ritalin increases the slow and steady release of dopamine, therefore improving attention and focus for those in need of the increase. 'Individuals abuse Ritalin to lose weight, increase alertness and experience the euphoric feelings resulting from high doses' (U.S. Dept. of Justice, 2006). When abused, the tablets are either taken orally or crushed and snorted; some even dissolve the tablets in water and inject the mixture. Addiction occurs when it induces large and fast increases of dopamine in the brain (DOJ, 2006).

"**Adderall** is another stimulant used to treat ADHD as well as narcolepsy. Physical and psychological dependence may occur with this drug. Symptoms of Adderall overdose include dizziness, blurred vision, restlessness, rapid breathing, confusion, hallucinations, nausea, vomiting, irregular heartbeat, and seizures."[1]

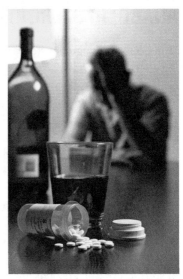

© Burlingham/Shutterstock.com

Depressants

"Depressants are sedatives or anxiolytic (anti-anxiety) drugs that depress the central nervous system. Benzodiazepines such as Valium and Xanax and barbiturates like Nembutal, Secobarbital, and Phenobarbital can be prescribed to relieve tension, induce relaxation and sleep, or treat panic attacks. All of these differ in action, absorption, and metabolism, but all produce similar intoxication and withdrawal symptoms. Depressants can produce both a physical and psychological dependence within two to four weeks. Those with a prior history of abuse are at greater risk of abusing sedatives, even if prescribed by a physician. If there is no previous substance abuse history, one rarely develops problems if prescribed and monitored by a physician. Depressants can be very dangerous, if not lethal, if used in combination with alcohol, leading to respiratory depression, respiratory arrest, and death. Some of the physiological effects of depressants include drowsiness, impaired judgment, poor coordination, slowed breathing, confusion, weak and rapid heartbeat, relaxed muscles, and pain relief. A major health risk associated with the use of depressants is the development of dependence to the drug, leading to serious side effects, such as stupors, coma, and death.

"The danger from prescription and over-the-counter drugs is often underestimated by students. Many assume that if the drug is legal and prescribed by a physician, even if for someone else, it must be safe. However, what they fail to realize is that medications and dosages are tailored to each patient and may not be appropriate in the manner they intend to use them."[1]

The proper disposal of prescription drugs is also important. They should not be discarded in the trash or flushed down the toilet. Many communities have designated dates when unused or expired prescription drugs can be brought in for proper disposal.

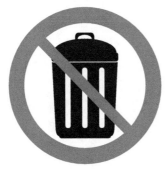

© veronchick84/Shutterstock.com

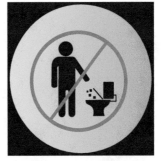

©MukeshKumar/Shutterstock.com

ANABOLIC STEROIDS

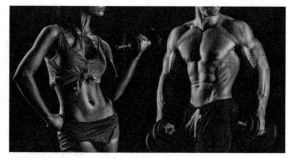

© Lebedev Roman Olegovich/Shutterstock.com

"Anabolic androgenic steroids are man-made and very similar to male sex hormones. The word anabolic means 'muscle building,' and androgenic refers to masculine. Legally, steroids are prescribed to individuals to treat problems occurring when the body produces abnormally low amounts of testosterone and problems associated with delayed puberty or impotence. Other cases for prescribed steroids use would involve individuals with whom a disease has resulted in a loss of muscle mass (NIDA, 2005). Although steroids are a banned substance in all professional and collegiate sports, most people who use steroids do so to enhance physical performance in sports or other activities. Some choose to use steroids to improve physical appearance or to increase muscle size and to reduce body fat. Some steroids can be taken orally or injected into the muscle. There are also some forms of steroid creams and gels that are to be rubbed into the skin. Most doses taken by abusers are ten to one hundred times the potency of normal doses used for medicinal purposes.

"Consequences from steroid abuse can cause some serious health issues. There can be some problems with the normal hormone production in the individual, which can be very severe and irreversible. Major side effects of steroid abuse can lead to cardiovascular disease, high blood pressure, and stroke because it increases the LDL cholesterol levels while decreasing the HDL levels. There can also be liver damage, muscular and ligament damage, as well as stunted bone growth. In addition to these problems, the side effects for males can be shrinkage of the testes and a reduction in sperm count. For females, steroid use can cause facial hair growth and the cessation of the menstrual cycle.

"Research also suggests some psychological and behavioral changes. Steroid abusers can become very aggressive and violent and have severe mood swings. Users are reported to have paranoid and jealous tendencies along with irritability and impaired judgment. Depression has also been linked to steroid use once the individual stops taking the drug, therefore leading to continued use. This depressed state can lead to serious consequences, and in some cases it has been reported to lead to suicidal thoughts (NIDA, 2005)."[1]

Are you a wise consumer?

Have you ever used a prescription medication that was not your own? If so, did you consider the possible side effects? Not everyone has the same body chemistry and if you were taking any other medication, even an over the counter drug, how would you know what the effects might be? Health literate individuals and wise consumers make informed decisions to avoid negative consequences.

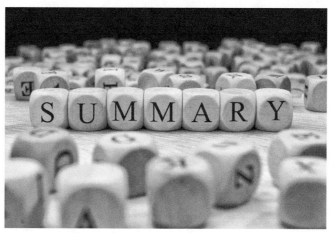

© Fabrik Bilder/Shutterstock.com

Students are faced with many decisions throughout their college experience. Social pressures can create instances where individuals feel that if they do not participate in certain behaviors, they might not be accepted. Knowing the potential consequences and making informed choices can not only prevent serious problems, it can also support long term goals. The improper use of drugs and alcohol can derail future plans and create significant health issues.

NOTES

Personal Reflections . . . so, what have you learned?

1. What is binge drinking and why is it so dangerous? If one of your friends was at a party and collapsed from drinking too much alcohol, what would you do?

2. What is the Good Samaritan law and why is it important?

3. What is changing about craft beer and why is it important for consumers to know?

4. Are E-cigarettes really safer? Why or why not? How do you feel when a person is smoking an E-cigarette next to you?

5. Should people who smoke pay more for insurance? Why or why not?

6. What about people who drink alcohol? Why or why not?

NOTES

RESOURCES ON CAMPUS FOR YOU!

Student Conduct

There are numerous campus resources available to students, as well as policies that outline university expectations across many areas. Listed in your Student Handbook are policies with respect to alcohol and tobacco use on campus. Additionally, students wishing to talk with a counselor concerning substance use will find the information at Health and Counseling services.

REFERENCES

American Heart Association (AHA). (2006). *Annual report.*

B-Well Health Promotion, Brown University. *Energy Drinks.* Retrieved 2016 from http://www.brown .edu/campus-life/health/services/promotion/nutrition-eating-concerns-eating-well-brown /energy-drinks.

Center on Addiction and Substance Abuse at Columbia University. Commission on Substances Abuse at Colleges and Universities.

Centers for Disease Control and Prevention. (2014). *Alcohol use in pregnancy.* Retrieved 2016 from http://www.cdc.gov/ncbddd/fasd/alcohol-use.html

Centers for Disease Control and Prevention. (2010). *Behavioral risk Factor surveillance system.*

Centers for Disease Control and Prevention. (2010). *National health interview survey.*

Centers for Disease Control and Prevention. (2010). *Smokeless tobacco.*

Centers for Disease Control and Prevention. (2012). *Secondhand smoke, 2012.*

Centers for Disease Control and Prevention. (2015). *Today's heroin epidemic.* Retrieved 2016 from www.cdc.gov/vitalsigns/heroin/index.html,

Center for Disease Control and Prevention. (2015). *Youth risk behavior survey.* Retrieved December 2015 from www.cdc.gov/healthyyouth/data/yrbs/index.htm.

Cobb, N.K., Byron, M.J., Abrams, D.B., & Shields, P. G. (2010). Novel nicotine delivery systems and public health: the rise of the "e-cigarette." *Am J Public Health*, 100, 2340–2.

Department of Health and Counseling Services, Winthrop University. *Influenza update.* Retrieved 2016 from http://www.winthrop.edu/hcs/default.aspx?id=22925

Department of Health and Counseling Services, Winthrop University. Retrieved 2016 from http://www.winthrop.edu/student-affairs/

Department of Health and Human Services, www.hhs.gov

Department of Justice, & National Drug Intelligence Center. (2006). *Ritalin fast facts.*

Everett, S. A., Lowry, R., Cohen, L. R., Dellinger, A. M. (1999). Unsafe motor vehicle practices among substance-using college students. *Accident Analysis.*

Ewing, J. (1984). Detecting alcoholism: the CAGE questionnaire. *Journal of the American Medical Association.*

Dennis, M. E., & Texas Commission on Alcohol and Drug Abuse. (2005). *Instructor manual, alcohol education program for minors.* Austin: TCADA.

Hallucinogens.com. *Psilocybin.* Retrieved 2016 from http://hallucinogens.com/psilocybin/

Hoeger, W. and Hoeger, S. (1999). *Principles and labs for fitness and wellness* (5th ed). Englewood, CO: Morton Publishing Company.

Johnston, L.D., O'Malley, P.M., Miech, R.A., Bachman, J.G., Schulenberg, J.E. (2014). Monitoring the future national results on drug use: 1975–2014: Overview, key findings on adolescent drug use. Ann Arbor, MI: Institute for Social Research, The University of Michigan.

Journal of the American Medical Association. (1994). Moderate alcohol intake and lower risk of coronary heart disease.

King, B.A., Alam, S. Promoff, G., Arrazola, R., & Dube, S.R. (2013). Awareness and ever use of electronic cigarettes among U.S. adults, 2010–2011. *Nicotine Tob,* 15, 1623–7.

McCusker, R., Goldberger, B., and Cone, E. (2006). The content of energy drinks, carbonated sodas, and other beverages. *Journal of Analytical Toxicology,* 30(2), 112–114. Doi:1093/30.2.112

McKinley Health Center. University of Illinois at Urbana-Champaign. (2005).

Miller, W., Tonigan, J., Longabaugh, R. (1995). Drinking inventory of consequences: An instrument for assessing adverse consequences of alcohol abuse. Test manual. Rockville, MD: National Institute on Alcohol Abuse and Alcoholism.

Miller, E. K., Erickson, C. A., & Desimone, R. (1996). Neural mechanisms of visual working memory in prefrontal cortex of the macaque. *Journal of Neuroscience.*

National Cancer Institute, & U.S National Institutes of Health. (2008).

National Institute on Alcohol Abuse and Alcoholism, & National Institutes of Health. *Statistics Snapshot of college drinking.*

National Institute on Alcohol Abuse and Alcoholism. Retrieved from 2016 http://niaaa.nih.gov /alcohol-health/special-populations-co-occurring-disorders/college-drinking

National Institute on Alcohol Abuse and Alcoholism, & National Institutes of Health. (2008). *Integrative genetic analysis of alcohol dependence using the genenetwork web resources.*

National Institute on Drug Abuse. Retrieved 2016 from http://www.drugabuse.gov/

National Institute on Drug Abuse. (2013). *Drug facts: cocaine.* Retrieved 2016 from http://www.drugabuse .gov/publications/drugfacts/cocaine,

National Institute on Drug Abuse. (2014). *Hallucinogens.* Retrieved 2016 from http://www.drugabuse.gov /drugs-abuse/hallucinogens

National Institute of Drug Abuse (NIDA), & U.S. Dept. of Health and Human Services. (2008).

National Institute on Drug Abuse. (2010). *The science of drug abuse and addiction. NIDA info facts: Hallucinogens.*

National Institute on Drug Abuse. (2010). *The science of drug abuse and addiction. NIDA info facts: Anabolic Steroids.*

National Institute of Drug Abuse (NIDA) (2001). Update on ecstacy. *NIDA Notes 16(5).*

National Traffic Safety Administration, & Traffic Safety Facts. (2012). *Annual assessment of alcohol related fatalities.*

NIDA for Teens. *Inhalants.* Retrieved 2016 from http://teens.drugabuse.gov/drug-facts/inhalants

Ray, O., Ksir, C. (1999). *Drugs, society, and human behavior* (8th ed). New York: WCB McGraw-Hill.

SAMHSA, National Clearinghouse for Alcohol and Drug Abuse, & www.health.org Centers for Disease Control and Prevention (CDC) (2006). Smoking and tobacco use. *Fast Facts.* Atlanta: Author.

Substance Abuse and Mental Health Service Administration. Retrieved 2016 from www.samhsa.gov.

Traffic Safety Facts 2013 Data. *Alcohol-impaired driving.* Retrieved 2016 from http://www-nrd.nhtsa.dot .gov/Pubs/812102.pdf

U.S. Food and Drug Administration. (2005). Prescription drug use and abuse: Complexities of addiction.

U.S. Food and Drug Administration. (2004). Oxycodone: FDA statement. statement on generic oxycodone hydrochloride extended release Tablets.

U.S. Food and Drug Administration, & Department of Health and Human Services. FDA issues regulation prohibiting sale of dietary supplements containing ephedrine alkaloids and reiterates its advice that consumers stop using these products.

Public Media. (2013). *DEA warns of new street drugs with friendly-sounding nicknames.* Retrieved 2016 from http://wusfnews.wusf.usf.edu/post/dea-warns-new-street-drugs-friendly-sounding-nicknames #stream/0

CREDITS

1. From *Health and Fitness: A Guide to a Healthy Lifestyle*, 5/e by Laura Bounds, Gayden Darnell, Kristin Brekken Shea, Dottiede Agnore. Copyright © 2012 by Kendall Hunt Publishing Company. Reprinted by permission.

Chapter 9 +

Human Diseases

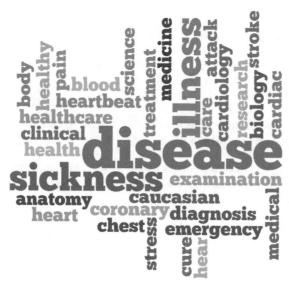

© dboystudio/Shutterstock.com

OBJECTIVES:

Students will be able to:

- Differentiate between communicable and non-communicable diseases.
- Discuss the major hypokinetic diseases afflicting Americans.
- List the six major cardiac risk factors and the three unalterable cardiac risk factors.
- Know the warning signs for a heart attack and stroke.
- Discuss three ways to combat obesity.
- Recognize the risk factors for cancer and describe the cancer warning signs.
- Identify four cancers that affect young adults; discuss prevention and risk factors.
- Differentiate between Type I and Type II diabetes and define the risk factors for each.
- Discuss ways to prevent other chronic illnesses, such as osteoporosis, asthma, anemia, lupus, and gastrointestinal disorders.
- Discuss strategies to avoid contraction of communicable diseases and identify the symptoms and treatment for each disease.

American Heart Association's (AHA) Risk for Disease Questionnaire

History

"You have had:

_____ Heart attack

_____ Heart surgery

_____ Cardiac catheterization

_____ Coronary angioplasty (PTCA)

_____ Pacemaker/implantable cardiac defibrillator/rhythm disturbance

_____ Heart valve disease

_____ Heart Failure

_____ Heart transplantation

_____ Congenital heart disease

Symptoms

_____ Chest discomfort from exertion

_____ Unreasonable breathlessness

_____ Dizziness, fainting, blackouts

_____ Take heart medications

Other health issues

_____ Diabetes

_____ Asthma or another lung disease

_____ Burning or cramping in lower legs when walking short distances.

_____ Musculoskeletal problems that limit physical activity

_____ Concerns about the safety of exercise.

_____ Take prescription medication(s)

_____ Pregnancy

> If you marked any of these statements in this section, AHA recommends you get a physician's clearance before activity.

Cardiovascular risk factors

_____ You are a man older than 45 years.

_____ You are a woman older than 55 years, you have had a hysterectomy, or you are postmenopausal.

_____ You smoke, or quite within the previous 6 mo.

_____ Your blood pressure is greater than 140/90.

_____ You don't know your blood pressure.

_____ You take blood pressure medication.

_____ Your blood cholesterol level is >200 mg/dL.

_____ You don't know your cholesterol level.

_____ You have a close blood relative who had a heart attack before age 55 (father or brother) or age 65 (mother or sister).

_____ You are physically inactive (i.e., you get less than 30 min. of physical activity on at least three days per week).

_____ You are more than 20 pounds overweight

> If you marked two or more of the statements in this section, AHA recommends checking with your doctor before starting a regular exercise program.

_____ None of the above is true."[3]

> You should be able to exercise safely without consulting your physician or other healthcare provider in a self-guided program or almost any facility that meets your exercise program needs.

Source: American Heart Association, Inc.

NON-COMMUNICABLE DISEASES

Non-communicable diseases are not transmitted person to person. These diseases can develop from many sources, some of which include genetic predisposition, behaviors such as excessive sun exposure, smoking, unhealthy eating habits, and/or lack of exercise.

Cardiovascular Disease (CVD)

"The cardiovascular system is responsible for delivering oxygen and other nutrients to the body. The major components of the cardiovascular system are the heart, blood, and the vessels that carry the blood. Cardiovascular disease (CVD) is a catch-all term that includes several disease processes including various diseases of the heart, stroke, high blood pressure, congestive heart failure, and atherosclerosis. The heart muscle may become damaged or lose its ability to contract effectively. The vessels that supply the heart with oxygen may become blocked or damaged and subsequently compromise the heart muscle. Finally, the peripheral vascular system (all of the vessels outside the heart) may become damaged and decrease the ability to provide oxygen to other parts of the body. The great news is that from 1998 to 2008, deaths due to cardiovascular disease declined 30.6% (AHA, 2012). Americans are also on the whole, living longer,

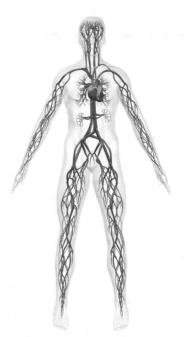

© Sebastian Kaulitzki/Shutterstock.com

as life expectancy increases. The bad news is that many of the risk factors for CVD are lifestyle-related and therefore preventable, and Americans are much more likely to die from CVD than anything else. MyLifeCheck.org is a part of a campaign to increase awareness of positive attributes of health.

"CVD and stroke are largely preventable for a significant part of the lifespan. High blood pressure, high cholesterol, and smoking continue to put people at risk of heart attack and stroke. To address these risk factors, the Centers for Disease Control and Prevention is focusing many of its efforts on the 'A B C's' of heart disease and stroke prevention: appropriate Aspirin therapy, Blood pressure control, Cholesterol control, and support for Smoking cessation for those trying to quit and, even more generally, comprehensive tobacco prevention and control efforts. (CDC, 2012)."[1]

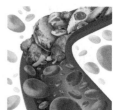

© Lightspring/Shutterstock.com

WHAT ARE THE RISK FACTORS OF CARDIOVASCULAR DISEASE?

"A risk factor for a disease is something that increases your risk of developing that disease. Risk factors can be behavioral, environmental, or genetic.

- **Cigarette Smoking**—Smokers have two to four times the risk of developing cardiovascular disease than do nonsmokers (AHA, 2014). Cigarette smoking is the most 'potent' of the preventable risk factors. Former U.S. Surgeon General C. Everett Koop claims that cigarette *smoking is the number one preventable cause of death and disease in the United States* and the most important health issue of our time. Smoking accounts for 50 percent of female deaths due to heart attack before the age of 55 (Rosato, 1994).

- **Hypertension (High Blood Pressure)**—The AHA (2015) reports that approximately 80 million American adults have high blood pressure. *Hypertension is the most important modifiable risk factor for stroke.*

- **Cholesterol**—Dietary cholesterol contributes to blood serum cholesterol (cholesterol circulating in the blood), which can contribute to heart disease. Every 1 percent reduction in serum cholesterol can result in a 2–3 percent reduction in the risk of heart disease (AHA, 2014). To lower cholesterol, reduce intake of dietary saturated fat, increase consumption of soluble fiber, maintain a healthy weight, do not smoke, and exercise regularly.

- **Inactivity**—Aerobic exercise on a regular basis can favorably influence the other modifiable risk factors for heart disease. Consistent, moderate amounts of physical activity can promote health and longevity. The Surgeon General's report (Satcher, 1996) states that as few as 150 extra calories expended daily exercising can dramatically decrease CVD risk.

What is your risk? Mark any of the following that apply to you.

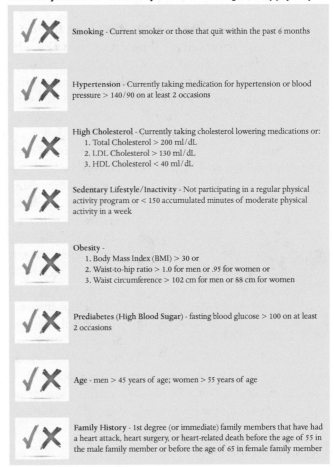

Smoking - Current smoker or those that quit within the past 6 months

Hypertension - Currently taking medication for hypertension or blood pressure > 140/90 on at least 2 occasions

High Cholesterol - Currently taking cholesterol lowering medications or:
1. Total Cholesterol > 200 ml/dL
2. LDL Cholesterol > 130 ml/dL
3. HDL Cholesterol < 40 ml/dL

Sedentary Lifestyle/Inactivity - Not participating in a regular physical activity program or < 150 accumulated minutes of moderate physical activity in a week

Obesity -
1. Body Mass Index (BMI) > 30 or
2. Waist-to-hip ratio > 1.0 for men or .95 for women or
3. Waist circumference > 102 cm for men or 88 cm for women

Prediabetes (High Blood Sugar) - fasting blood glucose > 100 on at least 2 occasions

Age - men > 45 years of age; women > 55 years of age

Family History - 1st degree (or immediate) family members that have had a heart attack, heart surgery, or heart-related death before the age of 55 in the male family member or before the age of 65 in female family member

Illustrations © Arak Rattanawijittakorn/Shutterstock.com

- **Obesity**—Highly correlated to heart disease, mild to moderate obesity is associated with an increase in risk of CVD. Fat distribution around the mid-section produces a higher risk than fat distribution around the hips and lower body.

- **Diabetes**—At least 65 percent of diabetics die of some form of CVD (CDC, 2012). Exercise is critical to help increase the sensitivity of the body's cells to insulin. 18.3 million Americans have diabetes (AHA, 2012.)

- **Stress**—Although difficult to measure in concrete form, stress is considered a factor in the development and acceleration of CVD. Without stress-management techniques, constant stress can manifest itself in a physical nature in the human body. Stress contributes to many of today's illnesses.

- **Age**—Risk of CVD rises as a person ages.

- **Gender**—Men have a higher risk than women until women reach postmenopausal age.

- **Heredity**—A family history of heart disease will increase risk."[1]

Measuring your risk: If you said yes to two or more of the above risk factors, you have a moderate-high risk of developing CVD over your lifetime. It's time to make some changes!!

WHO IS AT RISK FOR CVD?

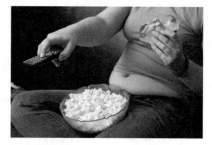

© esolla/Shutterstock.com

"There are an estimated 82,600,000 Americans that have some form of CVD. Many factors can predispose a person to be at risk for CVD. Sedentary living, habitual stress, smoking, poor diet, high blood pressure, diabetes, obesity, high cholesterol, and family history can all increase risk. Advancing age increases risk. Males typically have a higher risk than women until women are post-menopausal, then risk evens out. Misconceptions still exist that CVD is not a real problem for women. Because more women have heart attacks when they are older, the initial heart attack is more likely to be fatal. It is important for women to realize that CVD is an equal opportunity killer. Just like men, more women die from heart disease than anything else.

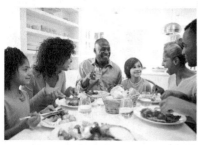

© Monkey Business Images/Shutterstock.com

"Certain populations have an inherently higher health risk such as African Americans and Hispanics. Genetic predisposition is a strong factor; familial tendencies toward elevated triglycerides, fat distribution (abdominal fat accumulation denotes a higher health risk than hip/thigh accumulation of fat), and high low-density lipoprotein cholesterol (LDL-C) levels increase risk. LDL-C is a blood lipid that indicates a higher cardiac risk. Saturated fat intake tends to increase LDL cholesterol. Dr. William Franklin of Georgetown University Medical School in Washington claims that anyone who has a close relative who has had a heart attack should begin monitoring his heart with regular stress tests when he is 45. If your father died in his 40's of a heart attack, then you should be concerned a decade earlier in your 30's. Variables such as age, gender, race, and genetic makeup may place you at a higher or lower risk but cannot be changed. These can be termed unalterable risk factors."[1]

Does Exercise Help?

"A growing body of evidence, however, indicates physical inactivity is more critical than excess weight in determining health risk. Longitudinal studies such as the ongoing research by epidemiologist Steven Blair, previously of the Cooper Institute in Dallas, Texas, and information from the ongoing Harvard alumni study indicate that lifestyle is more significant than weight. **Fitter people have lower death rates regardless of weight.** Indeed, the mortality rate for low fit males is more than 20% higher than for those that are

Spotlight on . . .

Family History

It is critically important that every person know and understand as much about their family history as they can. Family history is not exclusive to blood relatives. Looking closely at genes, habits, and environment of you and your family can help you to identify areas of concern for your health. Start with the immediate family members, move to grandparents, and finally to aunts, uncles, and cousins. Don't rule out your close friends with whom you spend a great amount of time. Realize that habits and environments can include those that we spend time with beyond our family members.

Check out the Web-based tool "My Family Health Portrait" at https://familyhistory.hhs.gov/FHH/html/index.html?_ga=1.135790840.878283.1456872088

high fit. While this effect is smaller for women, the decrease in mortality rate for high fit females is more than 6% compared to those who are lower fit. Increasing lifestyle activity and walking regularly, spending less time on the couch, and doing something active daily can have a positive impact on health."[1]

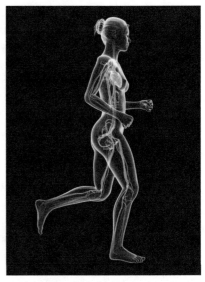

© Sebastian Kaulitzki/Shutterstock.com

TYPES OF CARDIOVASCULAR DISEASE

Arteriosclerosis & Atherosclerosis

"**Arteriosclerosis** is a term used to describe the thickening and hardening of the arteries. Healthy arteries are elastic and will dilate and constrict with changes in blood flow, which allows proper maintenance of blood pressure. Hardened, non-elastic arteries do not expand with blood flow and can increase intra-arterial pressure causing high blood pressure. Both high blood pressure and arteriosclerosis increase the risk of an **aneurysm**. With an aneurysm, the artery loses its integrity and balloons out under the pressure created by the pumping heart, in much the same way as an old garden hose might if placed under pressure. If an aneurysm occurs in the vessels of the brain, a stroke might occur. Aneurysms in the large vessels can place a person at risk of sudden death. Maintaining normal elasticity of the arteries is very important for good health. Exercise helps to manage symptoms and the factors that contribute to cardiac risk.

"**Atherosclerosis** is a type of arteriosclerosis. Atherosclerosis is the long-term buildup of fatty deposits and other substances such as cholesterol, cellular waste products, calcium, and fibrin (clotting material in the blood) on the interior walls of arteries. This may create a partial or total blockage (called an occlusion) that may cause high blood pressure, a heart attack, or stroke. This process can occur in any vessel of the body. If it occurs outside of the brain or heart, it is termed **peripheral vascular disease**. Within the heart the gradual narrowing of the coronary arteries to the myocardium, or heart muscle, is called **coronary artery disease**. *Atherosclerosis is a disease that can start early in childhood.* The rate of progression of the disease depends on family history and lifestyle choices. Exercise helps manage symptoms as well as increase coronary collateral circulation."[1]

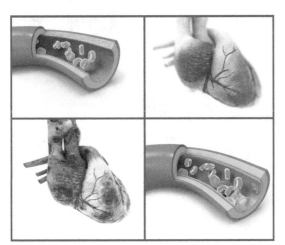

© Giovanni Cancemi/Shutterstock.com

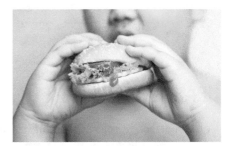

© kwanchai.c/Shutterstock.com

Hypertension

"**Hypertension**, or high blood pressure, is often called the "silent killer" because typically there are no symptoms. Because hypertension is asymptomatic, it is important to get your blood pressure checked on a regular basis. In 2009, the estimated prevalence of hypertension (a blood pressure reading of 140/90 mm or higher) was one in 3 adults. High blood pressure is associated with a shortened life span. A higher percentage of men than women have HBP until 45 years of age. From ages 45 to 54 and 55 to 64, the percentages of men and women with HBP are similar. After that, a much higher percentage of women have HBP than men (AHA, 2014). High blood pressure causes the heart to work harder. Chronic, untreated hypertension can lead to aneurysms in blood vessels, heart failure from an enlarged heart, kidney failure, atherosclerosis, and blindness.

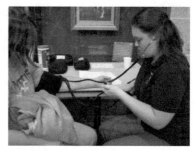

© Winthrop University

"The top number is the **systolic** reading, which represents the arterial pressure when the heart is contracting and forcing the blood through the arteries. The bottom number is the diastolic reading, which represents the force of the blood on the arteries while the heart is relaxing between beats. In 2017 new blood pressure guidelines were issued. Based on readings, the blood pressure categories are normal, elevated, or hypertension (stage 1 or stage 2). Normal blood pressure is less than 120/80 mm Hg. Elevated blood pressure includes a reading from 120–129/<80 mm Hg. Blood pressure readings of 130–139 (systolic) mm Hg or 80–89 (diastolic) mm Hg is categorized as Stage 1 hypertension, and readings of >140 (systolic) or >90 (diastolic) mm Hg is categorized as Stage 2 hypertension. Classifications are determined by at least two readings obtained on two separate occasions. If you are considered elevated or hypertensive, it is time to take action by modifying your lifestyle. Any reading consistently over 120/80 mm Hg could indicate a high risk. With persons over 50 years old, a systolic reading of 140 or above is a more important CVD risk factor than the diastolic reading (Whelton et al., 2017). Hypertension cannot be cured, but it can be successfully treated and controlled. Most people with hypertension have additional risk factors for cardiovascular disease. Some of the risk factors for high blood pressure include Hispanic or African American heritage, older age, family history, a diet high in fat and sodium, alcoholism, stress, obesity, and inactivity. Exercise has been shown to help symptoms of high blood pressure in mild to moderate hypertension."[1]

Did you know . . .

Teens, Sleep, and Blood Pressure in the News

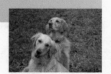

Courtesy of Shelley Hamill

A new study finds that teens who get too little sleep or erratic sleep may elevate their blood pressure. "Our study underscores the high rate of poor quality and inadequate sleep in adolescence coupled with the risk of developing high blood pressure and other health problems which may lead to cardiovascular disease," says Susan Redline, M.D., professor of medicine and pediatrics and director of University Hospital's Sleep Center at Case Western Reserve University in Cleveland, Ohio. Researchers say technology in bedrooms (phone, games, computers, and music) may be part of the problem (AHA, 2016).

HEART ATTACK

"A heart attack or **myocardial infarction** occurs when an artery that provides the heart muscle with oxygen becomes blocked or flow is decreased. The area of the heart muscle served by that artery does not receive adequate oxygen and becomes injured and may eventually die. The heart attack may be so small as to be imperceptible by the victim, or so massive that the victim will die. It is often reported that heart attack victims delay seeking medical help with the onset of symptoms. Every minute counts! In one study, men waited an average of three hours before seeking help. Women waited four hours. It is important to seek medical help at the first sign of a heart attack. Women who smoke and take oral contraceptives are ten times more likely to have a heart attack (Payne and Hahn, 2000). In addition to the classic symptoms of heart attack, women were more likely than men to report throat discomfort, pressing on the chest, and vomiting."[1]

Women & Heart Attacks

We now understand that men and women can experience heart attacks differently. Women, especially those under the age of fifty-five, who suffer a heart attack are less likely to feel the classic chest pain or pressure that their male counterparts. Women report more atypical symptoms, such as shortness of breath or pain in the neck, shoulder, arms, back, abdomen, or stomach. Women are also less likely to seek medical attention immediately following a heart attack, which increases their chance of heart damage and death from a heart attack. For these reasons, women have lower survival rates from a heart attack than males of the same age.

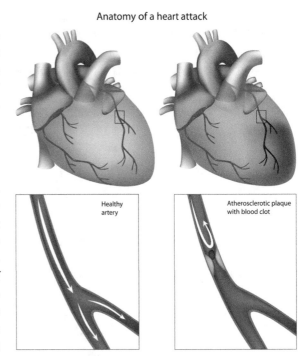

Anatomy of a heart attack

Healthy artery

Atherosclerotic plaque with blood clot

© Alila Medical Media/Shutterstock.com

Spotlight on . . .

Heart Attack Symptoms and Warning Signs

If you think you're having a heart attack, call 911 or your emergency medical system immediately.

Some heart attacks are sudden and intense—the "movie heart attack," where no one doubts what's happening—but most heart attacks start slowly, with mild pain or discomfort. Often people affected aren't sure what's wrong and wait too long before getting help. Here are signs that can mean a heart attack is happening:

- **Chest discomfort.** Most heart attacks involve discomfort in the center of the chest that lasts more than a few minutes, or that goes away and comes back. It can feel like uncomfortable pressure, squeezing, fullness, or pain.
- **Discomfort in other areas of the upper body.** Symptoms can include pain or discomfort in one or both arms, the back, neck, jaw, or stomach.
- **Shortness of breath.** This feeling often comes along with chest discomfort. But it can occur before the chest discomfort.
- **Other signs:** These may include breaking out in a cold sweat, nausea, or lightheadedness.

If you or someone you're with has chest discomfort, especially with one or more of the other signs, don't wait longer than a few minutes (no more than five) before calling for help. Call 911 and get to a hospital right away.

Calling 9-1-1 is almost always the fastest way to get lifesaving treatment.

Other than the previously mentioned symptoms, women may experience chest pressure or pain, dizziness, and unexplained feelings of fatigue, anxiety, or weakness. If someone is experiencing any of these signs or symptoms, get them to a doctor quickly. Additionally, have the person take full strength aspirin immediately. Aspirin has blood-thinning properties that can help prevent fatal clots from forming (AHA, 2012).

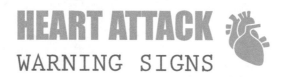

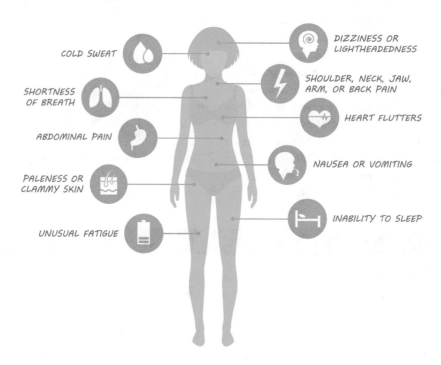

© eveleen/Shutterstock.com

Did you know . . .

The "ABCs" of heart disease and stroke prevention

Aspirin therapy

Blood pressure control

Cholesterol control

Smoking cessation

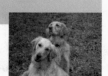

Courtesy of Shelley Hamill

The American Heart Association projects that by 2030, 40.5% of the U.S. population will have some form of CVD, costing the healthcare system an estimated $1 trillion every year. (AHA, 2012).

ISCHEMIC STROKE

UNSTABLE PLAQUE IN THE CEREBRAL ARTERY
ATHEROSCLEROSIS

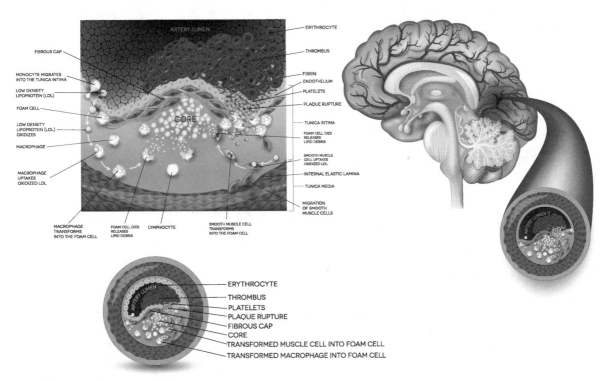

© Tefi/Shutterstock.com

Stroke

"Do you know the warning signs of a stroke? There is a public awareness campaign to increase knowledge of stroke warning signs and symptoms. Stroke, or more recently called **'brain attack,'** is the third leading cause of death affecting 795,000 Americans per year (AHA, 2015). This occurs when the vessels that supply the brain with nutrients become damaged or occluded and the brain tissue dies because of insufficient oxygen. The cerebral artery, the main supply of nutrients to the brain, can be narrowed due to atherosclerosis. The conditions that precipitate stroke may take years to develop. Stroke has the same risk factors as heart disease. African-Americans have nearly twice the risk for a first-ever stroke than Caucasians and a much higher death rate from stroke (AHA, 2015). African Americans also have a high incidence of stroke risk factors such as high blood pressure. On the average, someone in the United States has a stroke every

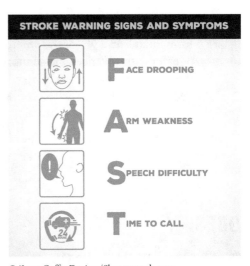

© iLoveCoffeeDesign/Shutterstock.com

forty seconds, and every three to four minutes someone dies of a stroke (AHA, 2015). One-third of all stroke victims die, one-third of stroke victims suffer permanent disability, and one-third of stroke victims gradually return to their normal daily routines (Bishop and Aldana, 1999). Stroke is also a leading cause of serious disability. Various studies have shown significant trends toward lower stroke risk with moderate and high levels of leisure time physical activity."[1]

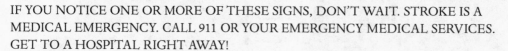

Spotlight on . . .

Stroke Symptoms/Warning Signs

IF YOU NOTICE ONE OR MORE OF THESE SIGNS, DON'T WAIT. STROKE IS A MEDICAL EMERGENCY. CALL 911 OR YOUR EMERGENCY MEDICAL SERVICES. GET TO A HOSPITAL RIGHT AWAY!

The American Stroke Association wants you to learn the warning signs of stroke:

- Sudden numbness or weakness of the face, arm, or leg, especially on one side of the body
- Sudden confusion, trouble speaking or understanding
- Sudden trouble seeing in one or both eyes
- Sudden trouble walking, dizziness, loss of balance or coordination
- Sudden, severe headache with no known cause

Be prepared for an emergency.

- Keep a list of emergency rescue service numbers next to the telephone and in your pocket, wallet, or purse.
- Find out which area hospitals are primary stroke centers that have twenty-four-hour emergency stroke care.
- Know (in advance) which hospital or medical facility is nearest your home or office.

Take action in an emergency.

- Not all the warning signs occur in every stroke. Don't ignore signs of stroke, even if they go away!
- Check the time. When did the first warning sign or symptom start? You'll be asked this important question later.
- If you have one or more stroke symptoms that last more than a few minutes, don't delay! Immediately call 911 or the emergency medical service (EMS) number so an ambulance (ideally with advanced life support) can quickly be sent for you.
- If you're with someone who may be having stroke symptoms, immediately call 911 or the EMS. Expect the person to protest—denial is common. Don't take "no" for an answer. Insist on taking prompt

For stroke information, call the American Stroke Association at 1-888-4-STROKE. For information on life after stroke, ask for the Stroke Family Support Network.

OBESITY

"Since 1979 the World Health Organization (WHO) has classified obesity as a disease. 'Obesity is a complex condition, one with serious social and psychological dimensions, that affects virtually all age and

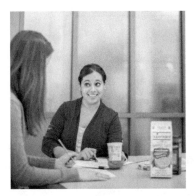

© Winthrop University

socioeconomic groups and threatens to overwhelm both developed and developing countries. As of 2000, the number of obese adults has increased to over 300 million' (WHO, 2008). 'Globesity' may be the new term coined for the world's heavy populations. While malnutrition still contributes to an estimated 60 percent of deaths in children ages five and under globally, in the United States the excess body weight and physical inactivity that leads to obesity cause more than 112,000 deaths each year, making it the second leading cause of death in our county.

"Obesity causes, contributes to, and complicates many of the diseases that afflict Americans. Obesity is associated with a shortened life, serious organ impairment, poor self-concept, and a higher risk of cardiovascular disease and diabetes, as well as colon and breast cancer. Fat distribution is related to health risk (Canoy, 2007). 'Apples' describe male-fat patterned distribution with fat accumulating mostly around the torso. 'Pears' describe female-fat patterned distribution with fat accumulating mostly on the hips and upper thighs. Apples have a higher health risk especially if they have visceral fat located around internal organs."[1]

Causes of Obesity

"Is it your genes or your fast-food lunches every day? Most likely it is both. Since you cannot change who your parents are, change your lifestyle habits. Physical inactivity is certainly a major, if not the primary, cause of obesity in the United States today (Wilmore, 1994). Most often caloric intake exceeds caloric expenditure. Glandular disorders affect 2 percent of the obese population. Genetically we are predisposed to a certain somatotype, fat distribution, size, and weight. In every person, body weight is the result of many factors; genetic, metabolic, behavioral, environmental, cultural as well as socioeconomic influences (Surgeon General, 2005). An individual's lifestyle choices can help to modify these tendencies. Nineteen out of twenty overweight teenagers will be overweight adults (Texas A&M University Human Nutrition Conference, 1998)."[1]

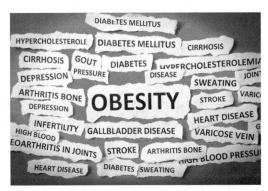

© Aliwak/Shutterstock.com

Did you know . . .

Health Risks of Obesity

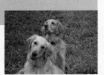

Courtesy of Shelley Hamill

Each of the diseases listed below is followed by the percentage of cases that are caused by obesity.

Colon cancer 10%   Breast cancer 11%   Hypertension 33%

Heart disease 70%   Diabetes 90% (Type II, non-insulin-dependent)

As these statistics show, being obese greatly increases the risk of many serious and even life threatening diseases.

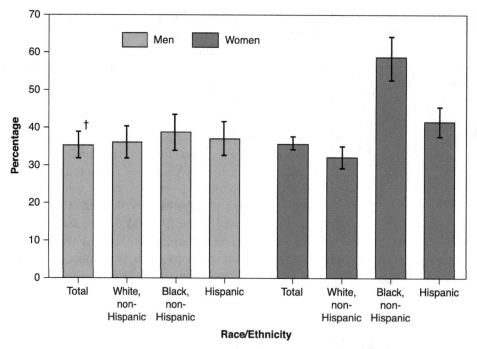

Source: National Health and Nutrition Examination Survey, 2009–2010.

© Kendall Hunt Publishing Company

Figure 9.1 Prevalence of Obesity Among Adults Aged ≥20 Years, by Race/Ethnicity and Sex—National Health and Nutrition Examination Survey. United States, 2009—2010

Spotlight on . . .

Childhood Obesity

About one in three children and teens in the U.S. are overweight or obese. Overweight kids have a 70–80 percent chance of staying overweight their entire lives. Obese and overweight adults now outnumber those at a healthy weight; nearly seven in ten U.S. adults are overweight or obese. Excess weight at young ages has been linked to higher and earlier death rates in adulthood. Perhaps one of the most sobering statements regarding the severity of the childhood obesity epidemic came from former Surgeon General Richard Carmona, who characterized the threat as follows:

> "Because of the increasing rates of obesity, unhealthy eating habits, and physical inactivity, we may see the first generation that will be less healthy and have a shorter life expectancy than their parents."

Obesity has also risen dramatically in adults. Today over 144 million Americans, or 66 percent of adults age 20 and older, are overweight or obese (BMI at or above 25). That is nearly seven out of every 10 adults. Additionally, 33 percent (over 71 million) of adults are classified as obese (BMI at or above 30). Obese Americans now outnumber overweight Americans, which means that individuals who are above a healthy weight are significantly, not slightly, above a healthy weight. Some experts project that by 2015, 75 percent of adults will be overweight, with 41 percent obese.

Source: American Heart Association, Inc.

Physiological Response to Obesity

"For an obese person, more blood vessels are needed to circulate blood. The heart has to pump harder, therefore increasing blood pressure. Extra weight can be tough on the musculoskeletal joints, causing problems with arthritis, gout, bone and joint diseases, varicose veins, gallbladder disease, as well as complications during pregnancy. Obese individuals often are heat intolerant and experience shortness of breath during heavy exercise. Obesity increases most cancer risks (Bishops and Aldana, 1999)."[1]

CANCER

"Cancer is characterized by the spread of abnormal cells that serve no useful purpose. Tumors can be either benign, having a slow and expanding type of growth rate, remaining localized, and being well differentiated; or malignant, growing rapidly, infiltrating (crowding out and replacing normal cells), metastasizing (spreading to other parts of the body via the circulatory or lymphatic system) and being poorly differentiated. There are four classifications of cancers according to the type of cell and organ of origination:

HUMAN CELL STRUCTURE

Cytoplasm
Nucleus
Nucleolus

Normal   Cancer

© Becris/Shutterstock.com

1. Carcinoma cancers originate in epithelium (layers of cells that cover the body and line organs and glands). These are the most common.
2. Sarcomas begin in the supporting or connective tissues including bones, muscles, and blood vessels.
3. Leukemias arise in the blood-forming tissues of bone marrow and spleen.
4. Lymphomas form in the lymphatic system."[1]

Risk Factors

"Risk factors include a family history, race and culture, viruses, environmental and occupational hazards, cigarette smoking, alcohol consumption, poor dietary habits, and psychological factors that compromise the immune system. Heredity or family history is thought to account for 10 percent of all cancers with the most likely sites for inherited cancers involving the breast, brain, blood, muscles, bones, and adrenal gland.

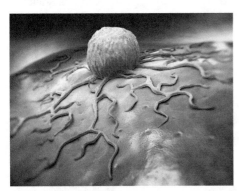

© Tatiana Shepeleva/Shutterstock.com

Research has revealed a variety of internal and external agents that are believed to cause cancer. These agents are termed carcinogens and include occupational pollutants (nickel, chromate, and asbestos), chemicals in food and water, certain viruses, and radiation (including the sun).

"Be certain to contact a physician if you experience any of these signs. With any cancer, early detection is the key to treatment and survival. A common misconception is that cancer is a death sentence. However, the forms of cancer with the highest incidence and mortality rates are those directly related to lifestyle factors that can be changed or eliminated. Due to dramatic improvements in diagnosis and treatment, more cancer patients are being cured and their quality of life is greatly improved. Treatment usually involves one or the combination of the following procedures:

- Surgery—removal of the tumor and surrounding tissue
- Radiation—X-rays that are aimed at the tumor to destroy or stop the growth
- Chemotherapy—an intravenous administration of fifty or more drugs combined to kill the cancerous cells
- Immunotherapy—activating the body's own immune system with interferon injections to fight the cancerous cells"[1]

"The seven warning signs of cancer are:

1. Change in bowel or bladder habits
2. A sore that does not heal
3. Unusual bleeding or discharge
4. Thickening or lump in the breast, testes, or elsewhere
5. Indigestion or difficulty swallowing
6. Obvious change in a wart or mole
7. Nagging cough or hoarseness."[1]

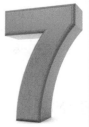

© martan
/Shutterstock.com

Can Cancer Be Prevented?

"Healthy lifestyle practices such as not smoking—30 percent of all cancer deaths are attributed to smoking (Donatelle, 2010); those smoking two or more packs a day are fifteen to twenty-five times more likely to die of cancer than nonsmokers (Hales, 2011)—exercising regularly, and avoiding sun exposure are simple yet essential ways to decrease your risk of cancer. A diet low in fat (less than 30 percent of total calories) but high in fruits, vegetables (at least five servings per day), and whole grains are the best nutritionally for reducing cancer risk. Avoid smoke-filled areas. Second hand or environmental tobacco smoke (ETS) can increase the risk among nonsmokers. Researchers have found the risk of cancer to increase threefold with as little as three hours of exposure per day. Avoid environmental carcinogens whenever possible. Follow safety precautions if employed in or living near factories that create smoke or dust.

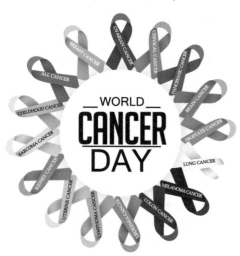

© suns design/Shutterstock.com

"It is theorized that 80 percent of cancers can be prevented with positive lifestyle choices. Avoiding tobacco and over-exposure to sunlight are two major examples. Eating a varied diet, consuming antioxidants, having a positive attitude, and participating in regular physical activity are simple choices that can have a large impact on cancer prevention. Thirty-five percent of the total cancer death toll is associated with diet (Rosato, 1994), and fit individuals may have a decreased risk of reproductive organ cancers (Bishop and Aldana, 1999). Cancer is the second leading cause of death in the United States, accounting for about 23 percent of all deaths yearly (Hoeger et al., 2009)."[1]

Does Exercise Help?

"Recognition of the potential of exercise to prevent cancer came in 1985 when the American Cancer Society began recommending exercise to protect against cancer. Regular activity has been shown to reduce risk of colon cancer. Active

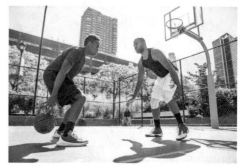

© oneinchpunch/Shutterstock.com

people have lower death rates from cancer than inactive people—50 to 250 percent lower. Colon, breast, rectal, and prostate cancers each have an established link with inactivity.

"It is also thought that exercise can boost immunity that can help kill abnormal cancer cells (Bishop and Aldana, 1999). Dr. Steven Blair at the Institute for Aerobics Research in Dallas, Texas, has done long-term epidemiological studies that show rate of death due to cancer is significantly lower in patients with elevated levels of fitness. It must also be noted that people who are active tend to also participate in other healthy behaviors, such as eating a varied diet low in fat and high in fiber. These other behaviors may also influence cancer risk and help those with cancer lead more fulfilling and productive lives. The American Cancer Society reports that people with healthy lifestyles (non-smokers, regular physical activity, and sufficient sleep) have the lowest cancer mortality rates."[1]

TABLE 9.1 Physical Activity and Cancer

Cancer Type	Effect of Physical Activity
Colon	Exercise speeds movement of food and cancer-causing substances through the digestive system, and reduces prostaglandins (substances linked to cancer in the colon).
Breast	Exercise decreases the amount of exposure of breast tissue to circulating estrogen. Lower body fat is also associated with lower estrogen levels. Early life activity is deemed important for both reasons. Fatigue from therapy is reduced by exercise.
Rectal	Similar to colon cancer, exercise leads to more regular bowel movements and reduces "transit time."
Prostate	Fatigue from therapy is reduced by exercise.

TYPES OF CANCER

Lung Cancer

"Lung cancer is the number one cause of cancer deaths in the United States (CDC, 2015). The major cause of lung cancer is cigarette smoking, accounting for 85 percent of all lung cancer deaths, making it one of the most preventable forms of cancer. Smoking cessation decreases the death rate of lung cancer in half. Other risk factors include asbestos exposure, secondhand smoke, radiation exposure, and radon exposure. Early detection of lung cancer is difficult, resulting in only 15 percent of cases being discovered early. With early detection, there is a 43 percent chance of surviving twelve months; however, the overall five-year relative survival rate is only 16 percent. Symptoms include a nagging or persistent cough, blood in the sputum, chest pain, shortness of breath, recurring bronchitis or pneumonia, weight loss, loss of appetite, and/or anemia."[1]

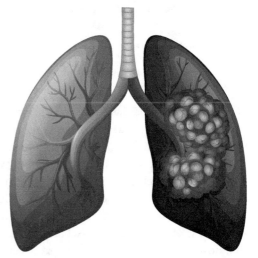

© BlueRingMedia/Shutterstock.com

Skin Cancer

"Overexposure to the ultraviolet (UV) rays of the sun is the primary culprit in these cases. Ninety percent occur on parts of the body not usually covered with clothes, including the face, hands, forearms, and ears. The two most common types of skin cancers are basal cell carcinoma and squamous cell carcinoma (non-melanomas). Both are usually treated successfully with surgery, especially if detected early. Subsequent tumors are likely in persons previously treated for these types of cancer. The fatality rate for these cancers is less than one percent. Monthly skin self-exam (SSE) can reveal cancerous changes at an early stage. Use a systematic approach. During this exam, look for abnormal growth of cells. If you notice any of these warning signs see your physician immediately."[1]

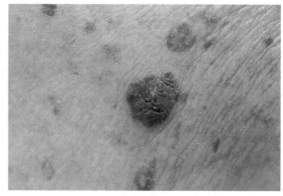

© charnsitr/Shutterstock.com

SIGNS AND SYMPTOMS OF SKIN CANCER

Abnormal
1. Asymmetry
2. Uneven borders
3. Color variation
4. Diameter (greater than 6 mm)
5. Evolving (change in size, shape and color)

Normal mole
1. Symmetry
2. Even borders
3. Color uniform
4. Diameter (smaller than 10 mm)
5. Normal mole

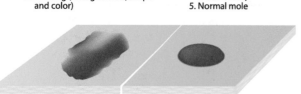

© Designua/Shutterstock.com

PROTECTED SKIN
WITH A SUNSCREEN LOTION

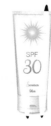
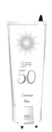

© Tefi/Shutterstock.com

Breast Cancer

"One in eight women will develop breast cancer in her lifetime (American Cancer Society, 2016). Risk factors include: age 40 years or older, family history or personal history of breast cancer, early onset of menstruation (before age 12), having no children, having a first child at a late age (after age 30), late menopause (after age 55), exposure to radiation, obesity, and certain types of benign breast disease (premenopausal women). Early detection is the best way to reduce the mortality rate among breast cancer patients. It is recommended by the American Cancer Society that women 20 years of age and older perform a breast self-examination once a month. Any persistent lumps, swelling, thickening or distortion of the breast, pain or tenderness of the nipple, or discharge of blood or fluid from the nipple should be reported immediately. A diagnostic X-ray, called a mammogram, can detect a tumor two or three years before it can be detected by a self-exam. The American Cancer Society recommends all women begin routine mammograms by the age of 40, and physicians recommend that women at high risk (with a family history) have mammograms every six to twelve months beginning between the ages of 25 and 35. With early diagnosis and a localized tumor, there is an 89 percent chance of surviving five years."[1]

SYMPTOMS OF BREAST CANCER

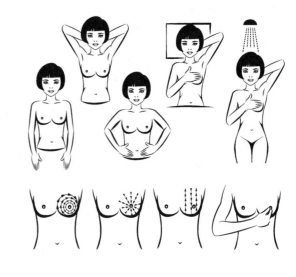

DIMPLED OR DEPRESSED SKIN

VISIBLE LUMP

NIPPLE CHANGE EX. INVERSION

BLOODY DISCHARGE

TEXTURE CHANGE

COLOR CHANGE

© eveleen/Shutterstock.com

© eveleen/Shutterstock.com

"Breast self-exam (BSE) is a method utilized in an effort to promptly detect lumps located in the breast. Early detection increases survival. During this exam, one looks for masses within the soft tissue of the breast or changes in the breast appearance. Due to the varying texture, size, and sensitivity of one's breast, it is important to do the self-exam at the same time each month. The following is a guideline to determine the proper timing:

- Women with menstrual cycles—one week after the beginning of the menstrual period when the breasts are usually not tender
- After menopause or hysterectomy—choose a day that is easy to remember, such as the first day of the month."[1]

Cervical Cancer

"Cervical cancer is representative of abnormal growth and maturation of the cervical squamous epithelium. Typically there are no symptoms in the early stages. Eventually individuals with cervical cancer will have uterine bleeding, cramps, infections, and pain in the abdominal region. Risk factors include: first vaginal intercourse at an early age, multiple sexual partners, cigarette smoking, and infections with certain types of human papilloma viruses. Due to early detection with the Pap smear, cancer of the cervix is rare and easily treated in women who have regular exams. It is recommended that all women begin Pap tests no later than three years after first intercourse or starting at age 21, whichever comes first. This procedure should continue until an individual reaches the age of 70, at which point the physician may recommend discontinuing Pap smears."[1]

Testicular Cancer

"In 2016, the American Cancer Society estimated about 8,720 new cases of testicular cancer will be diagnosed and about 380 men will die of testicular cancer. The incidence rate of testicular cancer has been increasing in the United States and many other countries for several decades. The increase is mostly in seminomas. Experts have not been able to find reasons for this increase. Lately, the rate of increase has slowed.

"Testicular cancer is not common; about 1 of every 263 males will develop testicular cancer at some point during his life. The average age at the time of diagnosis of testicular cancer is about 33. This is largely a disease of young and middle-aged men, but about 7% of cases occur in children and teens, and about 7% occur in men over the age of 55. Because testicular cancer usually can be treated successfully, a man's lifetime risk of dying from this cancer is very low: about 1 in 5,000 (American Cancer Society, 2016).

"Men with undescended testicles in childhood seem to be at greatest risk. Other risks may include: family history, inguinal hernia, testicular trauma, mumps orchitis, elevated testicular temperature, vasectomy, or exposure to electromagnetic fields. Testicular self-exams should be performed monthly to detect any enlargement or thickening of the testes. The cure rate if detected early is close to 80 percent. Testicular self-exam (TSE) can detect cancer in early stages when disease is more curable. Exams should begin at age 15. Self-examination should be performed every month in order to detect any changes. The best time to perform the exam is after taking a warm bath or shower when the skin of the scrotum is relaxed."[1]

Testicular Cancer

Healthy   **Testicular Cancer**

Pampiniform (venous) plexus

Testicular artery

Epididymis

Ductus (vas) deferens

Testis

Tumor

© joshya/Shutterstock.com

Google Challenge!

How can the way we "potty" affect our risk for colon cancer?

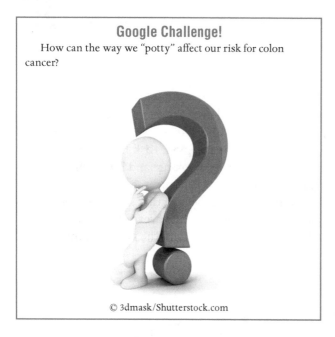

© 3dmask/Shutterstock.com

Colon and Rectum Cancers

"Colon and rectum cancers are the third leading types of cancer in men and women, claiming about 100,000 lives a year (American Cancer Society, 2016). The majority of cases occur in men and women over the age of 50. Risk factors include a family or personal history of colorectal cancer or polyps (growths) and ulcerative colitis. High fat, low-fiber diets have also been shown to increase the risk. Symptoms include bleeding from the rectum, blood in the stool, or a change in bowel habits (recurring constipation or diarrhea). Digital rectal exams, stool blood tests, and proctoscopic exams can detect early stages of colorectal cancer."[1]

Oral Cancers

"Each year, more than 48,330 new cases of cancer of the oral cavity and pharynx are diagnosed and over 9,570 deaths due to oral cancer occur. The five year survival rate for these cancers is only about 60 percent (ACS, 2016) http://www.cdc.gov/oralhealth/oral_cancer/. Oral cancer is related directly to a person's behavior. The major behavioral risk factors include cigarette, pipe, or cigar smoking, excessive alcohol use, and chewing tobacco use. Particularly vulnerable are persons who drink and smoke. Early symptoms include: a bleeding sore that will not heal, a lump or thickening, a red or white patch (lesion) that will not go away, a persistent sore throat, difficulty chewing, swallowing, or moving of the tongue or jaws. A cure is often achieved easily with early detection."[1]

TABLE 9.2 Preventing Cancer through Diet and Lifestyle

Type	Decreases Risk	Increases Risk	Preventable by Diet
Lung	Vegetables, fruits	Smoking; some occupations	33–50%
Stomach	Vegetables, fruits; food refrigeration	Salt and salted food	66–75%
Breast	Vegetables, fruits	Obesity; alcohol	33–50%
Colon/rectum	Vegetables; physical activity	Meat; alcohol; smoking	66–75%
Mouth/throat	Vegetables, fruits; physical activity	Salted fish; alcohol; smoking	33–50%
Liver	Vegetables	Alcohol; contaminated food	33–66%
Cervix	Vegetables, fruits	Smoking	10–20%
Esophagus	Vegetables, fruits	Deficient diet; smoking; alcohol	50–75%
Prostate	Vegetables	Meat or meat fat; dairy fat	10–20%
Bladder	Vegetables, fruits	Smoking; coffee	10–20%

Here are some tips issued by a panel of cancer researchers:
- Avoid being underweight or overweight, and limit weight gain during adulthood to less than eleven pounds.
- If you don't get much exercise at work, take a one-hour brisk walk or similar exercise daily, and exercise vigorously for at least one hour a week.
- Eat eight or more servings a day of cereals and grains (such as rice, corn, breads, and pasta), legumes (such as peas), roots (such as beets, radishes, and carrots), tubers (such as potatoes), and plantains (including bananas).
- Eat five or more servings a day of a variety of other vegetables and fruits.
- Limit consumption of refined sugar.
- Limit alcoholic drinks to less than two a day for men and one a day for women.
- Limit intake of red meat to less than three ounces a day, if eaten at all.
- Limit consumption of salted foods and use of cooking and table salt. Use herbs and spices to season foods.

Sources: World Cancer Research Fund; American Institute for Cancer Research, 2003, © Kendall Hunt Publishing Company

DIABETES

"**Diabetes** is a disorder that involves high blood sugar levels and inadequate insulin production by the pancreas or inadequate utilization of insulin by the cells (Wilmore, 1994). Diabetes is becoming more common in the United States. In 2008, CDC estimated that 23.6 million Americans, or 7.8 percent of the

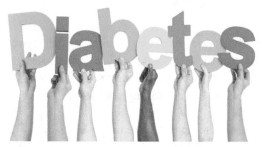

© Rawpixel.com/Shutterstock.com

population, had diabetes and another 57 million adults had prediabetes (CDC, 2011). There are three types of diabetes, Type I, Type II, and gestational.

"Type I or insulin-dependent diabetes is typically associated with childhood or adolescent onset. In this form of diabetes the pancreas does not produce insulin, and the individual requires regular injections. The signs and symptoms of Type I diabetes appear suddenly and dramatically. Symptoms include fatigue, irritability, abnormal hunger and thirst, frequent urination, and weight loss (Floyd et al., 2007). This type of diabetes is only seen in about 5 percent of all diabetics and is considered the more serious of the two forms.

"Type II or non-insulin-dependent diabetes is typically associated with adult onset and obesity. In this form of the disease the pancreas produces insulin, but the cells of the body are not able to use it effectively. The onset of Type II diabetes is more gradual than Type I. Some symptoms include drowsiness, blurred vision, itching, slow healing of cuts, skin infections, and numbness of fingers or toes (Floyd et al., 2007).

"Gestational diabetes is a form of glucose intolerance or insulin resistance that is typically diagnosed in some women late in pregnancy. This type of diabetes affects about 9.2 percent of all pregnant women in the United States each year (ADA 2014 or www.diabetes.org/gestational-diabetes.jsp.) Gestational diabetes can cause dangerously high blood sugar levels to occur in the pregnant female. This type of diabetes occurs more frequently among African Americans, Hispanic/Latino Americans, and Asians (Dabelea, Snell-Bergeon, Heartsfield, et al, 2005). It is also more common among obese women and women with a family history of diabetes.

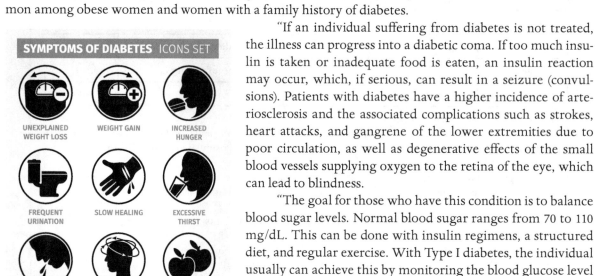

© Leyasw/Shutterstock.com

"If an individual suffering from diabetes is not treated, the illness can progress into a diabetic coma. If too much insulin is taken or inadequate food is eaten, an insulin reaction may occur, which, if serious, can result in a seizure (convulsions). Patients with diabetes have a higher incidence of arteriosclerosis and the associated complications such as strokes, heart attacks, and gangrene of the lower extremities due to poor circulation, as well as degenerative effects of the small blood vessels supplying oxygen to the retina of the eye, which can lead to blindness.

"The goal for those who have this condition is to balance blood sugar levels. Normal blood sugar ranges from 70 to 110 mg/dL. This can be done with insulin regimens, a structured diet, and regular exercise. With Type I diabetes, the individual usually can achieve this by monitoring the blood glucose level and adjusting the amount of insulin injected each day. In Type II diabetes, this can be accomplished with a controlled diet and regular exercise alone; in some instances oral hypoglycemic medication or insulin is required as well. The risk of developing diabetes can be reduced with regular activity, which reduces body weight and fat levels, and increases insulin sensitivity and glucose tolerance. Healthy

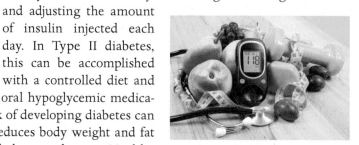

© ratmaner/Shutterstock.com

dietary habits also decrease the fat levels as well as obesity, therefore enhancing the body's ability to transport glucose into the muscles."[1]

Who Gets Diabetes?

"Eighty percent of the adults who develop Type II diabetes are obese (Surgeon General, 2005). The mortality rate is greater in diabetics with CVD—68% of people with diabetes die from some form of CVD. Each year, 1.6 million new cases of diabetes are diagnosed (AHA, 2012). Diabetes is the seventh leading cause of death in people over 40 (Corbin and Welk, 2009). Due to the surge in childhood obesity in the decade of the 90's, children are more at risk for diabetes. Diabetes is one of the most important risk factors for stroke in women. "[1]

Can Diabetes Be Prevented?

"Research shows that changing lifestyle habits to decrease risk for heart disease also decreases risk for diabetes. 'According to research, a seven percent loss of body weight and 150 minutes of moderate-intensity physical activity a week can reduce the chance of developing diabetes by 58 percent in those who are at high risk. These lifestyle changes cut the risk of developing Type II diabetes regardless of age, ethnicity, gender, or weight.' Type II diabetes may account for 90–95 percent of all diagnosed cases of diabetes (AHA, 2012). "[1]

Does Exercise Help?

"Exercise plays an important role in managing this disease, as exercise helps control body fat and improves insulin sensitivity and glucose tolerance. Exercise does not prevent Type II diabetes; however, exercise does help manage the disorder. "[1]

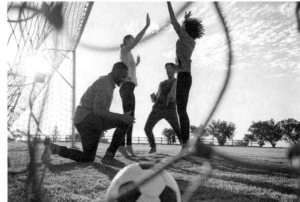

© Monkey Business Images/Shutterstock.com

OSTEOPOROSIS

"**Osteoporosis** is a disease characterized by low bone density and structural deterioration of bone tissue, which can lead to increased bone fragility and increased risk of fractures to the skeletal structure. Osteoporosis is sometimes called the 'silent disease' because there are often no symptoms as bone density decreases. "[1]

Who Gets Osteoporosis?

"For 53 million Americans, osteoporosis is a major public health threat (NIH, 2015). Considered to afflict mostly women, this disease can affect males as well. Of the women with osteoporosis, 80 percent are postmenopausal. One out of two women and one out of eight men over 50 will get osteoporosis in their lifetime. Risk increases with age. Have you observed older women who seem to slump? Many women with low bone density have kyphosis (also called dowager's hump), or a rounding of the upper back. The head tilts forward because often the cervical vertebrae in the upper spine actually suffer compression fractures. This keeps older women from being able to stand up straight or to get a full breath. Small, thin-boned women are at higher risk, and there may also be a genetic factor. If there are people in a family with weak, thin bones then relatives with the same body type may have an inherently higher risk. Post-menopausal Caucasian and Asian women are at the highest risk. It is unknown why these particular groups are more susceptible to osteoporosis. African Americans have bone that is 10 percent more dense than Caucasians. Others at risk include those with poor diets, especially if calcium and vitamin D are low over a long period of time. It is estimated that 75 percent of adults do not consume enough calcium on a daily basis. An inactive lifestyle contributes greatly. A history of excessive use of alcohol or cigarette smoking can also increase risk. Another growing group of high-risk individuals is the eating disordered. Many active young women suffer stress fractures, which can be a sign of osteoporosis (NIH, 2015). "[1]

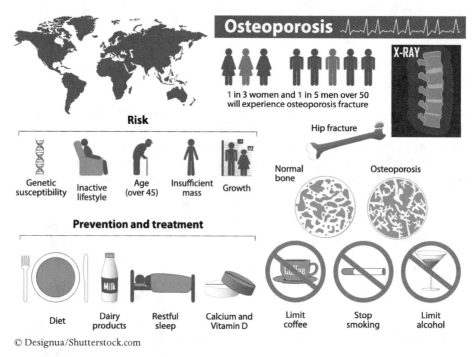

© Designua/Shutterstock.com

Can Osteoporosis Be Prevented?

"The good news is that osteoporosis can be both prevented and treated. Regular physical activity reduces the risk of developing osteoporosis. A lifetime of low calcium intake is associated with low bone mass (www.osteo.org). Adequate calcium intake is critical for optimal bone mass. Growing children, adolescents, and pregnant and breast-feeding women need more calcium. It is estimated by the National Institutes of Health that less than 10 percent of girls age 10–17 years are getting the calcium they need each day. A varied diet with green

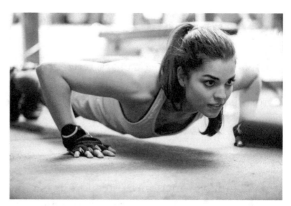

© antoniodiaz/Shutterstock.com

leafy vegetables and plenty of dairy will help ensure good calcium intake. Many calcium-fortified foods are now available. A varied diet will also ensure adequate intake of vitamin D, which aids in prevention. It is also advisable to limit caffeine and phosphate-containing soda, which may interfere with calcium absorption. Prolonged high-protein diets may also contribute to calcium loss in bone. A high-sodium diet is thought to increase calcium excretion through the kidneys. For post-menopausal women, some physicians consider hormone replacement therapy to help strengthen bones. Weight bearing exercise such as walking, running, tennis, and basketball is an excellent way to strengthen bones to help prevent osteoporosis."[1]

Did you know . . .

Current Recommendations to Decrease Osteoporosis Risk

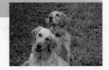

Courtesy of Shelley Hamill

- Engage in daily weight-bearing aerobic activity
- Weight training (the ACSM recommends ten–twelve reps, two sets two times weekly)
- Vitamin D (well-balanced diet and adequate exposure to sunlight)
- Estrogen replacement therapy (for some women, especially post-menopausal women)

ASTHMA

"Asthma is a respiratory disorder that involves difficulty breathing, wheezing, and/or coughing due to the constriction of the bronchial tubes. An individual will typically notice a wheezing sound when they are trying to breathe, while coughing and/or when experiencing difficulty breathing. In some cases those who suffer from asthma can stop an attack by simply removing themselves from an irritant such as cigarette smoke. Most of the time asthma attacks require some type of medical intervention, and, in rare cases, death can result from lack of treatment. Antihistamines, corticosteroids, and bronchodilation drugs are usually successful in reducing the bronchospasm."[1]

Pathology of Asthma

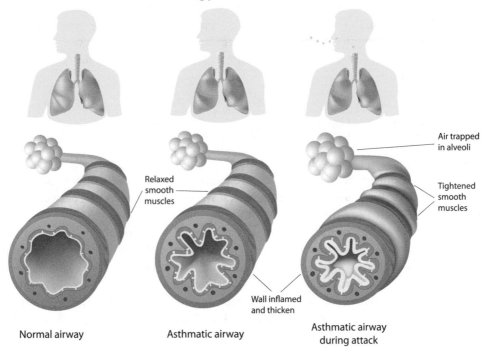

Normal airway   Asthmatic airway   Asthmatic airway during attack

© Alila Medical Media/Shutterstock.com

ANEMIA

"Anemia means 'without blood.' It is a condition in which the quantity or quality of red blood cells is insufficient. Normal red blood cells contain hemoglobin, which carries oxygen to organs and tissues. Anemic individuals have a reduced oxygen carrying capacity. Anemias can be the result of too little iron, loss of blood (including heavy menstrual bleeding or frequent blood donations), insufficient red cell production or genetic abnormalities. Symptoms include fatigue, infection, and/or trouble healing. There are four types of anemias known: iron-deficiency anemia, pernicious anemia, aplastic anemia, and sickle-cell anemia."[1]

LUPUS

"Lupus is a chronic inflammatory disease that occurs when your body's immune system attacks your own tissues and organs. There are four different types of lupus. They are: systemic lupus erythematosus (SLE), cutaneous lupus erythematosus (CLE), drug-induced lupus, and neonatal lupus.

"With an autoimmune disease, the body cannot tell the difference between foreign substances such as viruses and bacteria and its own cells and tissues. When this happens the body begins attacking itself with auto-antibodies. This causes inflammation,

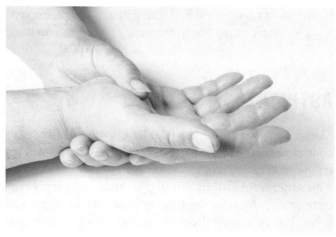

© blackboard1965/Shutterstock.com

pain, and damage in different parts of the body. Signs of inflammation include swelling, redness, pain, and warmth. If this inflammation is chronic, as with SLE, it can cause long-term damage. Signs and symptoms of a lupus flare include: aching all over, swollen joints, loss of appetite, recurring nose bleeds, sores on the skin, headache, nausea or vomiting, puffy eyelids, persistent fever over 100 degrees, prolonged fatigue, skin rashes, anemia, pain in the chest with deep breaths, excessive protein in urine, sensitivity to sun, hair loss, abnormal blood clotting problems, seizures, or mouth ulcers which last more than two weeks."[1]

GASTROINTESTINAL DISORDERS

"Ulcers, which are open sores, can develop in the lining of the stomach (gastric ulcers) or small intestine (duodenal ulcers) and are due to the corrosive effect of excessive gastric juices. Conventional theory blames lifestyle factors such as stress and diet. However, new research has identified a link between the bacterium Helicobacter pylori (H. pylori) and the formation of ulcers. One theory suggests that an infection caused by this bacterium leads to an inflammation of the stomach lining, which results in increased susceptibility of the stomach to stressors such as smoking, alcohol, high-fat diets, and/or anxiety. The most prominent symptom is a burning pain in the upper abdomen that is related to the digestive cycle. A bleeding ulcer, although not common, can be fatal. Excessive weight loss and anemia can result from an untreated ulcer. Medications that reduce stomach acid and relieve symptoms, lifestyle changes such as eating small, frequent meals, avoiding high-fat foods, cigarettes, alcohol, caffeine, and taking antacids can all reduce the effects of ulcers. One in five men and one in ten women suffer from peptic ulcers. Risk factors include: a stressful lifestyle, cigarette smoking, heavy use of alcohol, caffeine, or painkillers containing aspirin or

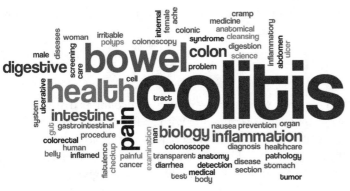

© ibreakstock/Shutterstock.com

ibuprofen, advanced age, and family history.

"Irritable bowel syndrome (IBS) (spastic colon or irritable colon) is a common problem resulting from intestinal spasms. Symptoms include episodes of abdominal cramping, nausea, pain, gas, loud gurgling bowel sounds, and disturbed bowel function. No biochemical or structural abnormalities have been identified as the cause; therefore, no standard medical treatment exists for IBS. Common interventions include reducing emotional stress, eating high- fiber diets, or taking stool softeners, laxatives, and drugs to reduce intestinal spasms. "[1]

COMMUNICABLE DISEASES

"Communicable diseases are those diseases that are transmitted from person to person. These diseases can be transmitted directly by physical contact, which can include coughing or sneezing, or indirectly by contaminated water or infected insects. "[1]

HIV/AIDS (Non-Sexual Contraction)

"HIV/AIDS can be contracted through blood transfusions, sharing needles, and/or the exchange of blood or breast milk from a mother to her unborn or newborn child. The groups that have been found to be at higher risk include IV drug users and those individuals who received a blood transfusion before 1985. More information on HIV/AIDs can be found in Chapter 7. "[1]

Mononucleosis

"Mononucleosis, also known as 'the kissing disease' because it is transmitted by saliva exchange, is primarily a self-limited (one that does not need treatment and will go away on its own) infection of young adults. The majority of cases occur in the 15 to 30 age range. This disease is most frequently caused by the Epstein-Barr virus (EBV); however, other viruses including cytomegalovirus (CMV) and the bacterium Toxoplasma gondii have been implicated (McCance and Huether, 2009). The virus attacks lymphocytes (cells found in blood and lymph tissues), which causes proliferation of cells in the immune system. This results in swelling of the lymph nodes, which is a prominent feature of this illness. After infection, there is an incubation period of thirty to fifty days (McCance and Huether, 2009). Initially, there are mild symptoms of headache and fatigue. This is followed by

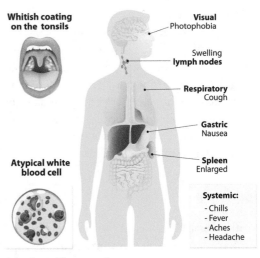

Mononucleosis

Whitish coating on the tonsils

Atypical white blood cell

Visual Photophobia

Swelling **lymph nodes**

Respiratory Cough

Gastric Nausea

Spleen Enlarged

Systemic:
- Chills
- Fever
- Aches
- Headache

© Designua/Shutterstock.com

fever, lymph node enlargement (primarily those in the neck), and sore throat, which is the most common symptom and can be quite severe. "[1]

Hepatitis

"Hepatitis means 'inflammation of the liver.' There are various causes, such as alcohol or drug-induced inflammation; however, the most common cause of hepatitis is infection with a virus. At the current time, there are six types of viruses known to cause hepatitis (A, B, C, D, E, and G). Descriptions of hepatitis have been found by Hippocrates as far back as the fifth century BC. The first recorded cases were believed to be transmitted by the smallpox vaccine contaminated with infected human lymph tissue given to German shipyard workers in 1883.

"The course of hepatitis can vary from asymptomatic infection (which is completely cleared by the immune system and unknown to the infected person) to rapid liver failure and death, or a slower process with cirrhosis and/ or liver cancer. In early hepatitis there is an inflammation of the liver due to the response of the immune system in an attempt to eradicate the virus. The damaged liver produces scar tissue as it attempts to heal itself, which can lead to cirrhosis (causing the liver to shrink and harden). This makes the liver unable to perform its life-sustaining functions. The individual who is chronically infected with hepatitis B or C is at a higher risk for the development of liver cancer. Unfortunately, chronic hepatitis is often asymptomatic until irreversible liver damage has occurred. "[1]

Meningitis

"Meningitis is an inflammation of the membranes that cover the spinal cord and the brain. Meningitis is usually caused by a viral (the most common type) or bacterial infection. It is important to determine which type of infection is causing the meningitis. If the meningitis is from a viral source, typically it will be less severe and resolve on its own. The best course of action if you have contracted viral (aseptic) meningitis is bed rest, drink plenty of fluids, and take medicine to relieve fever and headaches. If the meningitis is from a bacterial source, it can result in blindness, deafness, permanent brain damage, learning disability, or even death. Most often bacterial meningitis can be treated successfully with antibiotics if caught early. "[1]

Common Cold

"The common cold is caused by several different viruses that are spread by droplets from sneezing or coughing, or touching surfaces where the virus is present such as hands, money, or door handles. Symptoms include congestion, sneezing, sore throat, coughing, and a low-grade fever. There is no treatment for the common cold; however, the symptoms can be treated to help the infected individual feel more comfortable until the virus has run its course. Gargle with saltwater at the onset to relieve symptoms and possibly reduce the severity of the illness. "[1]

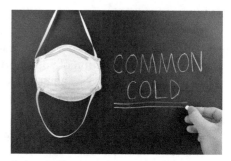

© simez78/Shutterstock.com

Influenza

"Influenza (flu) is a viral infection of the nose, throat, bronchial tubes, and lungs. The flu is spread in a similar manner as the common cold. Symptoms include high fever, chills, headache, muscle and joint ache, coughing, and fatigue. As with the common cold, there is no treatment for the flu; however, medication can be taken to ease the symptoms. The following reduce the risk of contracting colds and/or flu:

- Wash hands often.
- Keep hands away from your eyes, nose, and mouth.
- Drink at least eight glasses of water a day.
- Get enough rest (six to eight hours a night).
- Use Kleenex instead of handkerchiefs.
- Get enough vitamin C.
- Receive a flu shot."[1]

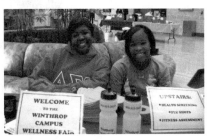

© Winthrop University

TABLE 9.3 Is It a Cold or the Flu?

Symptoms	Cold	Flu
Fever	Rare	Characteristic, high (102–104°F); lasts 3–4 days
Headache	Rare	Prominent
General Aches, Pains	Slight	Usual; often severe
Fatigue, Weakness	Quite mild	Can last up to 2–3 weeks
Extreme Exhaustion	Never	Early and prominent
Stuffy Nose	Common	Sometimes
Sneezing	Usual	Sometimes
Sore Throat	Common	Sometimes
Chest Discomfort, Cough	Mild to moderate; hacking cough	Common; can become severe
COMPLICATIONS	Sinus congestion or earache	Bronchitis, pneumonia; can be life-threatening
PREVENTION	None	Annual vaccination; antiviral medicines– see your doctor
TREATMENT	Only temporary relief of symptoms	Antiviral medicines–see your doctor

Source: From the National Institute of Allergy and Infectious Diseases, www.niaid.nih.gov Nov 2008.

Are you a healthy consumer?

Since we are so driven for survival, we sometimes consume products that we think might be beneficial in preventing disease. Most of the decisions of our consumer behavior is driven by ads, claims, and testimonies that are not often grounded in science or research support. While there are some products that are effective in helping prevent disease and improve health, make sure that your consumer behaviors are based on science and research rather than fads and false claims.

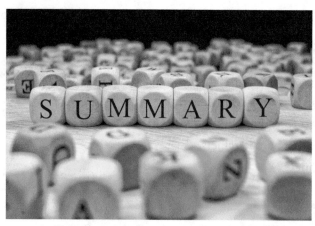

© Fabrik Bilder/Shutterstock.com

Throughout this chapter we have discussed many human diseases that can affect an individual's life. Chronic diseases, such as cardiovascular disease, stroke, obesity, cancer, diabetes, osteoporosis, and asthma, are common within America. We also discussed communicable diseases, such as colds and flu, among others. Being informed of your risk is important in your efforts to prevent disease. Understanding how quality of life is affected through disease can be a powerful motivator.

Personal Reflections . . . so, what have you learned?

1. List the eight risk factors for cardiovascular disease. Do any apply to you currently? Are any risk factors within your family that you should be aware of and work to prevent?

2. What are the signs and symptoms of a heart attack in men and women? What are the signs and symptoms of a stroke?

3. How is obesity related to chronic disease?

4. What are the seven warning signs of cancer? What are three methods of cancer prevention that you practice regularly? What is at least one other cancer prevention strategy you could employ?

5. What are three differences between a cold and a flu?

NOTES

RESOURCES ON CAMPUS FOR YOU!

Health & Counseling Services

Follow these Centers for Disease Control and Prevention tips to stay healthy

- Avoid touching your eyes, nose, or mouth. Germs spread this way.
- Cover your nose and mouth with a tissue when you cough or sneeze. Throw the tissue in the trash after you use it.
- Try to avoid close contact with sick people.
- Wash your hands often with soap and water, especially after you cough or sneeze. Alcohol-based hand cleaners are also effective.

> **More information on Human Diseases can be found at:**
>
> Centers for Disease Control (CDC) American Heart Association (AHA)
>
> American Cancer Society (ACS) American Diabetes Association (ADA)
>
> World Health Organization (WHO) U.S. Department of Health and Human Services
>
> National Breast Cancer Foundation

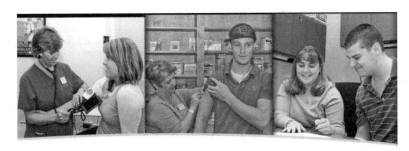

© Winthrop University

REFERENCES

American Cancer Society. (2016). Retrieved from www.cancer.org

American Diabetes Association (ADA). (2005). Retrieved from www.diabetes.org/gestational-diabetes.jsp

American Heart Association (AHA). (2015). *About high blood pressure.* Retrieved from http://www.heart.org/HEARTORG/Conditions/HighBloodPressure/AboutHighBloodPressure/About-High-Blood-Pressure_UCM_002050_Article.jsp#.Vtb7gH-LdHQ

American Heart Association (AHA). (2016). *Poor teen sleep habits may raise blood pressure, lead to CVD.* Retrieved from http://heartinsight.heart.org/Spring-2016/The-Importance-of-Sleep/

American Heart Association (AHA). (2015). *Heart disease and stroke statistics–2012 update.* Retrieved from www.aha.com

American Heart Association (AHA). (2015). *My life check- Life's simple 7.* Retrieved from www.mylifecheck.org

American Heart Association (AHA). (2014). *Understand your risk for high blood pressure.* Retrieved from http://www.heart.org/HEARTORG/Conditions/HighBloodPressure/UnderstandYourRiskforHighBloodPressure/Understand-Your-Risk-for-High-Blood-Pressure_UCM_002052_Article.jsp#.VtcM5X-LdHQ

Canoy, M.P. et al. (2007). Abdominal fat distribution predicts heart disease, *Circulation.*

Centers for Disease Control (CDC). (2015). *Lung cancer statistics.* Retrieved from http://www.cdc.gov/cancer/lung/statistics/index.htm

Centers for Disease Control and Prevention (CDC). (2014). *Number of Ccvilian, non-institutionalized persons with diagnosed diabetes, United States, 1980–2014.* Retrieved from www.cdc.gov/diabetes/statistics/prev/national/figpersons.htm

Centers for Disease Control and Prevention (CDC). (2013). *Oral cancer.* Retrieved from www.cdc.gov/oralhealth/topics/cancer.htm

Corbin, C. and Welk, G. (2009). *Concepts of physical fitness* (15th ed). New York: McGraw-Hill.

Dabelea, D., Snell-Bergeon, J.K., Heartsfield, C.L. et al. (2005). Increasing prevalence of gestational diabetes mellitus (GDM) over time and by birth cohort. *Diabetes Care, 28,* 579–584.

Donatelle, R.J. and Davis, L.G. (2007). *Access to health* (10th ed). Boston: Benjamin Cummings.

Donatelle, R.J. (2010). *Access to health* (12th ed). San Francisco: Benjamin Cummings.

Floyd, P., Mimms, S., and Yelding, C. (2007). *Personal health: perspectives and lifestyles* (4th ed). Englewood, CO: Morton Publishing Company.

Greenberg, J. et al. (1998). *Physical fitness and wellness* (2nd ed). Boston: Allyn and Bacon.

Hales, D. (2011). *An invitation to health* (15th ed). Pacific Grove, CA: Brooks/Cole Publishing Company.

Hoeger, W.W.K., Turner, L.W., and Hafen, B.Q. (2009). *Wellness guidelines for a healthy lifestyle* (4th ed). Belmont, CA: Thompson Wadsworth.

McCance, K. and Huether, S. (2009). *S. Pathophysiology: The biologic basis for disease in adults and children* (6th ed). St. Louis, MO: Mosby-Year Book, Inc.

National Institute of Arthritis and Musculoskeletal and Skin Disease (NIA). (2015). *Osteoporosis.* Retrieved from http://www.niams.nih.gov/Health_Info/Bone/Osteoporosis/overview.asp

Otis, C.L. and Goldingjay, R. (2000). *The athletic woman's survival guide.* Champaign, IL: Human Kinetics Publishers.

Payne, W.A. and Hahn, D.B. (2000). *Understanding your health* (6th ed). St. Louis, MO: Mosby.

Rosato, F. (1994). *Fitness to wellness: The physical connection* (3rd ed). Minneapolis: West.

Satcher, D. (1996). *Surgeon General's report on physical activity and health.* Atlanta, GA: CDC.

Sesso, H.D. and Paffenbarger, R.S. (1956). The Harvard alumni health study, Harvard School of Public Health. Boston, MA.

Texas A&M University Human Nutrition Conference. (1998). College Station, TX.

U.S. Department of Health and Human Services (DHHS). (2004). *Surgeon General's report on bone health and osteoporosis: What it means to you.* Washington, DC: U.S. DHHS.

U.S. Department of Health and Human Services (DHHS). (2016). *Surgeon General's family health history initiative.* Washington, DC: U.S. DHHS.

Whelton PK, Carey RM, Aronow WS, Casey Jr DE, Collins KJ, Dennison Himmelfarb C, DePalma SM, Gidding S, Jamerson KA, Jones DW, MacLaughlin EJ, Muntner P, Ovbiagele B, Smith Jr SC, Spencer CC, Stafford RS, Taler SJ, Thomas RJ, Williams Sr KA, Williamson JD, Wright Jr JT. (2017). ACC/AHA/AAPA/ABC/ACPM/AGS/APhA/ASH/ASPC/NMA/PCNA Guideline for the Prevention, Detection, Evaluation, and Management of High Blood Pressure in Adults: Executive Summary, *Journal of the American College of Cardiology*, doi: 10.1016/j.jacc.2017.11.005.

World Health Organization (WHO). (2008). *Controlling the obesity epidemic.* Geneva: Author.

CREDITS

Chapter 10 + ───────────────

Safety Awareness

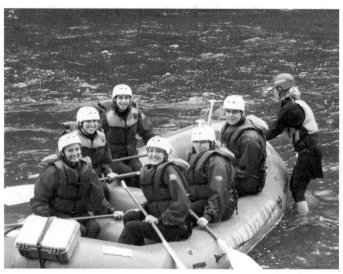

© Winthrop University

OBJECTIVES:

Students will be able to:

- Identify risk factors associated with unintentional injuries
- "Identify risks associated with drowsy driving.
- Identify the steps in disaster planning.
- Become aware of the prevalence of acquaintance rape.
- Become aware of the prevalence of family violence."[1]

© pockygallery/shutterstock.com

PRE-ASSESSMENT

1. Do you have an escape plan in place where you live if for some reason you would have to evacuate quickly? If so, what is it? Does it include your entire family including your pet(s)?

2. Do you have a first aid kit? Home and car? What are mandatory items in each?

3. Do you walk, jog, or run outdoors? If so, do you wear headphones? List 3 reasons why that might not be a good idea.

4. If you play sports or are involved in outside activities, do you use the safety gear required? Why or why not? Identify a few things you do where protective gear should be used and note what that would include.

Did you know . . .

Courtesy of Shelley Hamill

According to the Center for Disease Control (CDC, 2016):

- The number of emergency department visits in 2012 for unintentional injuries: 31.0 million;
- Number of deaths due to falls: 30,208;
- Number of deaths due to traffic accidents: 33,804;
- Number of deaths due to unintentional poisonings: 38,851.

"The purpose of this chapter is to provide information to help students make informed choices on personal safety and awareness issues. Being aware of possible hazardous situations may prevent injuries from occurring and save lives. The National Safety Council (NSC) defines an accident as 'that occurrence in a sequence of events which usually produces unintended injury, death, or property damage' (Bever, 1995)."[1] Accidents are the fourth leading cause of death in the United States after heart disease, cancer, stroke, and chronic obstructive pulmonary diseases (CDC). For people between the ages of 1 and 44, unintentional injuries were the leading cause of death In the United States in 2014. There were nearly 1,200 deaths due to unintentional injury in the 15-24-year-old aged group alone.

MOTOR VEHICLE SAFETY

"The leading cause of unintentional death is motor vehicle crashes."[1] In 2014, the 15–24 year-old age group had 6,531 deaths attributed to vehicular accidents (CDC). "One of the leading factors in motor vehicle crashes is driver inattention. According to the National Highway Traffic Safety Administration (NHTSA), nearly 80 percent of crashes involve some form of driver inattention. This signifies the importance of the driving task and that the need for attention is critical (NHTSA, 2010)."[1]

Distracted Driving

Distracted driving is any activity that could divert a person's attention away from the primary task of driving. All distractions endanger driver, passenger, and bystander safety. These types of distractions include:

- Texting
- Using a cell phone or smartphone
- Eating and drinking
- Talking to passengers
- Grooming
- Reading, including maps
- Using a navigation system
- Watching a video
- Adjusting a radio, CD player, or MP3 player

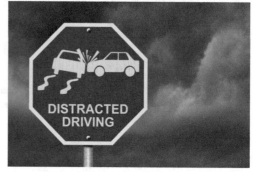

© karen roach/Shutterstock.com

But, because text messaging requires visual, manual, and cognitive attention from the driver, it is by far the most alarming distraction (NHTSA, 2013).

In 2013, 3,154 people were killed in motor vehicle crashes involving distracted drivers and approximately 424,000 people were injured (distraction.gov). Eleven percent of all drivers 15–19 years old involved in fatal crashes were reported as distracted at the time of the crashes. Drivers in their 20's make up 27% of drivers involved in fatal crashes (NHTSA, 2013).

"Operating a motor vehicle is the single most dangerous activity that we do on a daily basis and yet we feel confident that we can drive and do others things at the same time. We pride ourselves in our ability to multitask. We have been conditioned to think that we are more productive and successful if able to focus on more than one thing at a time. But can we truly multitask? John Medina, author of 'Brain Rules' says, 'Research shows that we can't multitask. We are biologically incapable of processing attention-rich inputs simultaneously.' The brain focuses on ideas and concepts one after another instead of both at the same time. The brain must let go of one activity to go to another, taking several seconds. According to Professor Clifford Nass at Stanford University, the more that you multitask, the less productive you become. When we operate a motor vehicle, many things can be considered distractions. Any secondary activity like texting, talking on a cell phone, putting on make-up, eating and drinking, adjusting your music or even your GPS can all cause problems while driving. Taking your eyes off the road for as little as two seconds can be dangerous. We have added more distractions by using our smart phones for Facebook, Twitter, Snapchat, and other social media."[1]

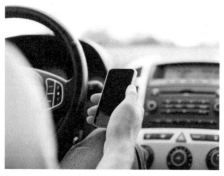

© Syda Productions/Shutterstock.com

Drowsy Driving

The risk, danger, and often tragic results of drowsy driving are alarming. Drowsy driving is the dangerous combination of driving and sleepiness or fatigue. This usually happens when a driver has not slept enough, but it can also happen due to untreated sleep disorders, medications, drinking alcohol, or shift work (CDC). This has become such a problem, the National Sleep Foundation declared November 1–8, 2015 as "Drowsy Driving Prevention Week." Drive alert and stay unhurt.

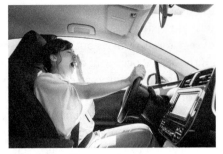
© chombosan/Shutterstock.com

No one knows the exact moment when sleep comes over their body. Falling asleep at the wheel is clearly dangerous, but being sleepy affects your ability to drive safely even if you don't fall asleep. Drowsiness:

- Makes drivers less able to pay attention to the road.
- Slows reaction time if you have to brake or steer suddenly.
- Affects a driver's ability to make good decisions.

"Young people are more prone to sleep-related crashes because they typically do not get enough sleep, stay up late, and drive at night. The National Sleep Foundation (NSF, 2007) has a few warning signs to indicate that a driver may be experiencing fatigue. These include not remembering the last few miles driven, drifting from their lane, hitting rumble strips, yawning repeatedly, having difficulty focusing, and having trouble keeping the head up. The NSF also offers these tips for staying awake while driving:

- Get a good night's sleep.
- Schedule regular stops.
- Drive with a companion.
- Avoid alcohol.
- Avoid medications that may cause drowsiness.

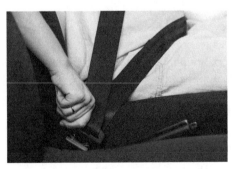
© Konstantin Kolosov/Shutterstock.com

"If anti-fatigue measures do not work, of course the best solution is sleep. If no motels are in sight and you are within one to two hours of your destination, pull off the road in a safe area and take a short twenty to thirty-minute nap. Most drowsy driving crashes involve males between the ages of 16–25 (NSF, 2008). Because of this growing problem, many colleges and universities are providing awareness programs to try to prevent this tragedy from occurring. In any kind of motor vehicle crash, a seat belt may save your life. The lap/shoulder safety belts reduce the risk of fatalities to front seat passengers of cars by 45 percent and for trucks by 60 percent. They also reduce the severity of injuries by 50 percent for cars and 65 percent for trucks (NSC, 2008). Air bags combined with safety belts offer the best protection. There has been an overall 14 percent reduction in fatalities since adding air bags to vehicles (NSC, 2008). Buckle up!"[1]

Motorcycles

There are over 9 million motorcycles registered in the United States (How many, 2012). "The increasing popularity with motorcycles and motor scooters is attributed to the initial low cost of purchase compared to automobiles, and good fuel efficiency, which is very important with the rising cost of gas. Motorcycles represent only three percent of registered vehicles but they represent 13 percent of the fatalities. Of the 35,900 occupant deaths in motor vehicle crashes, nearly 5,000 fatalities were motorcycle riders. Approximately 80 percent of the motor vehicle crashes result in death or serious injury. One of the main reasons motorcyclists are killed or injured is that an estimated 33 percent of motorcycle riders are not licensed or they are improperly licensed to operate a motorcycle. Most states require an education course uniquely for motorcycles to ensure riders have the knowledge and the skill to safely ride (NSC, 2011)."[1]

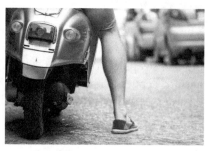

© Ekaterina Iatcenko/Shutterstock.com

"Another significant factor is protection. Because there is no protection provided by the motorcycle, the rider must rely on clothing, eye protection, and of course a helmet. According to the National Safety Council, as of 2010, twenty states have mandatory helmet requirements for all motorcyclists. Another twenty-seven states require only riders less than 18 years of age to wear helmets. And there are three states with no laws involving helmet usage. As in motor vehicle accidents, riding a motorcycle while under the influence of alcohol can decrease a rider's ability to operate the motorcycle safely. Almost 30 percent of riders killed annually are alcohol impaired. Alcohol diminishes reaction time, decision-making ability, and visual acuity. As with motor vehicles, all drivers or riders are impaired at .05 blood alcohol concentration (BAC)."[1]

Drivers of both motorcycles and automobiles must be attentive to those around them. Making sure to check lanes before changing and not riding in a driver's blind spot can help reduce crashes. During warmer weather, people who ride motorcycles are more likely to be on the road. May is Motorcycle Safety Awareness month and motorists are reminded to "share the road" and to be extra alert to help keep motorcyclists safe.

Bicycle Safety

Bicyclist injuries and fatalities have steadily increased since 2009. The five-year trend for bicyclist fatalities rose to 726 fatalities in 2012—the highest in five years. Additionally, 49,000 bicyclists were injured in 2012 (US Department of Transportation).

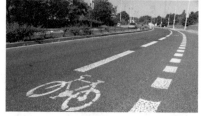

© Marsan/Shutterstock.com

"According to the CDC, 500,000 people are treated in emergency rooms, resulting in 700 deaths (CDC, 2011). Wearing a helmet reduces the risk of serious head injuries by as much as 85 percent and the risk of brain injury by as much as 88 percent (NHTSA, 2007). Helmets have also been shown to reduce injuries to upper and mid-face by 65 percent."[1]

Helmet Laws

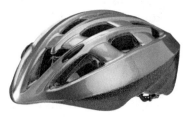

© Ljupco Smokovski/Shutterstock.com

Helmet laws affect both motorcyclists and bicyclists alike. In 2016, 19 states require motorcyclists to wear a helmet, 27 states have age requirement restrictions, and two require no helmets be worn (Bikersrights.com). For bicyclists, there is no federal law in the U.S. requiring bicycle helmets. States and localities below began adopting laws in 1987. At present, 22 states, including the District of Columbia, have state-wide laws, and more than 201 localities have local ordinances (Helmets.org).

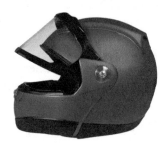

© AleksandrN/Shutterstock.com

HOME SAFETY

Poisoning

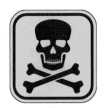

© Tribalium
/Shutterstock.com

Chemicals in and around the home can poison people or pets and can cause long-term health effects. Every 13 seconds, a poison control center in the United States answers a call about a possible poisoning. More than 90% of these exposures occur in the home. Poisoning can result from medicines, pesticides, household cleaning products, carbon monoxide, and lead (CDC).

The most common causes of poisoning among young children are cosmetics and personal care products, household cleaning products, and pain relievers. Common causes among adults are pain relievers, prescription drugs, sedatives, cleaning products, and antidepressants.

Pesticides are used in about three out of four U.S. homes. They are used to prevent or kill bugs or rodents. They can also poison people or pets. Children can swallow detergents, bleaches, and other cleaning products. Breathing fumes from these products can also harm people.

Carbon monoxide (CO) poisoning can be caused by poorly vented gas furnaces and appliances. CO is a colorless odorless gas and it can also be caused by gas generators used during electrical power outages and by indoor use of charcoal grills or portable stoves (CDC).

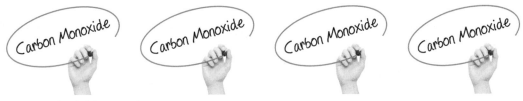

© Jacek Dudzinski/Shutterstock.com

To reduce the risk of carbon monoxide poisoning:
- "Don't use any gas-powered engines in an enclosed area.
- "Don't use a gas oven to heat your home.
- "Don't run the car in the garage.
- "Don't sleep in an enclosed room with a gas or kerosene heater."[1]
- In the event of a heavy snow, if you are sitting in your car make sure the tailpipe is not covered.

Of course, many people live in apartments or condominiums where units are connected. Though you may not have done any of the above things, your neighbors inadvertently may have. Make sure to have a working CO detector in your residence and check it at least once a year to make sure it is working and to change the batteries.

"The symptoms of CO poisoning are severe headache, mental confusion, dizziness, and other flu-like symptoms. If you experience these symptoms, get to a place with fresh air immediately and seek medical attention."[1]

Falls

"There are nearly 30,000 deaths each year in the United States that occur due to falls, as well as almost a million medically consulted injuries. The second leading cause of death due to injuries in the home is falls, resulting in over 16,900 deaths per year. The age groups most prone to death from falls are the elderly (65 and over) and the very young (between zero and four years old) (NSC, 2011). The National Safety Council estimates over eight million hospital visits were because of injuries resulting from falls."[1]

Though some aged groups may be more prone to falls, anyone can fall and there are a variety of contributing factors including:

- Walking while texting or reading texting (especially while using the stairs)
- Throw rugs or clutter
- Alcohol or drug use
- Slippery surfaces

If you have pets, make sure they are not underfoot when you are walking. Pay attention to where you are stepping and be aware of the conditions around you.

Spotlight on . . .

Elderly and Falls

According to the CDC:

- 1 out of 3 people over 65 fall each year
- Over 2.5 million older people are treated in emergency departments each year as a result of falls
- Each year over at least 250,000 older people are hospitalized for hip fractures
- More than 95% of hip fractures are caused by falling, usually by falling sideways.

Fires and Burns

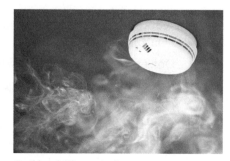

© nikkytok/Shutterstock.com

According to National Fire Protection Association (NFPA), in 2013 U.S. fire departments responded to an estimated 369,500 home structure fires. These fires caused 2,755 deaths, 12,200 civilian injuries, and $7.0 billion in direct damage. Home fires killed an average of eight people every day in 2013. Half of home fire deaths result from fires reported between 11 p.m. and 7 a.m. when most people are asleep.

One quarter of home fire deaths were caused by fires that started in the bedroom. Another quarter resulted from fires in the living room, family room or den. Cooking equipment is the leading cause of home fire injuries, followed by heating equipment. Smoking materials are the leading cause of home fire deaths.

Having a working smoke alarm is imperative. Working smoke alarms cut the risk of dying in reported home fires in half. When smoke alarms fail to operate, it is usually because batteries are missing, disconnected, or dead (NFPA). Additionally, having an appropriate fire extinguisher for home and auto is a good idea.

Everyone needs to have an escape plan in case of emergency. You should know multiple exit possibilities, how to "get below" the smoke so you can get out, and where to you will meet the rest of your household once you have escaped. You should also practice the plan with everyone to minimize confusion and if you have pets, make sure to include them in your plans!

Weather Related Concerns

Depending on what part of the country, or other country, you are from , Mother Nature can create situations that require people to take cover or evacuate. Extreme heat or cold, tornados, or thunderstorms are just a few of the weather events that can cause injury or death.

According to the National Weather Service (NWS) in 2014 there were:

- 26 fatalities and 154 deaths due to lightning strikes
- 30 fatalities and 233 deaths due to thunderstorm winds
- 20 fatalities and 107 deaths due to heat
- 57 fatalities and 26 deaths due to rip current
- 29 fatalities and 16 deaths to flash floods.

These are just a few examples of how serious the threat can be. Staying informed about the weather in our surroundings, taking cover when necessary, and having a plan in case of an emergency can reduce injury and save lives.

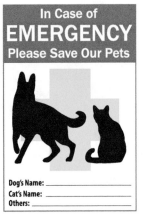

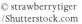

© strawberrytiger /Shutterstock.com

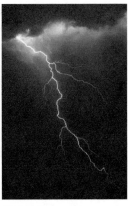

© Johan Swanepoel /Shutterstock.com

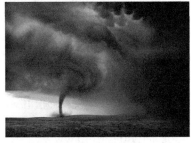

© solarseven/Shutterstock.com

Spotlight on . . .

Recreational Safety

There are many activities available to students, faculty and staff. Racket ball, outdoor equipment rental, even a climbing wall are just of few of the many possibilities. Your surrounding community may also offer bike trails, hiking trails, and different opportunities to participate in water sports. Let's not forget paintball, target shooting, and fencing, just to name a few. For each of these endeavors, safety needs and equipment should be addressed. Do you have the proper footwear, eye protection, head gear, or life vests needed? Have you had training on belay or can you swim? According to the CDC, every day ten people die from unintentional drowning; 80% of those who die from drowning are male, and 88% of people who died from boating accidents were not wearing life jackets (CDC, 2016). The Coalition to Prevent Eye Injuries reports that there are more than 600,000 eye injuries each year related to sports (Sports Eye Injuries, 2016). While everyone is encouraged to participate in whatever recreational activity fits your lifestyle, remember, *SAFETY* has to be included!

DISASTER PLANNING

"You never know where you might be when a natural disaster occurs. They can occur with little warning, and you could be at home, school, or work. What will you do if basic services like water and electricity are cut off? What if communication with family and loved ones is difficult? What will you do if you are asked to evacuate your home or are required to be confined there? You need to have a plan to effectively cope with the difficulties that come when a natural disaster takes place.

"FEMA, the Federal Emergency Management Agency, and the American Red Cross have created a four-step disaster planning program:

1. get informed,
2. make a plan,
3. assemble a kit,
4. maintain your plan and kit.

"First, get informed. Be aware of high-risk hazards for your local area. Do you live in an area known to be at high risk for tornadoes, earthquakes, or hurricanes? Educate yourself about community disaster plans and ask about disaster plans and procedures for schools, places of employment and other areas that you frequent. Understand community warning systems. How will your community warn its citizens of possible risks and how will communication occur after a disaster?

"Second, make a plan. Include the entire household in this process, especially children. Allow them to ask questions, offer input and practice this plan with them frequently. Include all caregivers who may be responsible for family members during a disaster as well. The focus of this plan is communication. If members of the household are separated during an emergency choose an out-of-town contact for everyone to call, if possible, to report their location and status. It is often easier to make a long-distance call from a disaster area than a local call. If you experience a disaster such as a fire, choose a location where all household members can meet in the immediate vicinity. A page of sample cards has been included in the notebook activities from www.ready.gov. Each member of the household should have this information handy.

"Next, discuss escape routes and safe places in the event of a natural disaster. Include plans for family members or guests with special needs, children, and pets to be protected during disasters.

"Next, assemble a disaster kit. These are supplies that may be used by your household to stay safe and more comfortable, during, and after a disaster. This kit should be assembled, stored in easy-to-carry containers, and reviewed at least once per year, or as your needs change. Figure 10.1 contains a list of common items."[1] First aid kits should be available in where you live, in your car, even a small kit might be useful in your backpack to deal with cuts or scrapes. There are many you can purchase commercially or put together your own.

"Last, you must maintain your plan. Make sure you review your plan on a regular basis. Conduct drills to work out any foreseeable problems. Restock food supplies. Check expiration dates and replace

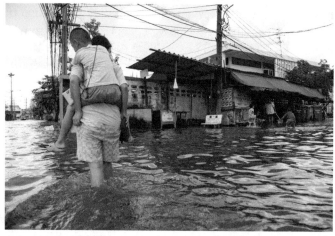

© think4photop/Shutterstock.com

Recommended Items to Include in a Basic Emergency Supply Kit:

- [ ] Water, one gallon of water per person per day for at least 3 days, for drinking and sanitation
- [ ] Food, at least a three-day supply of non-perishable food
- [ ] Battery-powered or hand crank radio and a NOAA Weather Radio with tone alert and extra batteries for both
- [ ] Flashlight and extra batteries
- [ ] First aid kit
- [ ] Whistle to signal for help
- [ ] Dust mask, to help filter contaminated air and plastic sheeting and duct tape to shelter-in-place
- [ ] Moist towelettes, garbage bags and plastic ties for personal sanitation
- [ ] Wrench or pliers to turn off utilities
- [ ] Can opener for food (if kit contains canned food)
- [ ] Local Maps

Courtesy of FEMA.

Figure 10.1

medications, food, and water as needed. Also, check batteries in smoke detectors, flashlights, and radios. During and after a natural disaster, the local, state, and federal governments and disaster relief agencies work to restore normal activity as soon as possible."[1]

Personal Safety

"Personal safety is something that affects our everyday lives, regardless of whom we are or where we live. Crime can happen to anyone at any time."[1] In 2015, the Federal Bureau of Investigation (FBI) reported that violent crime, including murder, rape, and assault increased across the board. And though property crime, including burglary and larceny were down, car break ends rose (FBI.org). And while we may not be able to prevent every possibility, there are some precautions we can take to reduce the risk of becoming a victim. Being aware of your surroundings and learning to avoid certain situations can reduce the likelihood of becoming a target.

An attacker looks for essentially three things when picking a victim:

1. Vulnerability
2. Accessibility
3. Availability

Practicing the following personal safety tips as you go about your daily activities may make you less attractive to a would be criminal.

- BE ALERT!! Know who is near you and what activities going on around you.
- Walk with authority, look ahead and scan your surroundings
- Do not walk in poorly lit areas.
- Avoid standing at a bus stop alone, especially at night.
- If approached by someone in a car, change your direction and enter a crowded store or business.
- Carry a cell phone and some type of safety device (i.e.: flashlight, whistle, pepper spray and etc.) when walking at night.
- Be alert to someone who asks for directions and/or continues to engage you in conversation.
- Obey all of the robber's orders. Keep all communication with the robber short and simple. Don't argue!
- Be identification conscious. Observe your attacker's personal appearance, type of weapon used, and type of vehicle so you can accurately describe them to police.
- Immediately report the incident to the police and do not hang up until the police arrive.

Car

- Keep doors and windows locked.
- Always park in well-lighted areas.
- If being followed, do not go home. Go to a police station or well populated area.
- Be aware of your surroundings at all times.

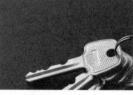

© Garsya/Shutterstock.com

Campus

- Avoid walking alone.
- Do not leave personal possessions unattended.
- Always notice other people—make eye contact.
- Avoid taking shortcuts through campus.
- Do not walk like a victim. Walk like you are on a mission.
- Always be aware of your surroundings.
- Trust your instincts. If someone or something makes you feel uncomfortable, get out of the situation.
- Use well-lighted stops if taking a bus.
- Have key in hand before reaching your room or car.
- Avoid jogging or walking alone.
- Hang up immediately once you realize the nature of a harassing call.
- Call a campus escort when on campus late at night."[1]

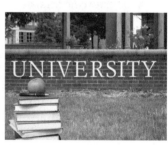

© AN NGUYEN/Shutterstock.com

College Campuses

While campus police do an excellent job of keeping the community safe, "many of the crimes on college campuses are crimes of opportunity. Theft is the most frequent crime on campus, yet it is the toughest challenge to convince students that their property can be taken. College students are typically very trusting, leaving their belongings unattended or inside vehicles in open view. Properly identifying your personal property such as backpacks, laptops, phones, and textbooks becomes extremely important. If you consider the amount of valuables you carry with you in a backpack, including wallet, cell phones, and possibly credit cards, the need for protection against theft becomes crucial. Reducing the opportunity and using common sense is the key to most crime prevention on college campuses."[1]

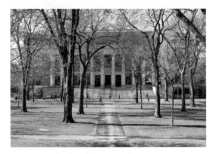

© Jorge Salcedo/Shutterstock.com

"It is also important to be cautious with the amount of personal information that you make available to the public whether it is on campus or over the Internet. Social networking sites like Facebook, Twitter, and Snapchat have become very popular, but they are not without safety concerns. With over 1.5 billion active users on Facebook alone, the risk of being victimized is very real. Choose the sites you post on carefully. Two main crimes can occur by using these types of sites: identity theft and unwanted attention/stalking.

"To protect yourself from identity theft choose strong passwords. Passwords that are lengthy contain letters, numbers, and symbols and use the entire keyboard are ideal. Always type the address directly into your browser or use personal bookmarks instead of accessing the site through an email or other Web page; you might be inadvertently typing your password into a fake site. Protect your personal information: your name, birthdate, and/or social security number can be used to create numerous kinds of accounts in your name.

"When you post information on the Internet, assume that it is permanent. Even if you remove it, the possibility exists that someone else has copied it to another location. Consider limiting the information you include on your profile. Information that can be used to locate you, such as your address, phone number, work, or class schedule, may be found and used by someone you don't want to see. And always use the privacy settings available with any site you choose to use. The less information given out, the less likely it will be used to harm you."[1]

Stalking

Stalking refers to harassing or threatening behavior that an individual engages in repeatedly such as following a person, appearing at a person's home or place of business, making harassing phone calls, leaving written messages or objects, or vandalizing a person's property.

Stalking is not a one-time event, but rather a series of threatening incidents that, if not responded to, may end in violence. Stalking often causes pervasive, intense fear and can be extremely disruptive for the victim.

Online stalkers (cyber stalkers) can easily disguise themselves by adopting several false identities and then

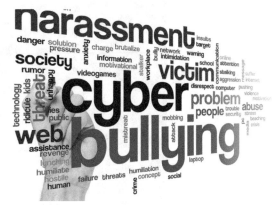

© ibreakstock/Shutterstock.com

harass the target through unsolicited emails, disturbing private or public messages on bulletin boards or in chat rooms, and communiqués of actual threats of harm. In addition, stalkers may pose as the victim online in order to incite others to harass and threaten the victim. Online stalking may lead to other forms of stalking.

Did you know . . .

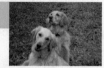

- 1 in 6 women and 1 in 19 men will be victims of stalking in their lifetimes
- 15% of college women report some kind of stalking
- Can involve repeated texts and phone calls, unwanted visits, being flashed, or being sent pornography
- Young women ages 18–19 experience the highest rates of stalking.
- 75% of stalkers are individuals that the victim knows (partner, former partner, or classmate)
- 61% of female victims and 44% of male victims were stalking by a current or former intimate partner
- 7.5 million people were stalked in one year in the U.S

Courtesy of Shelley Hamill

Remember: You have the right to break off a relationship at any time

What You Can Do

- **Once you have communicated** your disinterest, cut off all interaction and document any attempted contact.
- **Change your schedule and habits to avoid being alone.** Avoid being alone until the stalking ends, especially at night and when going from one place to another. Let others in your life know what is going on.
- **Contact** campus police and local authorities, or the Office of Victims Assistance.

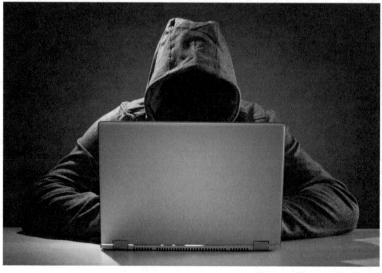

© Brian A Jackson/Shutterstock.com

Did you know . . .

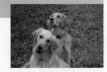

According to the Rape, Abuse, Incest Network:

- 1 in 4 college-aged women will be sexually assaulted.
- Anytime a person is forced physically or verbally to have sex against her or his own will, it is rape.

Courtesy of Shelley Hamill

- Contrary to popular thought, the majority of all sexual assaults (73%) are committed by someone known to the victim. A relative, friend, or acquaintance.
- Despite what others might say, you **DO** have recourse and **CAN** get help after an assault.
- If you are raped, not matter what the circumstances; remember that it is **NOT** your fault.
- Rape is **NOT** sex. It is an act of violence motivated by the rapist's need to dominate, control, and humiliate.
- Sexual assault can happen to anyone regardless of their race, class, age, appearance, or sexual orientation.
- Sexual trauma can be caused by rape, attempted rape, incest, unwanted sexual contact, and sexual harassment

Sexual Violence

"Sexual violence, including sexual assault and rape, is a serious and frightening crime committed against women, men, and children. Sexual violence is not about sex, it is about power. Perpetrators use this as an attempt to control a person using sex as a weapon. Rape can happen to anyone at any time. Most rape victims are women, but that does not exclude men as victims. According to the National Crime Victimization Survey, sexual assault is the fastest growing violent crime in the United States. It occurs with increasing frequency but remains the crime least often reported to the police. It is estimated that only about 10 to 15 percent of rape cases are reported and that in one out of seven reported rapes, the male is the victim.

"On college campuses, the majority of sexual assaults occur when the victim or attacker is under the influence of alcohol. The National Institute of Alcohol Abuse and Alcoholism (NIAAA) reported that drinking by college students contributes to an estimated 70,000 sexual assaults/date rapes each year. What does this mean? Impairment by alcohol or other drugs places an individual in a situation where their safety could be compromised. Alcohol affects the higher learning centers of the brain, making it difficult to focus on important information. This also makes it difficult for the individual to respond to negative situations in appropriate ways. The more aware and in control of your surroundings, the less likely you will become a victim.

"Most rapists plan their attack by familiarizing themselves with the victim's surroundings. In all rape cases, the attacker has the advantage from a surprise standpoint. Rapists commit the crime, not victims. There needs to be more prevention to eliminate crimes such as sexual assault from occurring."[1]

Acquaintance Rape

"Acquaintance rape is a particularly volatile issue on college campuses. The prevalence of date rape on campus is difficult to determine because victims are even less likely to report a rape by someone that they know. Studies indicate that as many as 25% of college women will experience an attempted or completed rape while in college (CDC, 2008) and the majority of the victims knew their attacker, a classmate, friend, previous partner, or acquaintance."[1] Remember, consent means you agree to participate in a behavior or activity and you must be in an unaltered state of mind. If you cannot give consent, it may be sexual assault. If you did not get consent, do no proceed with sexual activity.

"Safety Tips

- When at a party or club, do not leave beverages unattended or accept a drink from someone you do not know.
- When going to a party or club, go with friends and leave with friends.
- Be aware of your surroundings at all times.
- Do not allow yourself to be isolated with someone you do not know.
- Know the level of intimacy you want in a relationship and state your limits.
- Trust your instincts—if you are uncomfortable, get out of the situation.
- Have your own transportation—if you need to end the date, end it.
- When meeting someone new, meet in a public place."[1]

Spotlight on . . .

"Bystander Intervention

- If you see something, do something
- You may not be able to safely intervene but you could send an anonymous tip to campus police
- You can call 911
- You can report to the Dean of Students office
- Being an active bystander is a primary prevention model in eliminating sexual violence

We all have the responsibility to protect our campus community"[1]

Steps to Take if Rape Occurs

- Go to a friend's house or call someone you know to come over. You do not need to be alone!
- DO NOT shower or make any attempt to clean yourself; do not change clothes or remove any physical evidence of the attack.
- Call your local Rape Crisis Center for assistance and counseling. A counselor can also accompany you to the hospital.
- Seek immediate medical attention and notify the police.

Remember, as discussed in the chapter on healthy relationships, consent is crucial for preventing sexual coer-

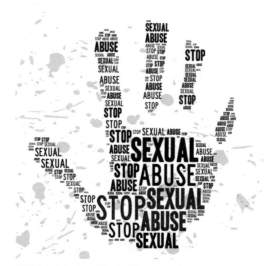

© Mohd Shahrizan Hussin/Shutterstock.com

cion and unwanted sexual behavior. Consent can and should be incorporated as an essential and fun part of sexual communication.

INTIMATE/FAMILY VIOLENCE

Women ages 16 to 24 experience the highest per capita rates of intimate violence. Intimate violence is defined as physical, sexual, or psychological harm caused by a current or former spouse or partner. Every day in the U.S. more than three women are murdered by their husbands or boyfriends (Domestic Violence Statistics, 2011).

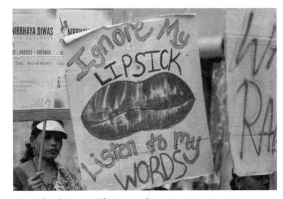

© arindambanerjee/Shutterstock.com

Another form of violence affecting our society is family violence. This includes partner violence, family violence, spouse abuse, child abuse, and battering. Family violence does not always have to be physical. "Psychological abuse can be equally as harmful and can progress into physical abuse. A few examples of family violence are name calling or put downs, isolation from family and friends, academic abuse, withholding money, threatening or physical harm, sexual assault, disrespect, abusing trust, sexual and reproductive abuse and harassment."[1]

Battering focuses on control of a relationship through violence, intimidation, or psychological abuse in an attempt to create fear in the victim. The violence may not happen often, but the fear of it happening is a terrorizing factor (FBI, 1990). "In most cases, victims are women; however, men can be victims, too. Often women are survivors of more severe physical violence over the course of the relationship."[1] In the U.S., intimate partners kill 1.5 million women each year. If you or a friend is the victim of family or intimate violence, seek help. Call the police or go to a shelter. Realize that the violence could even result in death, so action must be taken immediately.

ENVIRONMENTAL SAFETY

We have spent time discussing ways to protect people. Next we will cover suggestions on protecting our environment. While this could be a chapter by itself, thinking just a bit about things we could all do to help out and then implementing those strategies is important.

Reduce, Reuse, Recycle

The Environmental Protection Agency (EPA) defines sustainability as meeting the needs of the present without compromising the ability for future generations to meet their own needs. Easy ways to live green are to reduce, reuse, and recycle. The best way to have a positive effect on your environment is to get involved with programs through your campus or community. Simple things can make big differences. "Here are some suggestions:

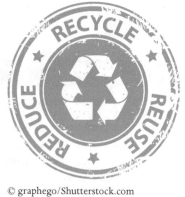

© graphego/Shutterstock.com

- Bring your own bags to the grocery store. It saves paper/plastic and the bags are reusable.
- When printing, use both side of the paper. It saves money.
- Think before you print—fewer copies save paper. Also consider using recycled paper.
- Drive less. Reduce your short trips around town and combine them for one day. Or better yet, ride your bike. It saves gas and money, and you get some exercise.
- Don't use paper or Styrofoam. Use reusable plates, cups, and water bottles. Make sure you use BPA-free plastic. Exposure to bisphenol A (BPA) may cause negative health effects.
- Conserve water by spending less time in the shower or turning off the water while brushing your teeth.
- Turn off your lights and computer. Unplug your phone charger and appliances when not in use. Lower your thermostat during the winter months and raise air conditioning temperatures in the summer, especially during the day when you are not home.
- Use fluorescent light bulbs—they use 50 percent less energy and last longer. However, remember to dispose of them properly because they do contain mercury.
- Carpool when you can or use the transit system, if available.
- Recycle, recycle, recycle—the amount of garbage we create is increasing. Our landfill sites are filling up fast. Waste has a negative effect on the environment and recycling helps to reduce the need for raw materials as well as using less energy. Locally you can recycle plastics, aluminum, clear and brown glass, and newspapers. Each building has recycling bins for disposing of various materials. Use them!
- Properly dispose of your used electronic devices such as cell phones and computers. A growing form of toxic waste is e-waste. With technology, e-waste now makes a significant portion of our waste. That waste contains heavy metals like mercury and lead, which can leach out of the landfills. Nearly 70 percent of all waste in our landfills comes from electronic equipment.
- Recycling your old phone keeps it and its (likely toxic) battery out of the landfill. Most phones contain metals like copper and silver. If these are recycled, it lessens the demand for mining new metals. The EPA states that recycling a million phones may reduce greenhouse gases by the same amount as taking 1,368 cars off the road for a year.
- Bringing your lunch to work or school can save money and save on the use of plastic and Styrofoam containers. If you spend about $7–8 each day on lunch, that can add up to almost $2,000 a year. Instead, make your lunch at home and

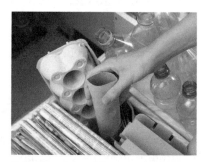

© Photographee.eu/Shutterstock.com

use reusable containers. Bringing your coffee from home in a reusable container can save you money as well.

- Buying used goods and selling your old goods can help save the landfills and save you money. Looking online is an easy way to find great items for less money. Selling your used items such as phones, furniture, or electronics online or in a garage sale could bring you some extra cash and save the landfills. You can also donate your items to a local charity to help others and keep the landfills clear.

"These are just a few ideas that you can use to make your environment a safer, greener place. Get educated! To find out how you can reduce carbon emissions or your carbon footprint, go to www .carbonfootprint.com."[1]

Are you a wise consumer?

There were many safety concerns addressed in this chapter. Some focused on natural occurrences and others identified activities we might chose to participate. Do you have a first aid kit? Do you wear the appropriate safety gear when participating in sport or outdoor activity? If you are engaging in outdoor activities, do you check the weather forecast before you go out? Are you being careful in your on-line communications to avoid hacking? All of these are things, among many others, that health literate people and wise consumers are aware pay attention to.

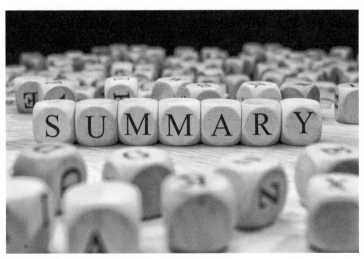

© Fabrik Bilder/Shutterstock.com

Safety is a huge topic. This chapter has only touched the surface on many of the more common safety concerns for college students. Take the time to be prepared, use proper safety equipment, know your surroundings, and plan ahead. While it is not possible to predict every possible risk, it is possible to mitigate many of them by thinking ahead.

NOTES